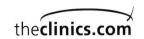

SURGICAL CLINICS
OF NORTH AMERICA

Recent Advances in the Management of Benign and Malignant Colorectal Diseases

GUEST EDITORS
Robin P. Boushey, BSc, MD, PhD, CIP, FRCSC
Patricia L. Roberts, MD

CONSULTING EDITOR
Ronald F. Martin, MD

August 2006 • Volume 86 • Number 4

SAUNDERS

An Imprint of Elsevier, Inc.
PHILADELPHIA   LONDON   TORONTO   MONTREAL   SYDNEY   TOKYO

W.B. SAUNDERS COMPANY
A Division of Elsevier Inc.

1600 John F. Kennedy Blvd., Suite 1800, Philadelphia, PA 19103-2899

http://www.theclinics.com

SURGICAL CLINICS OF NORTH AMERICA   **Volume 86, Number 4**
August 2006   **ISSN 0039–6109**
Editor: Catherine Bewick   **ISBN 1-4160-3914-7**

Reprints. For copies of 100 or more of articles in this publication, please contact the commercial Reprints Department Elsevier Inc., 360 Park Avenue South, New York, New York 10010-1710. Tel. (212) 633-3813, Fax: (212) 462-1935, email: reprints@elsevier.com

The ideas and opinions expressed in *The Surgical Clinics of North America* do not necessarily reflect those of the Publisher. The Publisher does not assume any responsibility for any injury and/or damage to persons or property arising out of or related to any use of the material contained in this periodical. The reader is advised to check the appropriate medical literature and the product information currently provided by the manufacturer of each drug to be administered to verify the dosage, the method and duration of administration, or contraindications. It is the responsibility of the treating physician or other health care professional, relying on independent experience and knowledge of the patient, to determine drug dosages and the best treatment for the patient. Mention of any product in this issue should not be construed as endorsement by the contributors, editors, or the Publisher of the product or manufacturers' claims.

Surgical Clinics of North America (ISSN 0039–6109) is published bimonthly by Elsevier Inc., 360 Park Avenue South, New York, NY 10010-1710. Months of publication are February, April, June, August, October, and December. Business and Editorial Offices: 1600 John F. Kennedy Blvd., Suite 1800, Philadelphia, PA 19103-2899. Customer Service Office: 6277 Sea Harbor Drive, Orlando, FL 32887-4800. Periodicals postage paid at New York, NY and additional mailing offices. Subscription prices are $200.00 per year for US individuals, $315.00 per year for US institutions, $100.00 per year for US students and residents, $245.00 per year for Canadian individuals, $385.00 per year for Canadian institutions, $260.00 for international individuals, $385.00 for international institutions and $130.00 per year for Canadian and foreign students/residents. To receive student/resident rate, orders must be accompanied by name of affiliated institution, date of term, and the *signature* of program/residency coordinator on institution letterhead. Orders will be billed at individual rate until proof of status is received. Foreign air speed delivery is included in all *Clinics* subscription prices. All prices are subject to change without notice. POSTMASTER: Send address changes to *Surgical Clinics*, Elsevier Periodicals Customer Service, 6277 Sea Harbor Drive, Orlando, FL 32887-4800. **Customer Service: 1-800-654-2452 (US). From outside of the US, call 1-407-345-1000.**

The Surgical Clinics of North America is also published in Spanish by McGraw-Hill Interamericana Editores S.A., P.O. Box 5-237 06500 Mexico D.F. Mexico; and in Portuguese by Interlivros Edicoes Ltda., Rua Comandante Coelho 1085, CEP 21250, Rio de Janeiro, Brazil; and in Greek by Paschalidis Medical Publications, Athens Greece.

The Surgical Clinics of North America is covered in *Index Medicus, EMBASE/Excerpta Medica, Current Contents/Clinical Medicine, Current Contents/Life Sciences, Science Citation Index*, and *ISI/BIOMED*.

Printed in the United States of America.

CONSULTING EDITOR

RONALD F. MARTIN, MD, Staff Surgeon, Department of Surgery, Marshfield Clinic, Marshfield, Wisconsin; Clinical Associate Professor of Surgery, University of Vermont, Burlington, Vermont; Lieutenant Colonel, Medical Corps, United States Army Reserve

GUEST EDITORS

ROBIN P. BOUSHEY, BSc, MD, PhD, CIP, FRCSC, Assistant Professor of Surgery; Clinical Investigator, Ottawa Health Research Institute, Cancer Centre Program; Director of Research, Division of General Surgery, Department of Colon and Rectal Surgery, Minimally Invasive Surgery Research Group, University of Ottawa, The Ottawa Hospital—General Campus, Ottawa, Ontario, Canada

PATRICIA L. ROBERTS, MD, Department of Colon and Rectal Surgery, Lahey Clinic, Burlington, Massachusetts

CONTRIBUTORS

ROBERT P. AKBARI, MD, Assistant Professor of Surgery, Temple University School of Medicine, Pittsburgh, Pennsylvania; Staff Surgeon, Division of Colon and Rectal Surgery, Western Pennsylvania Hospital, Pittsburgh, Pennsylvania

DAVID E. BECK, MD, Chairman, Department of Colon and Rectal Surgery, Ochsner Clinic Foundation, New Orleans, Louisiana

ROBIN P. BOUSHEY, BSc, MD, PhD, CIP, FRCSC, Assistant Professor of Surgery; Clinical Investigator, Ottawa Health Research Institute, Cancer Centre Program; Director of Research, Division of General Surgery, Department of Colon and Rectal Surgery, Minimally Invasive Surgery Research Group, University of Ottawa, The Ottawa Hospital—General Campus, Ottawa, Ontario, Canada

PETER A. CATALDO, MD, Associate Professor of Surgery, Department of Surgery, University of Vermont, College of Medicine, Burlington, Vermont

JOSE CINTRON, MD, Assistant Professor, Department of Surgery, University of Illinois, Chicago, Illinois

GEOFFREY P. DUNN, MD, FACS, Department of Surgery and Palliative Care Consultation Service, Hamot Medical Center, Erie, Pennsylvania

NAZLI ERBAY, MD, Assistant Professor of Radiology, Tufts University Medical School, Boston, Massachusetts; Department of Diagnostic Radiology, Lahey Clinic Medical Center, Burlington, Massachusetts

BRIDGET N. FAHY, MD, Surgical Oncology Fellow, Department of Surgery, Memorial Sloan-Kettering Cancer Center, New York, New York

JEAN PIERRE GAGNÉ, MD, FRCSC, Assistant Professor, Department of Surgery, Université Laval, Québec, Canada

ROBERT GRYFE, MD, PhD, FRCSC, Assistant Professor, Department of Surgery, University of Toronto, Toronto, Canada

WILLIAM R. JARNAGIN, MD, Associate Attending Surgeon, Associate Professor, Memorial Sloan-Kettering Cancer Center, Weill Medical College of Cornell University, New York, New York

ORIT KAIDAR-PERSON, MD, Research Fellow, Department of Colorectal Surgery, Cleveland Clinic Florida, Weston, Florida

GUILLAUME MARTEL, MD, CM, Division of General Surgery, Minimally Invasive Surgery Research Group, University of Ottawa, The Ottawa Hospital—General Campus, Ottawa, Ontario, Canada

NEELA NATARAJAN, MD, Department of Medical Oncology, Lahey Clinic Medical Center, Burlington, Massachusetts

BENJAMIN PERSON, MD, Clinical Fellow, Department of Colorectal Surgery, Cleveland Clinic Florida, Weston, Florida

ERIC C. POULIN, MD, MSc, FRCSC, FACS, Wilbert J. Keon Professor and Chair, Department of Surgery, University of Ottawa; Surgeon-in-Chief, Department of Surgery, The Ottawa Hospital, Ottawa, Canada

THOMAS E. READ, MD, FACS, FASCRS, Chief, Division of Colon and Rectal Surgery, Western Pennsylvania Hospital, Pittsburgh, Pennsylvania; Associate Professor of Surgery, Temple University School of Medicine, Pittsburgh, Pennsylvania

BRUCE E. SANDS, MD, MS, Medical Co-Director, Crohn's and Colitis Center; Director of Clinical Research, Gastrointestinal Unit; Associate Physician, Massachusetts General Hospital; Assistant Professor of Medicine, Harvard Medical School, Boston, Massachusetts

RICHARD M. SATAVA, MD, FACS, Professor, Department of Surgery, University of Washington Medical Center, Seattle, Washington

CHRISTOPHER D. SCHEIREY, MD, Assistant Professor of Radiology, Tufts University Medical School, Boston, Massachusetts; Department of Diagnostic Radiology, Lahey Clinic Medical Center, Burlington, Massachusetts

TODD D. SHUSTER, MD, Department of Medical Oncology, Lahey Clinic Medical Center, Burlington, Massachusetts

MARC SINGER, MD, Assistant Professor, Department of Surgery, University of Illinois, Chicago, Illinois

TAI M. TRAN, MD, Clinical Fellow, Tufts University Medical School, Boston, Massachusetts; Department of Diagnostic Radiology, Lahey Clinic Medical Center, Burlington, Massachusetts

CHRISTOPH WALD, MD, PhD, Assistant Professor of Radiology, Tufts University Medical School, Boston, Massachusetts; Department of Diagnostic Radiology, Lahey Clinic Medical Center, Burlington, Massachusetts

STEVEN D. WEXNER, MD, FACS, FRCS, FRCS(Ed), Chairman, Department of Colorectal Surgery, 21st Century Oncology Chair in Colorectal Surgery, Chief of Staff, Cleveland Clinic Florida, Weston, Florida; Professor of Surgery, Ohio State University Health Sciences Center at the Cleveland Clinic Foundation, Cleveland, Ohio; Clinical Professor of Surgery, University of South Florida College of Medicine, Tampa, Florida; Clinical Professor of Biomedical Science, Department of Biomedical Science, Charles E. Schmidt College of Medicine, Florida Atlantic University, Boca Raton, Florida.

CONTENTS

Recent advances in our knowledge of colorectal cancer genetics are
proving useful in its management. Accurate screening and counseling is now available for individuals at risk of rare inherited cancer
syndromes. The first two biologic-based therapies have recently
been introduced into clinical use, and molecular genetic-based chemopreventative strategies have been shown to modestly reduce
colorectal neoplasia risk. Our knowledge has produced significant
understanding of what genetic alterations define prognosis and
predict response to specific chemotherapeutic agents, and mass
genetic-based clinical screening efforts are being explored. Enthusiasm, however, must be tempered by the extraordinary cost that
often accompanies relatively modest gains. Finally, although
genetic-based therapy often receives the greatest attention, molecular genetics will likely have the greatest cost-effective impact in primary prevention and early diagnosis.

Screening of asymptomatic average-risk patients for the presence
of colon cancer and early detection in precursor stages is of great

interest to the general population. Comprehensive evaluation of symptomatic or high-risk patients represents another important clinical focus. Available techniques for total colon imaging, rectal cancer staging and the role of positron emission tomography are discussed.

Advances in Gastrointestinal Endoscopic Techniques 849
David E. Beck

Newer endoscopic techniques are being described at an increasing rate. It is important for surgeons to remain active in endoscopy and to participate in the development and evaluation of newer techniques. Newer diagnostic options include chromoscopy, which uses dyes; narrow band imaging and magnification endoscopy to assist in identifying lesions and guide biopsy or therapy; and colonic marking with tattoos or clipping. Colonic marking techniques are used frequently in current practice, whereas the other diagnostic options are mainly research tools. Therapeutic options include dilatation and colonic stents, advanced polypectomy techniques, lasers, and control of bleeding. With appropriate patient selection, these options are being offered with increased frequency.

Laparoscopic Colon Surgery: Past, Present and Future 867
Guillaume Martel and Robin P. Boushey

Since its inception, laparoscopic colon surgery has been limited by a significant learning-curve and issues as well as early concerns over port site metastases and the adequacy of oncologic resection. Recent randomized controlled trials have demonstrated the safety and feasibility of this approach for both benign and malignant colonic pathologies. Good evidence also exists to support several short-term postoperative benefits in laparoscopic resection compared with traditional laparotomy. Given the steep learning curve associated with laparoscopic colon surgery, technologies have been developed to assist surgeons in performing these procedures safely, prudently, and effectively. Some of these include sleeveless hand-assist devices, hemostatic instruments such as the ultrasonic scalpel and electrothermal bipolar vessel sealer, and improved laparoscopic camera systems, including "chip-on-a-stick," flexible, and three-dimensional laparoscopes.

Laparoscopic Rectal Surgery: Rectal Cancer, Pelvic Pouch Surgery, and Rectal Prolapse 899
Robert P. Akbari and Thomas E. Read

With the increasing popularity of minimally invasive approaches to surgery, laparoscopic techniques are being applied increasingly to more complex procedures. Surgeons who are interested in gaining skill and confidence with the techniques of rectal mobilization and resection initially should consider attempting procedures for benign disease. Patients who have rectal prolapse, who often have wide, accommodating pelvic anatomy, are the logical choice with whom to begin the laparoscopic rectal experience. Laparoscopic restorative proctocolectomy is more technically challenging. Laparoscopic proctectomy for rectal cancer probably should remain in the hands of well-trained, high-volume, experienced surgeons who have built a dedicated team for treatment of these patients, and who track their outcomes prospectively.

Transanal endoscopic microsurgery (TEM) has been used effectively to treat large rectal polyps and early rectal malignancy for more than 20 years in Europe. Until recently, only a few specialized centers offered TEM in the United States, where it is now gaining popularity. TEM is unique when compared with laparoscopy and other minimally invasive techniques that incorporate less invasive methods of performing old operations. Regional centers treating large volumes of rectal cancer are embracing TEM with early, encouraging results.

The use of robotics is slowly gaining acceptance in surgery by application to a few niche surgical procedures. There are great opportunities for colorectal surgery with such systems. More important than the technical advantages of dexterity enhancement, tremor reduction, and precision of robotics is the fundamental change in the approach of surgery as an Information Age technology. Viewing the surgical robot as an information system allows integration of the entire process of a surgical procedure. Such systems also provide the technology to perform surgery remotely through telemonitoring and telesurgery. Based upon these principles, three scenarios are proposed that will revolutionize the way that surgeons perform surgical procedures in the future and provide insight about how the operating room of the future will change.

There have been several recent advances in the treatment of common perianal diseases. Stapled hemorrhoidopexy is a procedure of hemorrhoidal fixation, combining the benefits of rubber band ligation into an operative technique. The treatment of anal fissure has typically relied upon internal sphincterotomy; however, it carries a risk of incontinence. The injection of botulinum toxin represents a new form of sphincter relaxation, without division of any sphincter muscle; morbidity is minimal and results are promising. For the treatment of fistula in a fistulotomy remains the gold standard, however, it carries significant risks of incontinence. Use of fibrin sealant to treat fistulae has been met with variable success. It offers sealing of the tract, and then provides scaffolding for native tissue ingrowth.

Patients who have severe fecal incontinence that is not responsive to conservative treatment may be divided broadly into two major categories of surgical approach. Overlapping sphincteroplasty, which is the most prevalent surgical procedure, may offer some benefit to patients who have anatomically identifiable anal sphincter defects, although recent data show that long-term results are moderate to poor. A second group includes incontinent patients who do not have a single, potentially correctable defect. These patients were traditionally treated by construction of a permanent stoma. Fortunately, recent advances in surgical technology have led to several techniques and several surgical alternatives to permanent stoma. This article reviews several of these newer, innovative treatment modalities for fecal incontinence.

This article reviews the basic principles of technical skills acquisition, the various methods of skill transfer, and a blueprint for integration of new skills into practice with special reference to laparoscopic colorectal surgery. Although much is based on evidence, a significant portion also is based on the experience that has been gained in teaching advanced laparoscopic skills to residents, fellows, and surgeons over the last 15 years.

Colorectal cancer (CRC) is a leading cause of cancer death in the United States. Patients who have untreated liver metastases from

CRC rarely survive 5 years and have a reported median survival of 6 to 13 months. The 5-year overall survival following resection of CRC liver metastases in current series is up to 58%. Unfortunately, most patients are not candidates for resection because of the extent or distribution of disease. Consequently, several alternate methods are being used to treat hepatic metastases from CRC, including microwave coagulation, radiofrequency ablation, and transplantation. This article provides a summary of the major studies that have been performed examining the modalities used in the management of hepatic metastases.

Until recently, 5-fluorouracil in combination with leucovorin was the most effective regimen available for patients who had metastatic colon cancer, and this also was the preferred regimen used in the adjuvant setting. The introduction of new chemotherapy agents (irinotecan, capecitabine, and oxaliplatin) and combination regimens, as well as the incorporation of new biologic agents (bevacizumab and cetuximab), has led to significant improvements in median survival for patients who have advanced stage disease. These newer regimens also are being used in adjuvant therapy for earlier stage disease, which is leading to significant improvements in disease-free survival rates. This article reviews the newer agents and combinations, their efficacy and toxicity based on recent clinical trials, and their current and future use in the metastatic and adjuvant settings.

Medical therapy for inflammatory bowel diseases has evolved rapidly over the last decade with the adoption of immune modulators such as 6-mercaptopurine, azathioprine, and methotrexate, and the introduction of infliximab, a chimeric antitumor necrosis factor alpha antibody. Greater explication of the immune and inflammatory mechanisms underlying Crohn's disease and ulcerative colitis has facilitated an abundance of treatments with novel targets and mechanisms of action. These include biologics such as monoclonal antibodies, soluble receptors, cytokines and peptides; and small molecules, including organic compounds and antisense oligonucleotides; medical devices; and live agents with immune-modulating properties. Many of these are likely to reach clinicians in the coming years, increasing the need to understand their mechanisms, potential for efficacy, and possible pitfalls.

FORTHCOMING ISSUES

RECENT ISSUES

SURGICAL
CLINICS OF
NORTH AMERICA

Surg Clin N Am 86 (2006) xv–xvii

Foreword

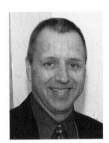

Ronald F. Martin, MD
Consulting Editor

I was recently at the annual meeting of the Society for Surgery of the Alimentary Tract, where I heard a very fascinating comment: "If surgeons were practicing evidence based surgery, the standard of care for all colectomies would be laparoscopic resection." I may be paraphrasing ever so slightly, but I wrote this down as quickly as I could in my notes. I also extend my apologies to the speaker who made the comment, because I was so taken by the statement that I momentarily forgot which of the speakers had uttered the sentence. The list of possibilities is narrow, however, since it occurred during the last day's session on the pros and cons of "straight" laparoscopic versus hand-assisted laparoscopic colectomy for various conditions. The very power of the sentence, though, floored me—to think that we as surgeons have enough *evidence* to establish a *technique* as representing a universal *standard of care* is quite astounding. It became a little less astounding as the session progressed and in each case the varied deliberators came to the conclusions: that if one were pushed, it would be difficult to demonstrate a significant meaningful difference between straight and hand-assisted laparoscopic colectomy and, moreover, one would be hard-pressed to show the same significantly meaningful difference between laparoscopic and open colon resection. It appeared to me that the one point everyone seemed to agree upon was that there were no data to suggest that laparoscopic procedures were inherently worse. Or as you will read in this issue, the data support the "noninferiorty" of laparoscopic colectomy.

When we began restructuring the *Surgical Clinics of North America* series, one of the goals was to try to redefine what constituted a general surgeon

doi:10.1016/j.suc.2006.07.002   *surgical.theclinics.com*

and what topics were of interest to practicing general surgeons. This issue, by Drs. Roberts and Boushey, certainly lends itself well to that line of thinking. I believe it is fair to say that the American Board of Surgery's position is that surgery of the colon and rectum is an expected core competency of those who are certified by the Board's examination process. Following that reasoning, the practice of colon and rectal surgery is a subset of general surgery, yet the data shown within this issue, as well as in many other publications, will demonstrate that surgeon volume and institutional volume (although more so surgeon volume) are independent predictors of superior patient outcomes. From that standpoint, we could make the argument that surgery of the colon and rectum should be left to those who have advanced training and higher individual volumes from a patient quality analysis.

Among the other topics in this issue that should be of interest to all surgeons is the introduction of new technology. How we train both the novice and the experienced surgeon to adopt new techniques, how we finance the incorporation of new devices, how we define and certify competency in these techniques are all basically unresolved issues in our discipline. Historically, the pace of technical change has been sufficiently slow to allow for a more general transition. Since the era of laparoscopy, let alone robotics, let alone tele-robtics, the pace has quickened to the point that natural adaptation is unlikely to completely suffice. Also, we find ourselves in a position of making large statements about small differences (see the opening paragraph). To me, the larger questions are what new problems are we actually solving? How much more (or less) will it cost us to solve them? Over what time frame should the transition take place? And what will be the likely more regional or global impact of these smaller changes?

For a large percentage of the work that is actually performed by general surgeons, one can find data indicating that it might be better and less costly if it were performed by specialists. Whether it is breast surgery, foregut surgery, colorectal surgery, vascular surgery or other areas, the data exist. And, not astonishingly, the reports are largely by specialists (I include myself—guilty as charged). The reality that we as a group have to contend with is this: if we eliminate the general surgeon in every case that might statistically be performed with better outcomes by a specialist, most of the general surgeons in our country would no longer be in business—and at this time, that would be a big problem.

New technology needs to be developed and needs to be disseminated and adopted. The role of the general surgeon will change, and needs to change. Perhaps the traditional model needs to be dispensed with entirely, requiring an overhaul of our postgraduate training model. But these changes will take some time. In the meantime, we need to focus on which of these changes make a huge difference and which make a small difference; which changes can be projected widely and which must be contained to specialty centers; which changes make the system stronger both professionally and financially; and over what time frame the changes should be implemented. At the end of the day, we are all here to serve the needs of our patients, individually and collectively, wherever they may live. It is unlikely that in the foreseeable future we will be able to say that we have enough evidence, based on a smaller or larger number of studies, to declare a universal standard of care. Surgery is still part science and part art, and we have been wrong before.

No matter what your opinion on the above, the articles contained in this issue will give almost any reader insight into the problems that we as general surgeons, colorectal surgeons, minimally invasive surgeons, and surgical oncologists routinely face. We are indebted to the contributors.

Ronald F. Martin, MD
Department of Surgery
Marshfield Clinic
1000 North Oak Avenue
Marshfield, WI 54449, USA

E-mail address: martin.ronald@marshfieldclinic.org

SURGICAL
CLINICS OF
NORTH AMERICA

ELSEVIER
SAUNDERS

Surg Clin N Am 86 (2006) xix–xx

Preface

Several advances in molecular biology, gastrointestinal endoscopy, diagnostic and interventional radiology, minimally invasive surgical techniques, and chemotherapeutics have improved our ability to manage patients with benign and malignant colorectal diseases. As with most new discoveries in medicine, recent changes in the treatment of various colorectal diseases have confronted varying opinions and controversy and have been slow to be adopted into routine practice.

In this issue of the *Surgical Clinics of North America*, we explore several recent advances in the workup and treatment of patients with benign and malignant colorectal diseases. The issue begins with a review of the genetics and recently identified genetic events and pathways associated with colorectal neoplasms. The clinical impact of such information as it relates to genetic counseling, diagnostic tests, prognosis, and potential novel therapeutics is reviewed.

The past decade has also seen the evolution of several nonsurgical endoscopic and radiological techniques aimed at removing the underlying pathologic process while minimizing unnecessary tissue manipulation and trauma. In many instances, this has replaced more-invasive surgical techniques and has resulted in quicker recovery without impacting the quality of care provided. This issue will examine various advances in both radiological imaging and therapeutics, as well as gastrointestinal endoscopic procedures that have, in many instances, replaced traditional surgical procedures.

A similar minimal-access approach has also been adopted by surgeons for treating various colorectal diseases. The laparoscopic colon era began in the 1990s with the successful and safe adoption of these techniques for the treatment of benign colonic conditions such as diverticular disease and benign polyps. Large multi-institutional trials performed in North America and Europe have consistently shown improved short-term outcomes, including reduced postoperative pain, reduced analgesia requirement, shorter hospital stay, and a quicker return of bowel function while preserving long-term oncologic outcomes in patients undergoing laparoscopic colon resection for cancer. We have included a discussion outlining the evidence, controversies, and technical aspects involved in laparoscopic colon surgery as well as a separate discussion highlighting the current status of laparoscopic rectal surgery for both benign and malignant conditions. Separate articles have also been devoted to discussing evolving technologies such as transanal endoscopic microsurgery, robotics and telemonitoring, and new techniques used in the treatment of common perianal diseases and fecal incontinence.

We recognize that one of the challenges associated with the introduction of new surgical techniques is their safe adoption by practicing surgeons. Consequently, we have included a separate article outlining effective strategies for transferring knowledge about new techniques and for acquiring the technical skills necessary for the widespread safe adoption of these techniques by practicing surgeons.

Because traditional multimodality therapy has resulted in overall poor survival and diminished quality of life in patients with advanced colorectal cancer, we felt that it was extremely important to highlight several advances that have occurred in treating these patients. Several newer interventions, including radiofrequency ablation, microwave coagulation, hepatic arterial chemotherapy, and newer systemic chemotherapeutics such as cetuximab, bevacizumab, and oxalaplatin are reviewed. We have also included a discussion on the use of several new and extremely promising immunomodulatory agents such as infliximab, anti-IL-12, and IFN alpha and beta currently being used or tested in the treatment of inflammatory bowel disease.

We are very fortunate to have been able to bring together such an experienced group of authors, who are truly leaders in there respective fields. We are grateful to them for generously contributing their time and expertise in the preparation of this issue. We would also like to thank Catherine Bewick of Elsevier for her tremendous commitment and tireless support in bringing this issue to publication. The current collection of articles provides the reader with the most recent knowledge regarding advances in the treatment of the patient with colorectal disease. We hope that it also stimulates the inquisitive nature of future generations of colorectal specialists.

Robin P. Boushey, BSc, MD, PhD, CIP, FRCSC
Department of Colon and Rectal Surgery
Division of General Surgery
Ottawa Health Research Institute
The Ottawa Hospital
University of Ottawa
501 Smyth Road, Room 2003
Ottawa, Ontario K1H 8L6, Canada

E-mail address: rboushey@Ottawahospital.on.ca

Patricia L. Roberts, MD
Department of Colon and Rectal Surgery
Lahey Clinic
41 Mall Road
Burlington, MA 01805, USA

E-mail address: Patricia.L.Roberts@lahey.org

SURGICAL
CLINICS OF
NORTH AMERICA

Surg Clin N Am 86 (2006) 787–817

Clinical Implications of Our Advancing Knowledge of Colorectal Cancer Genetics: Inherited Syndromes, Prognosis, Prevention, Screening and Therapeutics

Robert Gryfe, MD, PhD, FRCSC

*Department of Surgery and Samuel Lunenfeld Research Institute,
Mount Sinai Hospital, University of Toronto, 600 University Avenue,
Suite 455, Toronto, Ontario, Canada, M5G 1X5*

In the United States it is estimated that more than 145,000 individuals were diagnosed with colorectal cancer in 2005, and that more than 55,000 deaths were attributed to this disease [1]. It is likely that the genetics of no other cancer have been more intensely studied than those of colon and rectal cancer, and this is reflected by the approximately 1000 new scientific publications annotated annually in the National Center for Biotechnology and Information (NCBI) PubMed database (http://www.ncbi.nlm.nih.gov/entrez/) with both the medical subject headings (MeSH) of both "colorectal neoplasms" and "genetics." It is therefore impossible to cover the vast field of colorectal cancer molecular genetics in any single article. This article highlights the aspects of colorectal cancer genetics that are either currently relevant to clinical management or are anticipated to be so in the near future.

Cancer is fundamentally a genetic disease in which a number of genetic alterations present in a cancer cell allow for its uncontrolled growth, evasion of cell death, local invasiveness, and metastatic potential. Central to our understanding of colorectal carcinogenesis is the model proposed by Fearon and Vogelstein [2,3] that the pathological progression of adenoma to carcinoma is accompanied by distinct and reproducible genetic alterations such as APC gene inactivation, K-ras oncogene activation, and p53 mutation, and

The author's research is supported with funds provided by Eli Lilly Canada, Cancer Care Ontario, and the Canadian Institutes of Health Research.

E-mail address: rgryfe@mtsinai.on.ca

that these genetic events are believed to initiate colorectal neoplasia and lead to its orderly pathological progression. Further studies have confirmed this model and implicated many more genes in colorectal carcinogenesis [4]. Furthermore, a more complex genetic understanding of colorectal carcinogenesis has led to the identification of multiple alternate genetic and epigenetic pathways (ie, chromosomal instability, microsatellite instability, and methylator pathways) that appear to give rise to colorectal cancer [5].

To date, perhaps the greatest clinical advances have been recognized secondary to understanding inherited, germline genetic alterations that lead to relatively rare colorectal cancer syndromes; however, a better understanding of the somatic genetic changes that occur within colorectal cancer cells has also led to recent advances in sporadic colorectal cancer clinical management, and is anticipated to have great impact in the near future. The first portion of this article highlights clinical genetic issues relevant to the inherited cancer disorders of familial adenomatous polyposis (FAP), hereditary nonpolyposis colorectal cancer (HNPCC), Peutz-Jegehers syndrome (PJS), juvenile polyposis syndrome (JPS), and Cowden disease. In the second portion of this article, clinical genetic advances in sporadic colorectal cancer management, including the genetic basis of prognosis, response to therapy, screening, chemoprevention and novel therapeutics, are discussed.

Inherited colorectal cancer syndromes

Although approximately 20% of patients who have colorectal cancer or adenomatous polyps have a first-degree relative who has a history of these neoplasms, causative inherited genetic alterations have been identified in fewer than 5% of patients who have colorectal cancer [6]. Inherited syndromes that predispose to colorectal cancer are generally categorized based on the presence of large numbers of adenomatous polyps, few (if any) adenomatous polyps, or the presence of hamartomatous polyps (Table 1).

Table 1
Inherited colorectal cancer syndromes and their associated genes

Syndrome	Associated gene
Adenomatous polyposis syndromes	
Familial adenoamtous polyposis (FAP)	APC
MYH-associated polyposis (MAP)	MYH
Nonpolyposis syndrome	
Hereditary nonpolyposis colorectal cancer (HNPCC)	MSH2, MLH1, MSH6, PMS2
Hamartomatous polyp syndromes	
Peutz-Jeghers syndrome (PJS)	LKB1
Juvenile polyposis syndrome (JPS)	SMAD4, BMPR1A
Cowden disease, including Bannayan-Ruvalcaba-Riley syndrome	PTEN

Familial adenomatous polyposis and the APC and MYH genes

FAP is a rare, autosomal dominant disease that is typically associated with the development of hundreds to thousands of colorectal polyps. FAP accounts for less than 1% of all colorectal cancer, and occurs with a prevalence of approximately 1/8,000 births [6,7]. Adenomatous polyps usually arise during childhood or adolescence, and if left untreated, colorectal cancer will develop in young adulthood. An attenuated form of FAP has also been recognized. In attenuated FAP, the number of adenomatous polyps is decreased (<100), onset may be later, the location of these polyps may be more proximal in the colon, and cancers may not develop until 50 or 60 years of age [6–9].

In addition to colorectal neoplasms, the occurrence rate of several extracolonic tumors is increased in FAP. The FAP variant of Gardner syndrome has been characterized by colonic polyposis, osteomas, and dermoid cysts, whereas Turcot syndrome is distinguished by the occurrence of colorectal and brain neoplasms [6,9]. Extracolonic manifestations of FAP are of particular clinical relevance, because the widespread use of colonic endoscopy and prophylactic proctocolectomy has effectively decreased the likelihood of developing an advanced staged colorectal cancer. As such, periampullary cancer and desmoid tumors have become leading causes of death in individuals who have FAP [10].

The clinical management of FAP (like that of the other colorectal cancer syndromes) is complex and involves counseling, genetic testing, clinical screening, and treatment of multiple organ systems in not only the affected individual, but their at-risk relatives as well [9,11]. Practice parameters for FAP management have recently been published by the American Society of Colon and Rectal Surgeons, and include referral of individuals who have FAP, or those whose personal or family history make them at-risk for FAP, to specialized cancer registries and genetic counselors who specialize in the coordinated multidisciplinary management of these individuals [11]. Although no consensus exists on the lower limits of adenomatous polyp numbers that would raise suspicion for attenuated FAP, the occurrence of twenty or more synchronous polyps has often been used as a guideline [12].

The underlying genetic cause of FAP is a germline mutation in the APC gene [13,14]. In addition to the inherited germline APC mutations that lead to FAP, somatic mutations of the APC tumor-suppressor gene are believed to initiate most sporadic adenomatous polyps and colorectal cancers [3,4,15,16]. For this reason, APC has been dubbed the "gatekeeper" of colorectal neoplasia (Fig. 1). In FAP, a person is born having one mutated copy of the APC gene, and somatic inactivation of the second copy of the gene in a colonic epithelial cell leads to adenoma initiation [3]. In contrast, in sporadic polyps, both copies of APC must be inactivated by somatic events. In approximately 80% of cases of FAP there is a family history of the disease [6]. In the remaining 20% of cases, FAP occurs because of

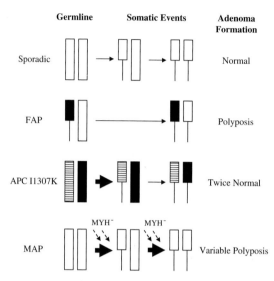

Fig. 1. APC gatekeeper inactivation in colorectal neoplasia. In sporadic cancer, both wild-type APC alleles (□) must undergo somatic mutation to initiate adenomatous polyp formation. In FAP, one APC allele carries a germline mutation (■) and polyp initiation occurs after somatic mutation of the second allele. In APC I1307K carriers, the germline APC variant (▤) undergoes mutation more readily than the wild-type sequence, but both APC alleles must be mutated somatically to lead to polyp initiation. In MYH-associated polyposis (MAP), both APC alleles must be somatically altered, but mutation rates of APC are increased due to the extrinsic forces of germline defects in base excision repair (MYH).

a new APC mutation arising shortly after conception, or when a family history is not evident because of adoption, nonpaternity, or lack of accurate knowledge.

To perform genetic testing for FAP, germline genetic analysis begins with an affected individual [6]. Before genetic testing, informed consent must be obtained. According to practice parameters published by The American Society of Clinical Oncology, before consenting, patients must be informed of [17]:

1. Information on the specific test being performed
2. Implications of a positive and negative result
3. Possibility that the test may not be informative
4. Options for risk estimation without genetic testing
5. Risk of passing a mutation to children
6. Technical accuracy of the test
7. Fees involved in counseling and testing
8. Risks of psychological distress
9. Risks of insurer or employment discrimination
10. Confidentiality issues
11. Options and limitations of medical surveillance and screening following testing

Despite the large size of the APC gene, several characteristics of the mutations observed in FAP have led to efficient detection strategies by which mutations are identified in 80% to 90% of classic cases of FAP [6]. Up to one third of germline APC mutations occur at "hotspot" codons 1061 and 1309 [16,18]. These can be assessed by a number of mutation specific methods that use polymerase chain reaction (PCR) amplification of these genomic DNA regions, such as direct sequencing, heteroduplex analysis, or single-strand conformational polymorphism analysis [6]. Approximately 95% of APC mutations lead to a predicted truncated protein (nonsense mutations) [18]. This has led to the development of an analysis technique known as the protein truncation test (PTT), in which RNA is used to synthesize protein in vitro [6,19]. If a nonsense mutation exists, a faster moving, smaller band is observed (as compared with the wild-type protein) when the PTT product is subject to gel electrophoresis.

Interestingly, mutational analyses in FAP have revealed significant genotype-phenotype correlations [16]:

1. Severe polyposis (> 5000 polyps) is associated with mutations between codons 1250 and 1464.
2. Attenuated polyposis (< 100 polyps) occurs when mutations are at extreme 5′ and 3′ ends of APC gene.
3. Congenital hypertrophy of the retinal epithelium (CHRPE) is associated with mutations between codons 457 and 1444.
4. Desmoid tumors are associated with mutations between codons 1403 and 1578.

Only after an APC mutation is found in an affected individual can unaffected, at-risk members of the same family be appropriately tested. At-risk analysis is site-specific—that is, the specific familial APC mutation is sought, not APC mutations in general [6]. If an at-risk individual does not carry the APC mutation observed in his FAP-affected relative, the at-risk relative is "negative," and can be counseled to receive "normal" population colorectal cancer screening [6,20]. If an APC mutation is not found in testing the initial affected individual, the test is "uninformative." All the first-degree relatives of a genetically uninformative individual who has FAP have a 50% chance of developing polyposis, and should therefore receive counseling and clinical screening. In the case of uninformative testing, linkage analysis may be useful if sufficient affected individuals are available for testing [6]. In FAP linkage analysis, a number of genetic markers near the APC gene are evaluated. Depending on the pattern of these markers in an at-risk individual as compared with multiple affected individuals in the same family, the likelihood for having inherited the disease-causing gene can be estimated. For clinical practicality, only likelihoods of greater than 95% or less than 5% are relevant.

An analysis of commercial APC tests ordered by US physicians in 1995 [20] revealed that fewer than 20% of patients received pretest genetic counseling, that written informed consent was not obtained in nearly 85%

of cases, and that the referring physician could not appropriately interpret test results more than 30% of the time. In the same study, testing was not indicated in 17% of cases, and a further 30% of physicians employed an incorrect testing strategy. These results underscore the potential complexity of FAP management, and the need to refer those affected or at-risk to centers specializing in the management of inherited colorectal cancer syndromes.

Individuals at-risk for FAP, as assessed by personal or family history or positive APC mutation analysis, are advised to begin clinical screening around puberty every 6 to 12 months by flexible sigmoidoscopy [9,11]. When polyps are detected, prophylactic surgery should be undertaken. The timing and extent of surgery depends on the severity of polyposis and whether or not there is rectal sparing. Surgical options include total proctocolectomy with pelvic pouch-anal anastomosis, abdominal colectomy with ileal-rectal anastomosis, or total proctocolectomy with ileostomy. For most cases of classic FAP, a pelvic pouch reconstruction is now the standard of care. Technical issues, including whether or not a mucosectomy is performed and whether or not a hand-sewn versus stapled anastomosis is created, are relatively patient-specific and remain the subjects of some debate. Postoperatively, lifetime endoscopic surveillance of the pelvic pouch, rectum, or ileostomy is required.

In addition to clinical colorectal screening, those who have or are at risk of FAP are recommended to undergo regular screening esophagogastroduodenoscopy starting at approximately 20 years of age [9,11]. The majority of FAP patients develop gastric or duodenal polyps. In contrast, approximately 5% develop duodenal or periampullary cancers. Duodenectomy or pancreaticoduodenectomy is advised in the case of persistent or recurrent severe dysplasia [9,11].

Treatment of desmoid tumors complicating FAP can be difficult [9,11]. Small, well-defined abdominal wall desmoids may be removed surgically. Intra-abdominal desmoids, particularly those involving the small bowel mesentery, should be treated according to their rate of growth and symptoms. Slow-growing, mildly symptomatic tumors may be treated with sulindac, tamoxifen, or vinblastine and methotrexate. Aggressive desmoid tumors may require high-dose tamoxifen, antisarcoma combination chemotherapy such as doxorubicin and dacarbazine, and possibly radiation.

In contrast to the truncating APC mutations observed in FAP, APC I1307K is a single nucleotide substitution (a nontruncating, missense mutation) that leads to a single amino acid difference in the approximate 3000 amino acids that constitute the APC protein [7,21,22]. The APC I1307K variant is carried by an estimated 6% of the Ashkenazi Jewish population, and approximately doubles the risk of developing colorectal polyps and cancers in heterozygous carriers [23]. This type of significant but relatively modest increased cancer risk is explained by incomplete penetrance—that is, those who have the genotype have a modestly increased risk of developing the phenotype. Given the previous successes in identifying the genetic cause of most highly penetrant colorectal cancer syndromes (such as FAP), it is likely that future advances in this field will be in identifying common, lower penetrant alleles, such as APC I1307K.

The APC I1307K variant creates a tract of eight consecutive adenine nucleotides [(A)$_8$] in the DNA sequence that encodes the APC gene, and is not believed to significantly alter the function of the APC protein [21,22]. Instead, the (A)$_8$ offers a nucleotide sequence that is more prone to somatic mutation than the wild-type sequence. Mechanistically, APC I1307K thus behaves like a mutation "hot spot" or a "premutation" (see Fig. 1). Importantly, unlike the highly penetrant, truncating APC mutations observed in FAP that almost universally lead to the development of polyps, the APC I1307K confers an approximate 10% to 15% lifetime risk of polyp or cancer development [22]. Moreover, APC I1307K carriers do not appear to develop colorectal cancer at a clinically significant younger age compared with those who have sporadic cancers [23]. Although the American College of Medical Genetics and American Society of Human Genetics do have guidelines for clinical APC I1307K genetic testing [24], existing literature suggests that neither a positive nor a negative result of this testing is predicted to change recommendations regarding clinical colorectal screening based on family history alone [25,26]. Specifically, a positive genetic test result confirms (but not alters) a recommendation for colonoscopic screening that may be modified based on family history and age of colorectal cancer onset alone. Similarly, a negative APC I1307K genetic result is insufficient to rule out the need for clinical screening should a significant family history exist.

In addition to APC mutations associated with FAP, a second genetic predisposition to colorectal polyposis and cancer has been identified with inherited mutations of the MYH gene [7,27–29]. In general, the polyposis observed in MYH carriers is less severe and is classified as attenuated. MYH participates in a DNA proofreading system known as "base-excision repair," and mutations of the MYH gene are thought to lead to somatic mutations of APC. In particular, specific G:C to T:A transversion mutations of the APC gene occur, which then give rise to colorectal neoplasia. For this reason the MYH gene is thought to be a "caretaker" gene, and increases mutation rate, as compared with the APC gene, which is a "gatekeeper" and initiates neoplasia directly (see Fig. 1).

The clinical genetics of MYH-associate polyposis are not as well-studied, and are more complex than those of APC-associated FAP [28,29]. Mutations of MYH appear to confer a codominant risk. Germline mutations of both MYH alleles (biallelic) are associated with the greatest risk of polyposis and cancer (similar to an autosomal recessive disease). In contrast, carriers of a single mutated copy of the MYH gene are at a moderately increased risk of developing polyps and cancers as compared with noncarriers (similar to an autosomal dominant disease with incomplete penetrance), but less so than biallelic MYH mutation carriers. Thus, MYH mutation carriers may present with attenuated polyposis, or cancer in the absence of synchronous adenomatous polyps. In addition to colorectal polyposis and cancer, adenomatous polyps of the duodenum and piloma-trixomas (benign cutaneous hair follicle neoplasms) have been reported in MYH mutation carriers [30,31]. In FAP cases that are uninformative for APC mutation, germline MYH mutational analysis should be undertaken, because up to one third of these individuals have been observed to harbor biallelic MYH mutations [28].

Hereditary nonpolyposis colorectal cancer, microsatellite instability, and DNA mismatch repair

HNPCC (also known as Lynch syndrome) is an autosomal dominant dis-order characterized by colorectal cancer in the absence of marked polyposis. HNPCC appears to account for approximately 2% to 4% of all colorectal cancer [6,7,32]. Although probands (the incident case) from HNPCC fami-lies are diagnosed with colorectal cancer at approximately 45 years, the ac-tual median age of colorectal cancer diagnosis in HNPCC now appears to be approximately 60 years [33].

In addition to colorectal cancer, numerous other cancers appear to occur at increased frequency in HNPCC kindreds (see Amsterdam II criteria, be-low) [34]. Most notably, the lifetime risks for endometrial or ovarian cancer in a female who has HNPCC are approximately 55% and 15% respectively [6,35]. Historically, Turcot syndrome (colorectal and brain cancers) can be a variant of HNPCC with glioblastoma multiforme, or FAP, where medulloblastoma is usually observed [36]. The HNPCC variant Muir-Torre syndrome is characterized by sebaceous gland adenomas or keratoacantho-mas and visceral cancers [37].

In HNPCC diagnosis is less straightforward than in FAP. In HNPCC, a more diverse range of cancers are observed, there is a lack of profound polyposis, and penetrance is lower than that observed in FAP. Individuals affected with HNPCC have an approximate 50% to 60% lifetime risk of de-veloping a colorectal cancer (compared with a near 100% chance of colorec-tal polyposis or cancer in FAP), and women who have HNPCC have an approximate 55% risk of developing endometrial cancer [6,35].

Clinically, HNPCC has been defined by the International Collaborative Group on Hereditary Nonpolyposis Colorectal Cancer (ICG-HNPCC) in terms of the following Amsterdam II criteria [32]:

1. Three or more relatives who have HNPCC-associated cancer (colorec-tal, endometrial, stomach, ovary, ureter or renal pelvis, brain, small bowel, hepatobilairy tract cancers or sebaceous tumors)
2. One affected individual should be a first-degree relative of the other two.
3. Two or more successive generations should be affected.
4. One or more of these cancers should be diagnosed before the age of 50 years.
5. FAP should be excluded.
6. Tumors should be verified by pathological examination.

Studies of large numbers of cancers have shown that certain characteristics appear more commonly in HNPCC compared with sporadic colorectal cancers. Colorectal cancers in HNPCC tend to arise proximal to the splenic flexure, and are associated with a variety of histological features, including tumor infiltrating lymphocytes, Crohn's-like lymphocytic reaction, mucinous, or signet ring differentiation, and a medullary growth pattern [32,34,38,39].

In addition to frequent differences in their clinical appearance, HNPCC tumors often display a molecular phenotype known as high-frequency microsatellite instability (MSI or MSI-H), also known as replication error positive, [RER+]) [16,40]. This molecular hallmark arises because the underlying genetic cause of HNPCC is a germline mutation in any one of several genes that participate in a DNA replication proofreading system known as mismatch repair [7,16,32,41]. As a "caretaker" system, a deficiency in mismatch repair leads to an increased mutation rate and secondary mutations in the genes, which then give rise to the various cancers observed in HNPCC [6,16]. Additionally, mismatch repair-deficiency causes "bystander" mutations in short, repetitive DNA repeats known as microsatellites (ie, cytosine-adenine dinucleotide repeats [(CA)n], or adenine mononucleotide repeats [(A)n]) (Fig. 2). It is estimated that the human

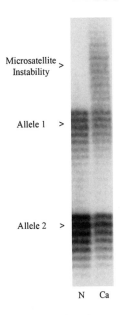

Fig. 2. Microsatellite instability. For a particular microsatellite locus, two consistent sets of (CA)n bands (allele 1 and 2) are amplified from DNA extracted from normal tissue (N). In contrast, allele 1 has undergone microsatellite instability expansion at this locus in DNA extracted from this individual's colorectal cancer (Ca).

genome contains hundreds of thousands of microsatellite repeat DNA regions, largely in noncoding (intronic) regions [42,43]. Microsatellite regions are highly polymorphic, and as such, microsatellite repeat numbers often differ among individuals, but are the same in all cells of any single individual. Instability of a microsatellite is apparent when the copy number of that particular microsatellite DNA region is different in a cancer when compared with normal tissue from that same individual; for example, $(CA)_5$ versus $(CA)_4$. MSI-H is defined as instability in two or more of the five National Cancer Institute-recommended panels of microsatellite loci [44]. Mutations of microsatellite DNA generally have no direct functional consequence on the cell, unless the microsatellite is located in the coding region of a gene [42,44].

To date, germline mutations in four mismatch repair genes—MLH1, MSH2, MSH6 and PMS2—appear to give rise to HNPCC [6,7,41]. The majority of HNPCC occurs because of MLH1 or MSH2 mutations. As with FAP, individuals who have HNPCC are born with one inactivated mismatch repair gene, and the second copy of this gene is then lost as a somatic event. In very rare instances, biallelic germline mismatch repair gene mutations have been identified in individuals who have severe cancer syndromes, leading to colorectal, hematological, and other cancers at very young ages [45].

Immunohistochemical analysis of paraffin-embedded specimens is now available for MLH1, MSH2, MSH6 and PMS2 [46]. In cases of MLH1-deficiency both MLH1 and PMS2 are immunohistochemically absent, because the PMS2 protein is rapidly degraded in the absence of MLH1. Similarly, in MSH2-deficiency both MSH2 and MSH6 protein expression are absent. In contrast, in the case of either PMS2 or MSH6-deficiency, only the gene of interest is not expressed. Although it is sensitive, immunohistochemistry testing may miss a proportion of mismatch repair protein deficiencies that arise because of functionally relevant substitution (missense) mutations that have been observed in 10% to 37% cases of HNPCC [41].

Based on the previously described clinical and genetic knowledge, the ICG-HNPCC now recommends that individuals fulfilling any of the following Revised Bethesda criteria be genetically assessed for HNPCC [32]:

1. Colorectal cancer diagnosed in a patient who is less than 50 years of age
2. Presence of synchronous, metachronous colorectal, or other HNPCC-associated tumors (as outlined in the Amsterdam II criteria), regardless of age
3. Colorectal cancer with the MSI-H histology (as described above) diagnosed in a patient who is less than 60 years of age
4. Colorectal cancer diagnosed in one or more first-degree relatives who has an HNPCC-related tumor, with one of the cancers being diagnosed under age 50 years
5. Colorectal cancer diagnosed in two or more first- or second-degree relatives who have HNPCC-related tumors, regardless of age

If the Revised Bethesda Criteria are met, the ICG-HNPCC recommends the following approach to genetic testing [32]:

1. The optimal approach to evaluation is microsatellite instability or immunohistochemical analysis of tumors, followed by germline MSH2/MLH1 testing in patients who have MSI-H tumors or tumors with a loss of expression of one of the mismatch repair genes.
2. After the mutation is identified, at-risk relatives should be referred for genetic counseling and tested if they wish.
3. An alternative approach, if tissue testing is not feasible, is to proceed directly to germline analysis of the MSH2/MLH1 genes.
4. If no mismatch repair gene mutation is found in a proband with an MSI-H tumor or a clinical history of HNPCC, the genetic test result is noninformative. The patients and the at-risk individuals (ie, relatives) should be counseled as if HNPCC were confirmed, and high-risk surveillance should be undertaken.
5. There is a need to assure patients of confidentiality to allay fears related to discrimination based on genetic status.

In addition to these recommendations, recent publications suggest that MSH6 and PMS2 immunohistochemistry should be performed if MSH2 and MLH1 expression are intact [46]. Furthermore, despite theoretical concerns, studies showing high sensitivity of mismatch repair protein immunohistochemistry as an initial screening tool for HNPCC detection raise the possibility that more laborious microsatellite testing may not be necessary in future clinical screening algorithms [46,47].

Mutational analysis in HNPCC is more complicated than in FAP because: (1) there are more genes to potentially screen; (2) mutations observed in the mismatch repair genes are less likely to occur at recurrent "hotspots"; (3) these mutations are more commonly nontruncating, missense mutations; and (4) these mutations are more commonly large genomic rearrangements, as compared with germline APC mutations [6,18,41]. If tumor tissue is available for analysis, the question of which mismatch repair gene to best assess initially can be screened using immunohistochemistry [47]. In certain populations, such as that of Finland, recurrent founder mutations account for a large percentage of HNPCC germline mutations, and thus genetic analysis begins with sequence-specific analysis for the specific founder mutation [48]. In most populations, founder mutations are not common, and genetic analysis incorporates methods to detect large genomic rearrangements and smaller genetic mutations [41,49]. Large genomic rearrangements account for 10% to 20% of MSH2 mutations and a lesser percentage of MLH1 mutations [6,41]. These mutations are effectively screened for using a recently developed assay known as multiplex ligation-dependent probe amplification (MLPA) [6,49]. In MLPA specific probes are hybridized to genomic DNA and then the probes (as opposed to the DNA) are amplified and quantified. Although germline mutations predisposing to HNPCC often lead to a truncated mismatch repair protein, 10% to 37% of mutations reported in MSH2, MLH1, and MSH6 are thought to be nontruncating, missense mutations [41,44]. Furthermore, germline mutations in HNPCC appear to be roughly equally distributed throughout all exons of the mismatch repair genes. Thus screening of these genes is optimally performed using full sequencing or other methods that may detect either missense or nonsense mutations. When detected, truncating, nonsense mutations are considered to be pathological; however, determining pathogenicity of sequence changes that lead to amino acid substitutions, splice-site changes, or in-frame nucleotide deletions/additions is less straightforward [50]. Predicting whether these alterations are variants of normal or disease-causing relies on a number of factors. Favoring disease causation would be: (1) a nonconservative amino acid substitution (versus conservative or semiconservative), (2) a change in an amino acid evolutionarily conserved between diverse species, (3) the absence of the genetic variant in normal populations, (4) cosegregation of the genetic alteration with disease, and (5) the association of the alteration with tumor MSI-H or lack of specific mismatch repair protein expression [44].

In addition to the high incidence of proximal colon cancer in HNPCC, it is believed that the timeframe of adenoma to carcinoma progression may be markedly accelerated as compared with sporadic colorectal cancer [51]. Thus, a polyp may progress to an invasive cancer in 2 to 3 years, rather than the 8 to 10 years this process is estimated to require in sporadic colorectal carcinogenesis. Mechanistically, this is believed to occur because of the rapid accumulation of somatic mutations associated with neoplastic initiation and progression secondary to mismatch repair deficiency [16]. Practically, this has led to the recommendation that those at risk of HNPCC undergo full colonoscopy, as opposed to flexible sigmoidoscopy, every 1 to 2 years beginning between ages 20 and 25 years [25]. Furthermore, because of the high incidence of endometrial or ovarian cancers in HNPCC, some authors recommend transvaginal ultrasonography, endometrial aspiration for pathological assessment, and plasma CA-125 (an ovarian cancer genetic marker) determination annually beginning at age 30 years in women at-risk for HNPCC [52].

Surgical recommendations in HNPCC remain controversial [11]. This primarily stems from a relative lack of high-level evidence to support or refute the theoretical advantages of prophylactic surgery or extended resection beyond what would normally be oncologically necessary. Given these relative uncertainties, proper counseling is critical to all decision-making and informed consent. The American Society of Colon and Rectal Surgeons recommendations for HNPCC include that individuals who fulfill the Amsterdam criteria and who are diagnosed with more than one advanced adenoma or a colon cancer be offered subtotal colectomy with ileorectal anastamosis or segmental colectomy, whereas those who have rectal polyps or a cancer may be offered total proctocolectomy with ileal-pouch anal anastomosis or anterior resection, assuming the sphincters can be saved

[11]. Prophylactic hysterectomy should be considered in women who have HNPCC undergoing other abdominal surgery or once their family is complete. Significant reduction in endometrial cancer, and to a lesser extent ovarian cancer, has been documented with prophylactic hysterectomy and bilateral salpingo-oopherectomy for women who have germline HNPCC mutations [53]; however, in this recent retrospective study, there was no standardized clinical screening in the group of women who did not undergo prophylactic surgery.

Interestingly, individuals whose family history satisfies the Amsterdam criteria for HNPCC but whose colon cancers do not display MSI-H appear to have a syndrome that is distinct from HNPCC, and has recently been referred to as "Familial Colorectal Cancer Type X" [54]. In a population-based study, Familial Colorectal Cancer Type X was nearly as common as HNPCC. However, as compared with HNPCC, the risk of colorectal cancer in Familial Colorectal Cancer Type X was observed to be more moderate and age of onset later. Furthermore, in Familial Colorectal Cancer Type X, the risk of extracolonic cancers such as endometrial cancer was not appreciably elevated [54]. These results have significant clinical screening and treatment implications, because currently individuals who fulfill the Amsterdam criteria are usually considered to have HNPCC and counseled as such.

Hamartomatous polyposis syndromes

Intestinal hamartomas are frequent in PJS, JPS, and Cowden disease (including Bannayan-Ruvalcaba-Riley syndrome). All these syndromes are very rare, with incidences below 1 per 100,000 [6,7].

PJS is an autosomal dominant disease characterized by perioral pigmentation, pathologically distinct Peutz-Jeghers–type hamartomatous polyps throughout the gastrointestinal tract, and an approximate 30% lifetime risk of colon cancer and 50% risk for breast cancer [6,7]. In PJS, patients are at risk for other extracolonic cancers, including pancreatic, gastric, small bowel, ovarian, uterine, and lung. Approximately 50% of PJS cases are believed to occur because of germline mutations of the STK11 gene [55,56].

Although solitary colonic juvenile polyps are believed to be one of the most common sources of lower gastrointestinal bleeding in children, multiple juvenile polyps are rarely observed [6,7,57]. JPS should be considered when more than three to five juvenile polyps are identified in the colon. The lifetime colon cancer risk in JPS approaches 60%, and patients are additionally at risk of developing stomach, small bowel, and pancreatic cancers. In approximately 50% of JPS cases, germline mutations of either the SMAD4 or BMPR1A genes, both involved in TGFβ signaling, are believed to confer an autosomal dominant risk [58,59]. In addition to genetic testing, colonoscopy, gastroscopy, and small bowel examination are recommended in PJS and JPS [6,57]. Endoscopic or surgical excision of large or symptomatic polyps is recommended.

Cowden disease is an autosomal dominant disease characterized by facial trichilemmomas, oral papillomas, multinodular goiter, fibrocystic breast disease, esophageal glycogenic acanthosis, and intestinal hamartomas [6,7]. Breast and thyroid cancer risk are most pronounced in Cowden disease, with colon cancer developing in up to 10% of patients. Germline mutations of the PTEN gene have been identified in the majority of patients who have Cowden disease, and also predispose to Bannayan-Ruvalcaba-Riley syndrome, which shares characteristics with Cowden disease and additionally includes slowed psychomotor development and pigmentary spotting of the penis [60,61].

In comparison to the "gatekeeper" function of the APC gene and the "caretaker" roles of the mismatch repair and MYH genes, the genes predisposing to hamartomatous polyposis have been dubbed "landscaper" genes [62]. In sporadic circumstances, non-neoplastic hamartomatous polyps are not believed to confer a significant cancer risk. In comparison, germline mutations and somatic inactivation of the STK11, SMAD4, BMPR1A, and PTEN genes in hamartomatous polyposis syndromes are believed to create an epithelial milieu (or landscape) at risk for neoplastic development.

Molecular genetic advances in sporadic colorectal cancer management

Numerous studies to date have focused on the clinical relevance of various genetic alterations in sporadic colorectal cancer management [63,64]. Genetic analyses of blood, stool, and tumors have been proposed as methods for primary polyp and cancer screening, monitoring for cancer response to therapy or recurrence, estimating prognosis and predicting response to adjuvant chemotherapy [64–66]. Furthermore, exploitation of cancer-specific genetic alterations has been proposed as a strategy for chemoprevention and colorectal cancer therapeutics [67,68]. Although some biologic-based chemotherapeutic agents have recently been adopted into colorectal cancer care, molecular genetic testing has not yet gained acceptance in the standard clinical management of sporadic colorectal cancer. Nonetheless, it does appear that genetic-based decision making will play a significant role in colorectal cancer management in the near future.

Genetic markers of prognosis and response to therapy

To date, the prognostic and predictive potential of dozens of genetic alterations in colorectal cancer have been explored [65]. Recently, a number of meta-analyses or systematic reviews of the scientific literature have been published evaluating the most promising of these molecular genetic markers.

Microsatellite instability

Tumor MSI-H is not only observed in the 2% to 4% of colorectal cancers that arise in the context of HNPCC, but is also observed in approximately

15% of sporadic colorectal cancers [2,42,43]. Sporadic MSI-H colorectal cancers appear to arise due to an epigenetic (nonmutational) phenomenon causing mismatch repair deficiency, as compared with the genetic (mutational) cause of mismatch repair deficiency and MSI-H observed in HNPCC [69]. In the majority of sporadic MSI-H colorectal cancers, the MLH1 gene has been silenced by promoter hypermethylation. Interestingly, hypermethylation and silencing of other genes such as p16 appear to be important in colorectal carcinogenesis and in a general sense, a cancer-specific methylation pathway (CpG island methylator phenotype, CIMP) has been proposed [70]. Although the vast majority of the 15% of sporadic colorectal cancers that display MSI-H are also CIMP, this epigenetic phenomenon is also observed in approximately 5% of the 80% to 85% of sporadic colorectal cancers that are microsatellite stable (Fig. 3) [71].

Arguably, MSI status has emerged the most consistent independent molecular genetic predictor of survival [38,72,73]. In a recent systematic review of the literature involving 32 studies and more than 7600 patients who had colorectal cancer [74], 17% were MSI-H, and the vast majority of the remaining 83% of cancers were microsatellite stable (MSS). A small number of cancers were observed to have an intermediate genotype referred to as low-frequency microsatellite instability (MSI-L). MSI-H was associated with a hazard ratio of 0.65 (95% CI, 0.59–0.71) of dying when compared with MSS cancers. That is, the risk of a patient who had MSI-H cancer dying was 65% that of a patient who had MSS colorectal cancer, even after controlling for pathological stage and other clinical predictors of survival.

Although cancer MSI-H status is associated with independent improved survival in patients who have colorectal cancer, it appears likely that patients who have MSI-H cancers do not derive the same benefit from

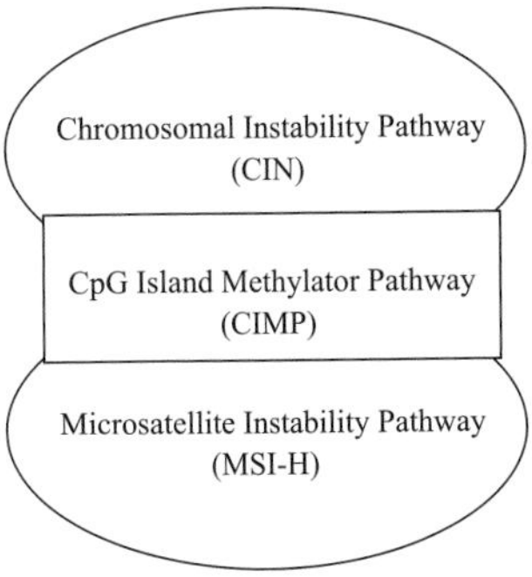

Cancer Characteristics	Sporadic Colorectal Cancer	Inherited Colorectal Cancer
CIN/MSS	80%	FAP <1%
CIMP/MSS	5%	not reported
CIMP/MSI-H	10-15%	rare[†]
MSI-H	rare[‡]	HNPCC 2-4%

Chromosomal Instability Pathway (CIN)
CpG Island Methylator Pathway (CIMP)
Microsatellite Instability Pathway (MSI-H)

Fig. 3. Genetic and epigenetic pathways of colorectal carcinogenesis. Colorectal cancer evolves through either the chromosomal instability (CIN) pathway, which is additionally characterized by microsatellite stability (MSS) or the microsatellite instability (MSI-H) pathway. The CpG island methylator pathway (CIMP) appears to overlap both MSI-H and CIN/MSS colorectal cancers. Percentages indicate estimated prevalence as a proportion of all colorectal cancer. [†]There have been two case reports of an HNPCC variant secondary to apparent germline CIMP [145]. [‡]Some sporadic MSI-H colorectal cancers may arise in the absence of CIMP [146].

fluorouracil (5-FU)-based adjuvant chemotherapy as patients who have
MSS colorectal cancers. In two studies of patients who had Stage II or III
colorectal cancer enrolled in randomized control trials of surgery alone compared with surgery plus adjuvant 5-FU-based chemotherapy [75,76], patients who had MSS were observed to benefit from 5-FU adjuvant
chemotherapy, whereas those who had MSI-H cancer did not benefit, and
may in fact have been harmed by the addition of 5-FU. A similar observation was noted in two recently published case series [77,78], but not in another [79], perhaps because of treatment biases not present in the
randomized control trials. Clinically, this suggests that 5-FU adjuvant chemotherapy should be withheld in the 15% to 20% of individuals who have
MSI-H colorectal cancer; however, the current observations are based on
retrospectively reanalysis of older clinical trials in the context of MSI-status.
Given the widespread acceptance of adjuvant 5-FU in Stage III colorectal
cancer and Stage II cancers with poor prognostic features, it appears that
new prospective randomized trials of MSI-status and 5-FU will only be possible in patients who have Stage II cancers without poor prognostic features
[80,81]. The ethical dilemma of withholding established 5-FU treatment may
be circumvented, however, if subgroup analyses of newer chemotherapeutic
agents such as irinotecan or oxaliplatin show specific benefit to patients who
have MSI-H colorectal cancer [65,82].

Chromosomal instability, p53, and DCC

Whereas 15% to 20% of colorectal cancers display MSI-H, the majority
of colorectal cancers are MSS [42,43]. In comparison with MSI-H colorectal
cancers, which display frequent micro-genetic (intragenic) mutations, most
MSS colorectal cancers display widespread alterations at the chromosomal
level. These macro-genetic alterations may be measured by techniques such
as flow cytometry, G banding cytogenetics, comparative genomic hybridiza-
tions (CGH), DNA allelotyping, or DNA fingerprinting [83]. Chromosomal
instability (CIN) measured by these methods may be characterized by abnormal chromosome number (aneuploidy) or gross changes within a chromosome such as allelic imbalance or loss of heterozygosity (LOH) [44,83].
MSI-H cancers rarely display CIN/LOH and are thus chromosomal stable,
and conversely, most MSS cancers do display CIN/LOH. In contrast to microsatellite status, no widely accepted consensus definition of CIN exists.
Furthermore, unlike MSI-H, which is known to be caused by an underlying
defect in DNA mismatch repair, no generalized mechanistic cause for CIN
has been discovered to date [84].

Consistent with the survival benefit observed for MSI-H, colorectal cancers displaying CIN as measured by either aneuploidy [85–87] or widespread
LOH [88] have been observed to be associated with poor survival; however,
this association has not been as consistently reported [63,64,83]. Furthermore, no meta-analysis or systematic review of the literature has been published summarizing colorectal CIN and survival. Thus, neither American

Society of Clinical Oncology, nor College of American Pathologists recommend the routine use of DNA content determination in colorectal cancer management [63,64].

In general, LOH is believed to eliminate either one or both copies of a tumor suppressor gene. Chromosomes 5q, 17p, and 18q all display considerable levels of LOH in colorectal cancer [89]. In the cases of 5q and 17p, the somatic genetic targets are believed to be the APC and p53 tumor suppressor genes, respectively [3,16]. In the case of 18q, debate continues as to whether the target is DCC, SMAD2, SMAD4, some combination of these putative tumor suppressor genes, or an as-yet-unidentified gene target [90].

Both 17p/p53 and 18q/DCC have been the focus of considerable research in colorectal cancer prognosis [91,92]. In the case of chromosome 17p, an intragenic mutation of the p53 gene commonly accompanies LOH, leading to inactivation of both copies of the p53 tumor suppressor gene [92,93]. Mutations of p53 (paradoxically) lead to stabilization of the mutant p53 protein, and can be detected by positive p53 expression by immunohistochemistry [94]. By comparison, the wild-type p53 protein is unstable and not visualized by immunohistochemistry. Approximately 45% to 55% of colorectal cancers harbor chromosome 17p LOH, p53 expression by immunohistochemistry, or p53 mutations by direct analysis, and there is strong correlation between these detection methods [92,94].

A recent systematic review of p53 abnormalities and colorectal cancer outcome from 241 publications involving nearly 19,000 patients [92] found that either p53 mutation or positive expression of p53 by immunohistochemistry was associated with a survival hazard ratio of approximately 1.24 to 1.43. Thus, the presence of a p53 mutation appears to confer an approximate 30% worse survival when compared with patients whose colorectal cancers do not have a p53 mutation. In neither this systematic review nor a recent reanalysis of three previous randomized trials of surgery alone versus surgery plus 5-FU-based adjuvant chemotherapy [95] was p53 status predictive of response to 5-FU adjuvant chemotherapy.

Chromosome 18q LOH and loss of DCC expression are observed in approximately 55% of colorectal cancers [91,96,97]. A recent meta-analysis of 17 studies of nearly 2200 patients [91] concluded that 18q LOH or loss of DCC expression were associated with a survival hazard ratio of 2.00 (95% CI 1.49–2.69) when compared with patients whose tumors did not show 18q LOH or had intact DCC expression. Thus, patients whose cancers display 18q LOH or DCC loss appear to have twice the risk of dying compared with those who do not show these molecular genetic features. This meta-analysis did not address the predictive impact of 18q LOH or DCC expression on response to 5-FU.

MSI status, p53 mutation, and DCC expression are nonrandomly associated with one another. MSI-H colorectal cancers infrequently harbor chromosome 17p or 18q LOH, p53 mutations, and usually express DCC [5,98,99]. Conversely, MSS/CIN cancers frequently display 17p or 18q

LOH, p53 mutations, and are often DCC-deficient. Thus future studies must address whether these survival associations previously identified are pathway-specific (ie, MSI-H versus MSS/CIN) or somatic target-specific (ie, DCC or p53 wild-type versus mutant).

Thymidylate synthase

Thymidylate synthase (TS) is an enzyme that catalyzes the methylation of deoxyuridine-5'-monophosphate (dUMP) deoxythymidine-5'-monophosphate (dTMP), providing the sole intracellular de novo source of thymidine [100]. The main mechanism of 5-FU is thought to be inhibition of TS. A recent meta-analysis of 20 studies with approximately 3500 patients [101] found that increased cancer TS expression was observed in approximately 50% of cancers and was associated with poorer patient survival. The combined hazard ratio for high TS expression was 1.74 (95% CI, 1.34–2.26), implying that patients whose tumors expressed high levels of TS had a 74% greater chance of dying compared with patients who had low TS expressing tumors. The association between TS expression and 5-FU responsiveness remains controversial. In the two largest trials to date to analyze TS expression in colorectal cancer patients randomized to surgery alone or surgery plus adjuvant 5-FU, one study of 862 patients [102] concluded that high TS expression compared with low was associated with 5-FU responsiveness (ie, improved survival of patients who received surgery plus 5-FU), whereas a second study of 706 patients [95] failed to demonstrate this association.

In addition to MSI-status, p53, DCC, and TS, numerous other genetic markers have been explored less extensively for their role in prognosis or as predictors of response to adjuvant or palliative chemotherapy [65,83,103–105]. Included in this list are chromosomal loci, tumor suppressor genes, oncogenes, and genes regulated by methylation believed to be involved directly in colorectal carcinogenesis, as well as genes whose product may be important specifically in pathways affected by 5-FU or newer colorectal cancer chemotherapeutic agents such as oxaliplatin, irinotecan, bevacizumab, or cetuximab. Although these studies have not yet led to specific recommendations for clinical management, it is likely that some of these genetic markers will make their way into the clinic in the near future [63,64]. Furthermore, new genomic and proteomic technologies offer the potential for interrogating whole genome [106,107] and proteome [108] associations with survival and response to therapy, and the future possibility of individualized molecular medicine.

Molecular genetic colorectal cancer screening

Given the common occurrence of adenomatous polyps and colorectal cancer in Western society, and the relative invasiveness of current screening procedures such as colonoscopy, the potential to identify cancer- or polyp-specific genetic markers from bodily fluids including blood or stool offers a potentially attractive avenue for sporadic cancer screening [66,109,110]. In general, both blood- and stool-based assays attempt to detect the same genetic alterations that are observed in colorectal cancers, via cells shed from the tumor into the bloodstream or gastrointestinal tract lumen. Currently, the most promising approach to genetic-based colorectal cancer screening appears to be stool-based DNA detection technologies [66,110]. Based on current research results, genetic-based screening for sporadic colorectal cancer should still be viewed as investigational. Despite this, commercial clinical DNA stool testing is currently available through licensed health care provider requisition in the United States (http://www.exactsciences.com/medical/pregen.html).

Detection of several different cancer genetic alterations from stool has been proposed as a possible clinical colorectal neoplasia screening strategy. Included within the genetic targets are APC, p53, and K-Ras mutations, as well as markers of MSI-H, LOH, and CIMP [66,110]. Another interesting strategy involves detection of intact long DNA within stool samples. The rationale for this lies in the fact that normal colonic epithelium exfoliates after undergoing apoptosis (programmed cell death), whereby the cell and its DNA are fragmented, and thus the presence of intact long DNA in stool is most likely to have originated from sloughed cancer or adenoma cells.

Overall detection from stool samples of any single genetic marker of neoplasia is only predicted to afford a sensitivity of approximately 40% [66,110]. In part this is because of the fact that no one alteration is present in all colorectal cancers and adenomas. Additionally, although concordance between stool sample and tumor testing is usually in the order of 80%, detection of a cancer DNA from stool is not perfect. To overcome these limitations, more recent efforts have involved panels of genetic markers. Using panels of tumor DNA markers for stool screening, sensitivities of 63% to 100% have been reported for colorectal cancer detection; however, virtually all studies of genetic-based screening in stool samples reported to date have involved a relatively small numbers of patients who had known cancer or adenomas.

Only one fully reported study to date has included a substantial average risk population [111]. A DNA fecal panel of 21 alterations from five different genetic markers was investigated in 2507 asymptomatic individuals. Thirty-one of these subjects had colorectal cancer, whereas 1051 had adenomas. Genetic stool screening sensitivity was only 51.6% for cancer and 10.5% for adenomas. The specificity of the test panel was 94.4%. Although fecal DNA testing outperformed fecal occult blood screening in this study, low sensitivities for both fecal DNA and occult blood testing mean that the majority of all neoplasms were not detected by either, and were discovered only by colonoscopic screening. Furthermore, given a relatively low prevalence of colorectal cancer in the general population, even a specificity of 94% is predicted to mean that just 2% of adults 50 to 59 years with a positive fecal DNA screen have colorectal cancer [112]. At present, fecal DNA screening is estimated to cost $400 to $800, and is predicted to cost at least three times as much per year of life gained compared with fecal occult blood testing. Thus, although promising, stool-based cancer DNA screening performance must improve and the cost must decrease if this technology is going to rival current colorectal cancer screening strategies.

Chemoprevention

A number of interventions with pharmaceuticals, vitamins, and minerals have been undertaken in high-, intermediate-, and average- risk populations to prevent formation of adenomatous polyps and colorectal cancer [67,113]. Although the absolute effect of all agents tested to date is modest, good scientific data do exist to support significant chemopreventative roles in colorectal neoplasia for nonsteroidal anti-inflammatories (NSAIDs), calcium carbonate, selenium and hormone replacement therapy (HRT).

Nonsteroidal anti-inflammatories

At present, NSAIDs are the most well-established agents in colorectal neoplasia chemoprevention, both in terms of the mechanism of effect and the risk reduction they afford [67,113]. The molecular basis of NSAID chemoprevention is primarily attributed to inhibition of cyclooxygenase (COX) enzymes in the conversion of arachidonic acid to prostaglandins [67,114,115]; however, in addition to inhibition of COX enzymes, NSAIDs may inhibit colorectal neoplasia through non-COX–mediated pathways [67,116]. For instance, aspirin has been shown to cause nuclear translocation of the NF-κB transcription factor and cancer cell apoptosis [116].

The COX enzyme comes in two isoforms: COX-1 and COX-2. COX-1 is a housekeeping protein that is constitutively expressed in many tissues, and is thought to lead to production of cytoprotective prostaglandins in the gastrointestinal tract [114,115]. In comparison, COX-2 expression is induced in response to growth factors, mitogens, and cytokines. It is through the inhibition of COX-2 by NSAIDs or specific COX-2 inhibitors that anti-inflammatory, analgesic and antipyretic effects are thought to occur [114,115].

Compared with normal colonic epithelium, COX-2 is overexpressed in approximately 50% of colorectal adenomas and in 85% of cancers [117]. It is hypothesized that this overexpression occurs as a result of transcription induction by oncogenic pathways. In support of this, wild-type p53 suppresses COX-2 expression, whereas mutant p53 leads to COX-2 overexpression [118]. Abundant experimental data also support the hypothesis that inhibition of COX-2 causes suppression of colorectal neoplasia. Preclinical in vivo evidence includes dose-dependent attenuation of the polyp phenotype in mouse models of FAP when these mice were crossed with heterozygote and homozygote COX-2 deficient mice [119] or were fed increasing doses of the COX-2 inhibitor celecoxib [120].

COX-2 overexpression is thought to drive tumorigenesis through multiple mechanisms [67,114,115]. COX-2 overexpression is associated with: (1) vascular endothelial growth factor (VEGF) secretion and angiogenesis; (2) increased expression of the BCL2 protein and resistance to apoptosis; (3) increased expression of metalloproteinases (MMPs) and CD44, and increased cancer cell invasiveness and metastasis; and (4) impairment of tumor infiltrating lymphocytes (TILs), circulating T-cells, and macrophages and host immunosuppression.

The most compelling evidence for NSAID chemoprevention of colorectal neoplasia comes from two double-blind, randomized-controlled trials. In one trial [121], 635 patients who had previously resected early colon cancer were randomized to aspirin 325 mg per day versus placebo for 3 years. Aspirin use was associated with a significant decrease of adenoma relative risk of 0.65 (95% CI, 0.46–0.91) on follow-up colonoscopy at a median of 12.8 months. Thirty percent of those on aspirin and 49% of those on placebo developed adenomas, and the time to detection of first adenoma was significantly longer in the aspirin group. In the second study [122], 1121 patients who had previous adenomas were randomized to aspirin 325 mg or 81 mg per day or placebo. In this trial, low-dose aspirin use was associated with a significantly reduced adenoma relative risk of 0.81 (95% CI, 0.69–0.96) and a relative risk of 0.59 (95% CI, 0.38–0.92) for advanced adenomas (≥ 1 cm in diameter, tubulovillous, villous, severe dysplasia, or invasive cancer) compared with placebo. Thirty-eight percent of individuals on aspirin 81 mg developed adenomas compared with 47% of those on placebo. No significant risk reduction was observed for those on aspirin 325 mg, 45% of whom developed adenomas.

Although modest but significant Level I evidence for colorectal neoplasia risk reduction has been demonstrated for nonspecific COX inhibition by aspirin, two recent chemoprevention trials with specific COX-2 inhibitors have been associated with significant increases in cardiovascular death and complications [123,123a]. In both trials, patients with previous colorectal adenomas were randomized to either placebo or one of the specific COX-2 inhibitors, celebrex or rofexoxib. In one trial [123], a total of 2035 patients who had previous adenomas were randomized to celebrex 200 mg twice daily, or 400 mg twice daily, or placebo. At approximately three years, a significant dose-response association was observed between celebrex use and death from myocardial infarction, stroke or heart failure with 3.4%, 2.3% and 1% cardiovascular mortality observed for those on celebrex 400 mg twice daily, 200 mg twice daily, and placebo, respectively. In the second chemoprevention trial [123a], a total of 2586 patients who had previous adenomas were randomized to rofecoxib 25 mg daily or placebo. Adverse thrombotic cardiovascular events, primarily myocardial infarctions and ischemic cerebrovascular events, were observed more often in those on rofecoxib (1.50 events per 100 patient-years) compared with those on placebo (0.78 events per 100 patient-years). A significantly increased relative risk of 1.92 (95% CI,

1.19–3.11) was observed after 18 months of rofecoxib use. Additionally, the rates of congestive heart failure, pulmonary edema, or cardiac failure may have been increased in those taking rofecoxib. Although cardiovascular events differed significantly in this trial, mortality from cardiovascular events was similar in those on rofecoxib compared to those taking placebo.

Chemoprevention in FAP has been an area of great interest [67]. The nonspecific COX inhibitor sulindac [124] and the COX-2 inhibitor celecoxib [125] have both been shown in several randomized, double-blind, placebo-controlled clinical trials to cause significant regression of existing polyps and to decrease new polyp formation in FAP patients [67,113,114]; however, there have also been case reports of FAP patients who had ileorectal anastomoses developing rectal cancers while on sulindac [126,127]. Furthermore, a 4-year randomized controlled trial failed to show an effect of sulindac on primarily prevention of polyps in at-risk patients who had APC mutations, but without polyposis at study enrollment [128]. Additionally, trials have not typically found that sulindac effectively treats duodenal adenomas [11]. For these reasons, NSAIDS and COX-2 inhibition should not be used as an alternative to surgery in FAP.

Calcium carbonate, selenium, and hormone replacement therapy

In addition to NSAIDs, Level I evidence exists for colorectal neoplasia chemoprevention with calcium carbonate, selenium, and HRT [67,113], although not all large placebo-controlled trials of these agents have demonstrated colorectal neoplasia risk reduction. Furthermore, in the case of HRT use, significant adverse health risks have been observed [129].

Unlike the COX-2 mediated effects of NSAIDs, the chemopreventative mechanisms of calcium carbonate, HRT, and selenium are poorly understood [67]. Calcium is believed to exert its antineoplastic effects through both luminal binding of mutagenic bile acids in addition to direct effects [130,131]. Extracellular calcium can activate a number of signaling pathways and intracellular calcium influences several nuclear proteins [130]. HRT is believed to directly and indirectly reduce bile acid production and inhibits insulin-like Growth Factor I [67,132]. Selenium is antioxidant [133]; however, at the present time, molecular genetic mechanisms linking calcium carbonate, HRT, and selenium and colorectal neoplasia chemoprevention remain largely speculative.

Genetic-based colorectal cancer treatment

One hope accompanying the complete sequencing of the human genome was the rapid development of genetic-based therapeutics for a myriad of diseases. In no disease were post-genomic clinical advances more anticipated than in cancer. To date two drugs, bevacizumab and cetuximab, have received United States Food and Drug Agency approval for use in colorectal cancer management [134].

Bevacizumab

Bevacizumab is a monoclonal antibody that targets and binds vascular endothelial growth factor-A (VEGF-A) [135]. This reduces the amount of VEGF ligand available to bind to its receptor, and prevents receptor activation. The VEGF pathway is believed to critical in cancer angiogenesis. Cancer cells secrete substances such as VEGF to recruit host vasculature to supply cancer growth.

Bevacizumab has been evaluated in first-line combination therapy for metastatic colorectal cancer. The first Phase III trial of bevacizumab [136] involved 813 patients who had metastatic colorectal cancer randomized to irinotecan, 5-FU, or leucovorin (IFL) plus placebo or bevacizumab. In this study, patients receiving IFL plus bevacizumab had significantly longer median survival compared with IFL alone, 20.3 versus 15.6 months. Additionally, patients receiving bevacizumab had longer progression-free survival, higher response rate, and longer median duration of response compared with those who did not. This benefit was accompanied by greater toxicity; grade 3 or 4 adverse events were observed significantly more often in patients receiving bevacizumab compared with those who did not, 85% versus 74%.

Two further Phase II and III trials have recently been reported using combination treatment with bevacizumab in metastatic colorectal cancer [137,138]. In the Phase III trial [137], 210 patients who had metastatic colorectal cancer were randomized to treatment with IFL or 5-FU, leucovorin (5-FU/LV), and bevacizumab, and a nonsignificant median survival advantage was observed for the 5-FU/LV and bevacizumab treatment group compared with IFL (18.3 versus 15.1 months). The toxicity was roughly equivalent in the two groups—Grade III/IV adverse events: 5-FU/LV and bevacizumab, 77.1%; IFL, 81.6%. In the other study [138], 237 patients who received 5-FU/LV or IFL were compared with 244 patients receiving 5-FU/LV and bevacizumab. Median survival for those receiving 5-FU/LV plus bevacizumab was 17.9 months, compared with 14.6 months in the patients who received 5-FU/LV or IFL. Grade III or IV adverse events were observed in 81% of those who received 5-FU/LV and bevacizumab, compared with 73% of patients who received 5-FU/LV or IFL. In summary, these clinical trials show that IFL plus bevacizumab offers the best survival in metastatic colorectal cancer [136,137], and 5-FU/LV and bevacizumab offer comparable survival to IFL with similar or less toxicity [138].

Cetuximab

Cetuximab is a monoclonal antibody that targets the epidermal growth factor receptor (EGFR) [135,139]. This competitively inhibits ligand binding of the receptor and EGFR activation. EGFR signaling is complex and has been shown to be involved in: (1) cancer cell proliferation; (2) degradation of extracellular matrix, tumor migration and invasion; and (3) endothelial proliferation and angiogenesis [139]. Inhibition of EGFR has proven a successful genetic target for cancer treatment, and in addition to cetuximab, two additional EGFR inhibitors, gefitinib and erlotinib, are in clinical use in non-small–cell lung and pancreatic cancer treatment [135].

One Phase III clinical trial using cetuximab in metastatic colorectal cancer has been reported to date [140]. This study aimed to demonstrate that the addition of cetuximab in second-line treatment of metatstatic disease could resensitize patients to a palliative chemotherapeutic agent that they had previously failed. As such, 329 patients who had progressed on irinotecan-based therapy were randomized to cetuximab alone or cetuximab with irinotecan. Significantly greater response rates (22.9% versus 10.8%) and median time to progression (4.1 versus 1.5 months) were observed in patients who received irinotecan and cetuximab compared with those who received cetuximab monotherapy. No significant difference in median survival (irinotecan and cetuximab, 8.6 months; cetuximab 6.9 months) was observed, however. Thus, although somewhat inconclusive in terms of efficacy, current results of cetuximab in colorectal cancer offer hope that the addition of cetuximab to first-line treatment will improve survival.

The cetuximab clinical trial discussed above did not observe a correlation between colorectal cancer EGFR expression and clinical response [140]. Furthermore, although EGFR overexpression has been observed in 25% to 82% of colorectal cancer specimens [139], oncogenic EGFR mutations (as opposed to protein overexpression) are rarely observed in colorectal cancers [141,142]. In contrast, EGFR gain of function mutations has been observed to predict response to the EGFR inhibitor, gefitinib, in non-small–cell lung cancer [143,144].

The introduction of biologic agents such as bevacizumab and cetuximab dramatically highlights the cost of such advances [134]. Eight weeks of 5-FU/LV are estimated to cost $63 to $304, and the addition of irinotecan or oxilaplatin brings this price to $9381 to $11889. The further addition of bevacizumab or cetuximab bring the drug cost of 8 weeks of therapy to a staggering $21,033 to $30,790. Obviously such costs for significant but relatively modest clinical gains will pose both financial and ethical challenges for the future.

Summary

Recent genetic advances in our knowledge of colorectal cancer genetics are beginning to pay translational dividends in the management of this common clinical problem. We are now able to accurately screen and counsel individuals at risk of rare inherited cancer syndromes. We have recently introduced two of what are sure to be numerous biologic-based therapies, and have shown that colorectal neoplasia risk can be modestly reduced by various chemopreventative agents. Finally, our advancing knowledge has led to significant inroads into understanding what genetic alterations define prognosis and predict response to specific chemotherapeutic agents, and we are beginning to explore the utility of this knowledge in mass genetic-based clinical screening efforts. Enthusiasm must be tempered, however, by the extraordinary cost that often accompanies relatively modest gains. Finally, although genetic-based therapy often receives the greatest attention, molecular genetics, will likely have the greatest cost-effective impact in primary prevention and early diagnosis.

Acknowledgments

I would like to acknowledge and thank Dr. Steve Gallinger for his help and thoughtful insights in the preparation of this manuscript.

References

[1] Jemal A, Murray T, Ward E, et al. Cancer statistics, 2005. CA Cancer J Clin 2005;55:10–30.
[2] Vogelstein B, Fearon ER, Hamilton SR, et al. Genetic alterations during colorectal-tumor development. N Engl J Med 1988;319:525–32.
[3] Fearon ER, Vogelstein B. A genetic model for colorectal tumorigenesis. Cell 1990;61: 759–67.
[4] Vogelstein B, Kinzler KW. Cancer genes and the pathways they control. Nat Med 2004;10: 789–99.
[5] Boland CR, Goel A. Somatic evolution of cancer cells. Semin Cancer Biol 2005;15:436–50.
[6] Burt R, Neklason DW. Genetic testing for inherited colon cancer. Gastroenterology 2005; 128:1696–716.
[7] de la Chapelle A. Genetic predisposition to colorectal cancer. Nat Rev Cancer 2004;4: 769–80.
[8] Knudsen AL, Bisgaard ML, Bulow S. Attenuated familial adenomatous polyposis (AFAP). A review of the literature. Fam Cancer 2003;2:43–55.
[9] King JE, Dozois RR, Lindor NM, et al. Care of patients and their families with familial adenomatous polyposis. Mayo Clin Proc 2000;75:57–67.
[10] Belchetz LA, Berk T, Bapat BV, et al. Changing causes of mortality in patients with familial adenomatous polyposis. Dis Colon Rectum 1996;39:384–7.
[11] Church J, Simmang C. Practice parameters for the treatment of patients with dominantly inherited colorectal cancer (familial adenomatous polyposis and hereditary nonpolyposis colorectal cancer). Dis Colon Rectum 2003;46:1001–12.
[12] American Gastroenterological Association medical position statement: hereditary colorectal cancer and genetic testing. Gastroenterology 2001;121:195–7.
[13] Kinzler KW, Nilbert MC, Su LK, et al. Identification of FAP locus genes from chromosome 5q21. Science 1991;253:661–5.
[14] Nishisho I, Nakamura Y, Miyoshi Y, et al. Mutations of chromosome 5q21 genes in FAP and colorectal cancer patients. Science 1991;253:665–9.
[15] Powell SM, Zilz N, Beazer-Barclay Y, et al. APC mutations occur early during colorectal tumorigenesis. Nature 1992;359:235–7.
[16] Kinzler KW, Vogelstein B. Lessons from hereditary colorectal cancer. Cell 1996;87:159–70.
[17] American Society of Clinical Oncology policy statement update: genetic testing for cancer susceptibility. J Clin Oncol 2003;21:2397–406.
[18] Laurent-Puig P, Beroud C, Soussi T. APC gene: database of germline and somatic mutations in human tumors and cell lines. Nucleic Acids Res 1998;26:269–70.
[19] Powell SM, Petersen GM, Krush AJ, et al. Molecular diagnosis of familial adenomatous polyposis. N Engl J Med 1993;329:1982–7.

[20] Giardiello FM, Brensinger JD, Petersen GM, et al. The use and interpretation of commercial APC gene testing for familial adenomatous polyposis. N Engl J Med 1997; 336:823–7.

[21] Laken SJ, Petersen GM, Gruber SB, et al. Familial colorectal cancer in Ashkenazim due to a hypermutable tract in APC. Nat Genet 1997;17:79–83.

[22] Gryfe R, Di Nicola N, Gallinger S, et al. Somatic instability of the APC I1307K allele in colorectal neoplasia. Cancer Res 1998;58:4040–3.

[23] Gryfe R, Di Nicola N, Lal G, et al. Inherited colorectal polyposis and cancer risk of the APC I1307K polymorphism. Am J Hum Genet 1999;64:378–84.

[24] Genetic testing for colon cancer: joint statement of the American College of Medical Genetics and American Society of Human Genetics. Joint Test and Technology Transfer Committee Working Group. Genet Med 2000;2:362–6.

[25] Winawer S, Fletcher R, Rex D, et al. Colorectal cancer screening and surveillance: clinical guidelines and rationale—update based on new evidence. Gastroenterology 2003;124:544–60.

[26] Smith RA, Cokkinides V, Eyre HJ. American Cancer Society guidelines for the early detection of cancer, 2003. CA Cancer J Clin 2003;53:27–43.

[27] Al-Tassan N, Chmiel NH, Maynard J, et al. Inherited variants of MYH associated with somatic G:C→T:A mutations in colorectal tumors. Nat Genet 2002;30:227–32.

[28] Sieber OM, Lipton L, Crabtree M, et al. Multiple colorectal adenomas, classic adenomatous polyposis, and germ-line mutations in MYH. N Engl J Med 2003;348:791–9.

[29] Croitoru ME, Cleary SP, Di Nicola N, et al. Association between biallelic and monoallelic germline MYH gene mutations and colorectal cancer risk. J Natl Cancer Inst 2004;96: 1631–4.

[30] Nielsen M, Franken PF, Reinards TH, et al. Multiplicity in polyp count and extracolonic manifestations in 40 Dutch patients with MYH associated polyposis coli (MAP). J Med Genet 2005;42:e54.

[31] Baglioni S, Melean G, Gensini F, et al. A kindred with MYH-associated polyposis and pilomatricomas. Am J Med Genet A 2005;134:212–4.

[32] Umar A, Boland CR, Terdiman JP, et al. Revised Bethesda guidelines for hereditary nonpolyposis colorectal cancer (Lynch syndrome) and microsatellite instability. J Natl Cancer Inst 2004;96:261–8.

[33] Hampel H, Stephens JA, Pukkala E, et al. Cancer risk in hereditary nonpolyposis colorectal cancer syndrome: later age of onset. Gastroenterology 2005;129:415–21.

[34] Rodriguez-Bigas MA, Boland CR, Hamilton SR, et al. A National Cancer Institute workshop on hereditary nonpolyposis colorectal cancer syndrome: meeting highlights and Bethesda guidelines. J Natl Cancer Inst 1997;89:1758–10.

[35] Dunlop MG, Farrington SM, Carothers AD, et al. Cancer risk associated with germline DNA mismatch repair gene mutations. Hum Mol Genet 1997;6:105–10.

[36] Hamilton SR, Liu B, Parsons RE, et al. The molecular basis of Turcot's syndrome. N Engl J Med 1995;332:839–47.

[37] Ponti G, Ponz de Leon M. Muir-Torre syndrome. Lancet Oncol 2005;6:980–7.

[38] Gryfe R, Kim H, Hsieh ET, et al. Tumor microsatellite instability and clinical outcome in young patients with colorectal cancer. N Engl J Med 2000;342:69–77.

[39] Kim H, Jen J, Vogelstein B, et al. Clinical and pathological characteristics of sporadic colorectal carcinomas with DNA replication errors in microsatellite sequences. Am J Pathol 1994;145:148–56.

[40] Aaltonen LA, Peltomaki P, Leach FS, et al. Clues to the pathogenesis of familial colorectal cancer. Science 1993;260:812–6.

[41] Peltomaki P, Vasen H. Mutations associated with HNPCC predisposition—update of ICG-HNPCC/INSiGHT mutation database. Dis Markers 2004;20:269–76.

[42] Ionov Y, Peinado MA, Malkhosyan S, et al. Ubiquitous somatic mutations in simple repeated sequences reveal a new mechanism for colonic carcinogenesis. Nature 1993;363: 558–61.

[43] Thibodeau SN, Bren G, Schaid D. Microsatellite instability in cancer of the proximal colon. Science 1993;260:816–9.
[44] Boland CR, Thibodeau SN, Hamilton SR, et al. A National Cancer Institute wworkshop on microsatellite instability for cancer detection and familial predisposition: development of international criteria for the determination of microsatellite instability in colorectal cancer. Cancer Res 1998;58:5248–57.
[45] Ricciardone MD, Ozcelik T, Cevher B, et al. Human MLH1 deficiency predisposes to hematological malignancy and neurofibromatosis type 1. Cancer Res 1999;59:290–3.
[46] Gill S, Lindor NM, Burgart LJ, et al. Isolated loss of PMS2 expression in colorectal cancers: frequency, patient age, and familial aggregation. Clin Cancer Res 2005;11:6466–71.
[47] Hampel H, Frankel WL, Martin E, et al. Screening for the Lynch syndrome (hereditary nonpolyposis colorectal cancer). N Engl J Med 2005;352:1851–60.
[48] Nystrom-Lahti M, Kristo P, Nicolaides NC, et al. Founding mutations and Alu-mediated recombination in hereditary colon cancer. Nat Med 1995;1:1203–6.
[49] Gille JJ, Hogervorst FB, Pals G, et al. Genomic deletions of MSH2 and MLH1 in colorectal cancer families detected by a novel mutation detection approach. Br J Cancer 2002;87:892–7.
[50] Raevaara TE, Korhonen MK, Lohi H, et al. Functional significance and clinical phenotype of nontruncating mismatch repair variants of MLH1. Gastroenterology 2005;129:537–49.
[51] de Vos tot Nederveen Cappel WH, Nagengast FM, Griffioen G, et al. Surveillance for hereditary nonpolyposis colorectal cancer: a long-term study on 114 families. Dis Colon Rectum 2002;45:1588–94.
[52] Burke W, Petersen G, Lynch P, et al. Recommendations for follow-up care of individuals with an inherited predisposition to cancer. I. Hereditary nonpolyposis colon cancer. Cancer Genetics Studies Consortium. JAMA 1997;277:915–9.
[53] Schmeler KM, Lynch HT, Chen LM, et al. Prophylactic surgery to reduce the risk of gynecologic cancers in the Lynch syndrome. N Engl J Med 2006;354:261–9.
[54] Lindor NM, Rabe K, Petersen GM, et al. Lower cancer incidence in Amsterdam-I criteria families without mismatch repair deficiency: familial colorectal cancer type X. JAMA 2005;293:1979–85.
[55] Hemminki A, Markie D, Tomlinson I, et al. A serine/threonine kinase gene defective in Peutz-Jeghers syndrome. Nature 1998;391:184–7.
[56] Jenne DE, Reimann H, Nezu J, et al. Peutz-Jeghers syndrome is caused by mutations in a novel serine threonine kinase. Nat Genet 1998;18:38–43.
[57] Chow E, Macrae F. A review of juvenile polyposis syndrome. J Gastroenterol Hepatol 2005;20:1634–40.
[58] Howe JR, Roth S, Ringold JC, et al. Mutations in the SMAD4/DPC4 gene in juvenile polyposis. Science 1998;280:1086–8.
[59] Howe JR, Bair JL, Sayed MG, et al. Germline mutations of the gene encoding bone morphogenetic protein receptor 1A in juvenile polyposis. Nat Genet 2001;28:184–7.
[60] Marsh DJ, Dahia PL, Zheng Z, et al. Germline mutations in PTEN are present in Bannayan-Zonana syndrome. Nat Genet 1997;16:333–4.
[61] Liaw D, Marsh DJ, Li J, et al. Germline mutations of the PTEN gene in Cowden disease, an inherited breast and thyroid cancer syndrome. Nat Genet 1997;16:64–7.
[62] Kinzler KW, Vogelstein B. Landscaping the cancer terrain. Science 1998;280:1036–7.
[63] Bast RC Jr, Ravdin P, Hayes DF, et al. 2000 update of recommendations for the use of tumor markers in breast and colorectal cancer: clinical practice guidelines of the American Society of Clinical Oncology. J Clin Oncol 2001;19:1865–78.
[64] Compton CC, Fielding LP, Burgart LJ, et al. Prognostic factors in colorectal cancer. College of American Pathologists consensus statement 1999. Arch Pathol Lab Med 2000;124:979–94.
[65] Allen WL, Johnston PG. Role of genomic markers in colorectal cancer treatment. J Clin Oncol 2005;23:4545–52.

[66] Davies RJ, Miller R, Coleman N. Colorectal cancer screening: prospects for molecular stool analysis. Nat Rev Cancer 2005;5:199–209.

[67] Hawk ET, Levin B. Colorectal cancer prevention. J Clin Oncol 2005;23:378–91.

[68] Pantaleo MA, Palassini E, Labianca R, et al. Targeted therapy in colorectal cancer: do we know enough? Dig Liver Dis 2006;38:71–7.

[69] Kane MF, Loda M, Gaida GM, et al. Methylation of the hMLH1 promoter correlates with lack of expression of hMLH1 in sporadic colon tumors and mismatch repair-defective human tumor cell lines. Cancer Res 1997;57:808–11.

[70] Toyota M, Ahuja N, Ohe-Toyota M, et al. CpG island methylator phenotype in colorectal cancer. Proc Natl Acad Sci USA 1999;96:8681–6.

[71] Samowitz WS, Albertsen H, Herrick J, et al. Evaluation of a large, population-based sample supports a CpG island methylator phenotype in colon cancer. Gastroenterology 2005;129:837–45.

[72] Samowitz WS, Curtin K, Ma KN, et al. Microsatellite instability in sporadic colon cancer is associated with an improved prognosis at the population level. Cancer Epidemiol Biomarkers Prev 2001;10:917–23.

[73] Benatti P, Gafa R, Barana D, et al. Microsatellite instability and colorectal cancer prognosis. Clin Cancer Res 2005;11:8332–40.

[74] Popat S, Hubner R, Houlston RS. Systematic review of microsatellite instability and colorectal cancer prognosis. J Clin Oncol 2005;23:609–18.

[75] Ribic CM, Sargent DJ, Moore MJ, et al. Tumor microsatellite-instability status as a predictor of benefit from fluorouracil-based adjuvant chemotherapy for colon cancer. N Engl J Med 2003;349:247–57.

[76] Barratt PL, Seymour MT, Stenning SP, et al. DNA markers predicting benefit from adjuvant fluorouracil in patients with colon cancer: a molecular study. Lancet 2002;360: 1381–91.

[77] Carethers JM, Smith EJ, Behling CA, et al. Use of 5-fluorouracil and survival in patients with microsatellite-unstable colorectal cancer. Gastroenterology 2004;126:394–401.

[78] Jover R, Zapater P, Castells A, et al. Mismatch repair status in the prediction of benefit from adjuvant fluorouracil chemotherapy on colorectal cancer. Gut 2006;55:848–55.

[79] Elsaleh H, Iacopetta B. Microsatellite instability is a predictive marker for survival benefit from adjuvant chemotherapy in a population-based series of stage III colorectal carcinoma. Clin Colorectal Cancer 2001;1:104–9.

[80] Figueredo A, Fine S, Maroun J, et al. Adjuvant therapy for stage III colon cancer after complete resection. Provincial Gastrointestinal Disease Site Group. Cancer Prev Control 1997; 1:304–19.

[81] Figueredo A, Germond C, Maroun J, et al. Adjuvant therapy for stage II colon cancer after complete resection. Provincial Gastrointestinal Disease Site Group. Cancer Prev Control 1997;1:379–92.

[82] Fallik D, Borrini F, Boige V, et al. Microsatellite instability is a predictive factor of the tumor response to irinotecan in patients with advanced colorectal cancer. Cancer Res 2003;63:5738–44.

[83] Vendrell E, Morales C, Risques RA, et al. Genomic determinants of prognosis in colorectal cancer. Cancer Lett 2005;221:1–9.

[84] Rajagopalan H, Nowak MA, Vogelstein B, et al. The significance of unstable chromosomes in colorectal cancer. Nat Rev Cancer 2003;3:695–701.

[85] Lanza G, Gafa R, Santini A, et al. Prognostic significance of DNA ploidy in patients with stage II and stage III colon carcinoma: a prospective flow cytometric study. Cancer 1998;82: 49–59.

[86] Bardi G, Fenger C, Johansson B, et al. Tumor karyotype predicts clinical outcome in colorectal cancer patients. J Clin Oncol 2004;22:2623–34.

[87] Risques RA, Moreno V, Ribas M, et al. Genetic pathways and genome-wide determinants of clinical outcome in colorectal cancer. Cancer Res 2003;63:7206–14.

[88] Kern SE, Fearon ER, Tersmette KW, et al. Clinical and pathological associations with allelic loss in colorectal carcinoma [corrected]. JAMA 1989;261:3099–103.

[89] Vogelstein B, Fearon ER, Kern SE, et al. Allelotype of colorectal carcinomas. Science 1989; 244:207–11.

[90] Riggins GJ, Thiagalingam S, Rozenblum E, et al. Mad-related genes in the human. Nat Genet 1996;13:347–9.

[91] Popat S, Houlston RS. A systematic review and meta-analysis of the relationship between chromosome 18q genotype, DCC status and colorectal cancer prognosis. Eur J Cancer 2005;41:2060–70.

[92] Munro AJ, Lain S, Lane DP. P53 abnormalities and outcomes in colorectal cancer: a systematic review. Br J Cancer 2005;92:434–44.

[93] Baker SJ, Fearon ER, Nigro JM, et al. Chromosome 17 deletions and p53 gene mutations in colorectal carcinomas. Science 1989;244:217–21.

[94] Baas IO, Mulder JW, Offerhaus GJ, et al. An evaluation of six antibodies for immunohistochemistry of mutant p53 gene product in archival colorectal neoplasms. J Pathol 1994; 172:5–12.

[95] Allegra CJ, Paik S, Colangelo LH, et al. Prognostic value of thymidylate synthase, Ki-67, and p53 in patients with Dukes' B and C colon cancer: a National Cancer Institute-National Surgical Adjuvant Breast and Bowel Project collaborative study. J Clin Oncol 2003;21: 241–50.

[96] Fearon ER, Cho KR, Nigro JM, et al. Identification of a chromosome 18q gene that is altered in colorectal cancers. Science 1990;247:49–56.

[97] Jen J, Kim H, Piantadosi S, et al. Allelic loss of chromosome 18q and prognosis in colorectal cancer. N Engl J Med 1994;331:213–21.

[98] Goel A, Arnold CN, Niedzwiecki D, et al. Characterization of sporadic colon cancer by patterns of genomic instability. Cancer Res 2003;63:1608–14.

[99] Konishi M, Kikuchi-Yanoshita R, Tanaka K, et al. Molecular nature of colon tumors in hereditary nonpolyposis colon cancer, familial polyposis, and sporadic colon cancer. Gastroenterology 1996;111:307–17.

[100] Formentini A, Henne-Bruns D, Kornmann M. Thymidylate synthase expression and prognosis of patients with gastrointestinal cancers receiving adjuvant chemotherapy: a review. Langenbecks Arch Surg 2004;389:405–13.

[101] Popat S, Matakidou A, Houlston RS. Thymidylate synthase expression and prognosis in colorectal cancer: a systematic review and meta-analysis. J Clin Oncol 2004;22: 529–36.

[102] Edler D, Glimelius B, Hallstrom M, et al. Thymidylate synthase expression in colorectal cancer: a prognostic and predictive marker of benefit from adjuvant fluorouracil-based chemotherapy. J Clin Oncol 2002;20:1721–8.

[103] Anwar S, Frayling IM, Scott NA, et al. Systematic review of genetic influences on the prognosis of colorectal cancer. Br J Surg 2004;91:1275–91.

[104] Adlard JW, Richman SD, Seymour MT, et al. Prediction of the response of colorectal cancer to systemic therapy. Lancet Oncol 2002;3:75–82.

[105] McDermott U, Longley DB, Johnston PG. Molecular and biochemical markers in colorectal cancer. Ann Oncol 2002;13(Suppl 4):235–45.

[106] Wang Y, Jatkoe T, Zhang Y, et al. Gene expression profiles and molecular markers to predict recurrence of Dukes' B colon cancer. J Clin Oncol 2004;22:1564–71.

[107] Ghadimi BM, Grade M, Difilippantonio MJ, et al. Effectiveness of gene expression profiling for response prediction of rectal adenocarcinomas to preoperative chemoradiotherapy. J Clin Oncol 2005;23:1826–38.

[108] Allal AS, Kahne T, Reverdin AK, et al. Radioresistance-related proteins in rectal cancer. Proteomics 2004;4:2261–9.

[109] Diehl F, Li M, Dressman D, et al. Detection and quantification of mutations in the plasma of patients with colorectal tumors. Proc Natl Acad Sci USA 2005;102:16368–73.

[110] Osborn NK, Ahlquist DA. Stool screening for colorectal cancer: molecular approaches. Gastroenterology 2005;128:192–206.

[111] Imperiale TF, Ransohoff DF, Itzkowitz SH, et al. Fecal DNA versus fecal occult blood for colorectal-cancer screening in an average-risk population. N Engl J Med 2004;351: 2704–14.

[112] Woolf SH. A smarter strategy? Reflections on fecal DNA screening for colorectal cancer. N Engl J Med 2004;351:2755–8.

[113] Raju R, Cruz-Correa M. Chemoprevention of colorectal cancer. Dis Colon Rectum 2006; 49:113–24 [discussion: 24–5].

[114] Brown JR, DuBois RN. COX-2: a molecular target for colorectal cancer prevention. J Clin Oncol 2005;23:2840–55.

[115] Dannenberg AJ, Altorki NK, Boyle JO, et al. Cyclo-oxygenase 2: a pharmacological target for the prevention of cancer. Lancet Oncol 2001;2:544–51.

[116] Stark LA, Din FV, Zwacka RM, et al. Aspirin-induced activation of the NF-kappaB signaling pathway: a novel mechanism for aspirin-mediated apoptosis in colon cancer cells. FASEB J 2001;15:1273–5.

[117] Eberhart CE, Coffey RJ, Radhika A, et al. Up-regulation of cyclooxygenase 2 gene expression in human colorectal adenomas and adenocarcinomas. Gastroenterology 1994; 107:1183–8.

[118] Subbaramaiah K, Altorki N, Chung WJ, et al. Inhibition of cyclooxygenase-2 gene expression by p53. J Biol Chem 1999;274:10911–5.

[119] Oshima M, Dinchuk JE, Kargman SL, et al. Suppression of intestinal polyposis in Apc delta716 knockout mice by inhibition of cyclooxygenase 2 (COX-2). Cell 1996;87:803–9.

[120] Jacoby RF, Seibert K, Cole CE, et al. The cyclooxygenase-2 inhibitor celecoxib is a potent preventive and therapeutic agent in the min mouse model of adenomatous polyposis. Cancer Res 2000;60:5040–4.

[121] Sandler RS, Halabi S, Baron JA, et al. A randomized trial of aspirin to prevent colorectal adenomas in patients with previous colorectal cancer. N Engl J Med 2003;348:883–90.

[122] Baron JA, Cole BF, Sandler RS, et al. A randomized trial of aspirin to prevent colorectal adenomas. N Engl J Med 2003;348:891–9.

[123] Solomon SD, McMurray JJ, Pfeffer MA, et al. Cardiovascular risk associated with celecoxib in a clinical trial for colorectal adenoma prevention. N Engl J Med 2005;352:1071–80.

[123a] Bresalier RS, Sandler RS, Quan H, et al. Cardiovascular events associated with rofecoxib in a colorectal adenoma chemoprevention trial. N Engl J Med 2005;352:1092–102.

[124] Giardiello FM, Hamilton SR, Krush AJ, et al. Treatment of colonic and rectal adenomas with sulindac in familial adenomatous polyposis. N Engl J Med 1993;328:1313–6.

[125] Steinbach G, Lynch PM, Phillips RK, et al. The effect of celecoxib, a cyclooxygenase-2 inhibitor, in familial adenomatous polyposis. N Engl J Med 2000;342:1946–52.

[126] Niv Y, Fraser GM. Adenocarcinoma in the rectal segment in familial polyposis coli is not prevented by sulindac therapy. Gastroenterology 1994;107:854–7.

[127] Thorson AG, Lynch HT, Smyrk TC. Rectal cancer in FAP patient after sulindac. Lancet 1994;343:180.

[128] Giardiello FM, Yang VW, Hylind LM, et al. Primary chemoprevention of familial adenomatous polyposis with sulindac. N Engl J Med 2002;346:1054–9.

[129] Rossouw JE, Anderson GL, Prentice RL, et al. Risks and benefits of estrogen plus progestin in healthy postmenopausal women: principal results fFrom the Women's Health Initiative randomized controlled trial. JAMA 2002;288:321–33.

[130] Lamprecht SA, Lipkin M. Chemoprevention of colon cancer by calcium, vitamin D and folate: molecular mechanisms. Nat Rev Cancer 2003;3:601–14.

[131] Bautista D, Obrador A, Moreno V, et al. Ki-ras mutation modifies the protective effect of dietary monounsaturated fat and calcium on sporadic colorectal cancer. Cancer Epidemiol Biomarkers Prev 1997;6:57–61.

[132] Borgelt L, Umland E. Benefits and challenges of hormone replacement therapy. J Am Pharm Assoc (Wash) 2000;40:S30–1.

[133] Duffield-Lillico AJ, Shureiqi I, Lippman SM. Can selenium prevent colorectal cancer? A signpost from epidemiology. J Natl Cancer Inst 2004;96:1645–7.

[134] Schrag D. The price tag on progress—chemotherapy for colorectal cancer. N Engl J Med 2004;351:317–9.

[135] Chung KY, Saltz LB. Antibody-based therapies for colorectal cancer. Oncologist 2005;10: 701–9.

[136] Hurwitz H, Fehrenbacher L, Novotny W, et al. Bevacizumab plus irinotecan, fluorouracil, and leucovorin for metastatic colorectal cancer. N Engl J Med 2004;350:2335–42.

[137] Hurwitz HI, Fehrenbacher L, Hainsworth JD, et al. Bevacizumab in combination with fluorouracil and leucovorin: an active regimen for first-line metastatic colorectal cancer. J Clin Oncol 2005;23:3502–8.

[138] Kabbinavar FF, Hambleton J, Mass RD, et al. Combined analysis of efficacy: the addition of bevacizumab to fluorouracil/leucovorin improves survival for patients with metastatic colorectal cancer. J Clin Oncol 2005;23:3706–12.

[139] Spano JP, Fagard R, Soria JC, et al. Epidermal growth factor receptor signaling in colorectal cancer: preclinical data and therapeutic perspectives. Ann Oncol 2005;16:189–94.

[140] Cunningham D, Humblet Y, Siena S, et al. Cetuximab monotherapy and cetuximab plus irinotecan in irinotecan-refractory metastatic colorectal cancer. N Engl J Med 2004;351: 337–45.

[141] Barber TD, Vogelstein B, Kinzler KW, et al. Somatic mutations of EGFR in colorectal cancers and glioblastomas. N Engl J Med 2004;351:2883.

[142] Tsuchihashi Z, Khambata-Ford S, Hanna N, et al. Responsiveness to cetuximab without mutations in EGFR. N Engl J Med 2005;353:208–9.

[143] Lynch TJ, Bell DW, Sordella R, et al. Activating mutations in the epidermal growth factor receptor underlying responsiveness of non-small-cell lung cancer to gefitinib. N Engl J Med 2004;350:2129–39.

[144] Paez JG, Janne PA, Lee JC, et al. EGFR mutations in lung cancer: correlation with clinical response to gefitinib therapy. Science 2004;304:1497–500.

[145] Suter CM, Martin DI, Ward RL. Germline epimutation of MLH1 in individuals with multiple cancers. Nat Genet 2004;36:497–501.

[146] Cunningham JM, Kim CY, Christensen ER, et al. The frequency of hereditary defective mismatch repair in a prospective series of unselected colorectal carcinomas. Am J Hum Genet 2001;69:780–90.

SURGICAL
CLINICS OF
NORTH AMERICA

Surg Clin N Am 86 (2006) 819–847

An Update on Imaging of Colorectal Cancer

Christoph Wald, MD, PhD*,
Christopher D. Scheirey, MD,
Tai M. Tran, MD, Nazli Erbay, MD

Department of Diagnostic Radiology, Lahey Clinic Medical Center,
41 Mall Road, Burlington, MA 01805, USA

For colon cancer, the second leading cause of death from malignancy in the United States, screening of asymptomatic average-risk patients for the presence of this disease and early detection in precursor stages is of great interest to the general population [1]. Comprehensive evaluation of symptomatic or high-risk patients represents another important clinical focus.

It has been demonstrated that timely recognition and removal of adenomatous polyps significantly decreases the risk of death from colorectal cancer in affected patients [2]. However, compliance with current recommendations of colon cancer screening in the general population remains low [3]. One can only speculate that compliance rates may improve with the advent of less onerous or less invasive examinations.

Despite the interest in colon cancer screening from a public health perspective, selection of the right time point and methodology for screening is difficult, because the incidence of cancer in nonadenomatous and small adenomatous colon polyps in elderly patients is high. The cost and risks of complications associated with an examination designed to detect clinically significant lesions need to be weighed against the derived survival benefit.

Total colon examination—available methods

Methods currently available for total colon examination include double-contrast barium enema (DCBE), endoscopic examination (colonoscopy),

---

* Corresponding author.
E-mail address: Christoph.Wald@lahey.org (C. Wald).

0039-6109/06/$ - see front matter © 2006 Elsevier Inc. All rights reserved.
doi:10.1016/j.suc.2006.06.001   *surgical.theclinics.com*

and more recently, cross-sectional imaging-based technology such as CT Colonography (CTC), also known as virtual colonoscopy or virtual endoscopy. The feasibility of magnetic resonance Colonography (MRC) for total colon assessment is also being evaluated, and will be discussed below.

Double-contrast barium enema

Dating back to the 1920s [4], radiographic examination of the colon with barium and air has been an important modality. Originally, it was the sole comprehensive colon examination, which was improved over time. Currently, it is one of several options. History and technique of the air contrast examination have been well described, and the reader is referred to a review article by Rubesin and colleagues [5] for more detailed information. With the advent and ever increasing use of endoscopic screening, the number of double-contrast enemas performed in the United States began to decrease steadily. Over time, this resulted in fewer and fewer radiologists capable of performing a technically adequate examination. In fact, the authors suspect that only a minority of radiology training programs in this country are currently able to offer residents sufficient exposure to become proficient in this interactive live fluoroscopic examination, the results of which are very examiner dependent. Such a trend was already suspected by Gazelle and colleagues [6] in their review of the issues surrounding screening for colorectal cancer in 2000.

Studies in the past have shown a wide range of diagnostic sensitivity and accuracy for air-contrast enema. The results vary depending on study population and lesion size. We do not know of any prospective study that looked at the accuracy of DCBE examination in a screening population. However, in symptomatic patients the reported sensitivity of double-contrast enema for the detection of cancer ranges from 85% to 90% [7–9]. Sensitivity for adenomas larger than 1 cm is reported to be 75% to 90%, whereas sensitivity for the detection of smaller lesions is reported to be only 50% to 80% [10,11]. Results observed in this particular subgroup of patients cannot be extrapolated to the screening population. Furthermore, judging the utility of an examination technique in context with colon cancer screening should take into account the low rate of progression of polyps < 1-cm diameter into colon cancer. The study by Winawer and colleagues [12] and the ensuing discussion among experts [13] may serve as an example of this complex and controversial issue.

Colonoscopy

Although colonoscopy is undoubtedly sensitive, one needs to remember that its success is also examiner dependent; in 5% to 15% of cases, endoscopists may not be able to reach the cecum for technical reasons [14–17].

Furthermore, there may be endoscopic blind spots due to haustral anatomy and convoluted arrangement of redundant bowel [18,19]. Nevertheless, colonoscopy offers the undisputed advantage of synchronous diagnostic and therapeutic intervention. However, this technique requires sedation, and carries a small but real risk of complications secondary to its invasiveness [15,17,20,21].

CT Colonography in colon cancer screening

After initial feasibility studies on CTC, the development of multidetector row CT scanners permitted radiologists to rapidly acquire volumetric datasets of patient anatomy at a high spatial resolution. Suitable computer software allows reconstruction and viewing of both two-dimensional (2D) and three-dimensional (3D) image representations of the colon and surrounding anatomy. CTC is minimally invasive (air or CO_2 insufflation per rectum is required), requires no sedation, and is less time consuming than an endoscopic examination. Currently, most centers have their patients undergo cathartic bowel preparation before both endoscopy and virtual colonoscopy. Individual technical aspects are discussed below.

Trials and reviews

At the time of the writing of this article, there are only two prospective multicenter trials on CTC in the average-risk asymptomatic screening population, which reported very different results.

In 2003, Pickhardt and colleagues [22] published results of a multicenter trial intended to assess the performance of CTC for the detection of colorectal neoplasia in an average-risk screening population. A total of 1233 asymptomatic adults (mean age, 57.8 years) underwent same-day CTC and optical colonoscopy. The sensitivity of virtual colonoscopy for adenomatous polyps was 93.8% for polyps at least 10 mm in diameter, 93.9% for polyps at least 8 mm in diameter, and 88.7% for polyps at least 6 mm in diameter. The sensitivity of optical colonoscopy for adenomatous polyps was 87.5%, 91.5%, and 92.3% for the three sizes of polyps, respectively. The specificity of virtual colonoscopy for adenomatous polyps was 96.0% for polyps at least 10 mm in diameter, 92.2% for polyps at least 8 mm in diameter, and 79.6% for polyps at least 6 mm in diameter. Two polyps were malignant; both were detected on virtual colonoscopy, and one of them was missed on optical colonoscopy before the results on virtual colonoscopy were revealed. The authors concluded that CT virtual colonoscopy with the use of a 3D approach is an accurate screening method for the detection of colorectal neoplasia in asymptomatic average risk adults, and compares favorably with optical colonoscopy in terms of the detection of clinically relevant lesions.

In 2004, Cotton and colleagues [23] published results of a multicenter trial in an asymptomatic screening population. One hundred four participants had lesions sized at least 6 mm. CTC detected 55.0% (95% confidence interval [CI], 39.9–70.0%) of lesions of at least 10 mm, compared with 100% for conventional colonoscopy. The specificity of CTC for detecting participants without any lesion was greater than 90%. CTC missed two of eight cancers. The accuracy of CTC varied considerably between centers, and did not improve as the study progressed. Authors concluded that CTC was not yet ready for widespread clinical application, and that techniques and training need to be improved.

In an attempt to clarify the situation, the American College of Radiology Imaging Network initiated another large multicenter trial, the results of which will not be available for another year or 2, as mentioned in a recent article by Ferrucci [24].

Two other recently published large comparative trials performed on symptomatic patients [25] and high-risk patients [26] yielded better sensitivity for colonoscopy than for double-contrast enema or CTC.

One may speculate that the observed differences in the performance of CTC is related to the differences in sophistication in postprocessing and interactive review (2D versus 3D review, different software products, use of stool tagging) and examiner experience, or a combination thereof [25,27].

In further attempts to establish the role of CTC, several authors have reviewed the literature on this technology. Most studies looked at performance of CTC in symptomatic patient cohorts; thus, the results and recommendations cannot simply be extrapolated to the asymptomatic screening population. Retrospective literature reviews are hampered by the lack of standards in performance and reporting of CTC trials. In a 2002 Lature review, Dachman [28] reported a wide range of sensitivity (8–100%) for detection of polyps larger than 1 cm. The author stated that because of wide technical variation (e.g., different bowel preparations, CT scanners, and interpretation software) used in the studies, meta-analysis of the results would not provide reliable statistics. Recently, Halligan and colleagues [29] reviewed a large number of studies performed between 1994 and 2004, and also found that reporting was highly variable, suggesting minimum reporting standards to overcome this problem. Based on a meta-analysis, the authors, Halligan and colleagues, concluded that CTC seemed sufficiently sensitive and specific in the detection of large and medium polyps, and especially sensitive in the detection of symptomatic lesions.

A US-based large prospective multicenter CTC trial is currently under way sponsored by ACRIN, the American College of Radiology Imaging Network, a National Cancer Institute-funded cooperative group, the results of which are expected for late 2006 or early 2007. The stated goal is the clinical validation of widespread use of CTC in a screening population for the detection of colorectal neoplasia in just under 2300 patients. It is widely expected that the results of this trial will determine whether CTC will become a reimbursable and recommended technique for colon cancer screening.

CT Colonography technique—too many choices?

The controversy about the true achievable sensitivity of CTC in screening asymptomatic and symptomatic patients results from differences in technical parameters. Many studies performed in recent years have looked at some of the variables and important ingredients of an optimal technique.

Retained fluid, liquid, and solid stool particles interfere directly with the test, either by masking of polyps or by creating false positive findings. Adequate bowel preparation is therefore vital for a highly sensitive study. However, it is well established that cathartic preparation presents a well-known barrier to colorectal cancer screening compliance [30]. A study comparing CTC after noncathartic preparation and with colonoscopy performed 3 to 7 days later yielded an average sensitivity of 95.5% (95% CI, 92.1–99%) for the identification of colorectal polyps ≥8 mm [31]. Patients had to comply with a low-residue diet and ingested Gastrografin with meals for fecal tagging purposes. However, as Pickhardt pointed out in a commentary [32], this approach is not suitable if same-day colonoscopy/polypectomy is desired.

The use of laxatives for bowel preparation proved to be a major barrier for patient compliance [33]. With regard to laxatives, preparations containing magnesium citrate or sodium phosphate seem to be preferred because they result in less fluid retention than polyethylene solutions [34,35]. Low-residue diet in the days before the study is also helpful, and may reduce the need for aggressive laxative therapy [36]. Labeling stool with oral barium or iodine-containing substances is an important adjunct technique in dealing with the issue of fecal residue, avoiding too many false-positive results in CTC [22,27,37]. The utility of stool tagging is demonstrated in Fig. 1A–D.

Adequate colonic insufflation is another important technical factor; either room air or CO_2 are applied to the patient. There is no consensus as to which agent yields better distension [38]. In an article by Barish and colleagues [38], many of the above variables of performing CTC in clinical practice are discussed, moreover, the authors believe that spasmolytics are not routinely necessary to achieve adequate results. Most clinical practices today will have access to multidetector row CT scanners that are indispensable for state-of-the-art CTC. These modern scanners achieve fast anatomic coverage at superior resolution. Scanning is performed in supine and prone positioning to help differentiate mobile fecal residue, and so on, from fixed pathology, and to shift intraluminal fluid, allowing for inspection of otherwise obscured portions of colon [39–43]. CTC can be performed at 40% to 50% dose reduction in modern scanners, using thin collimation acquisition parameters [44].

Last, adequate image viewing with use of various 2D and 3D display methods and fast 3D rendering on specialized offline workstations play an important role in CTC. A combination of the various displays seems to be most accurate. Faster computers and improved software allow expeditious review in a 3D mode with 2D problem solving. Polyps are more

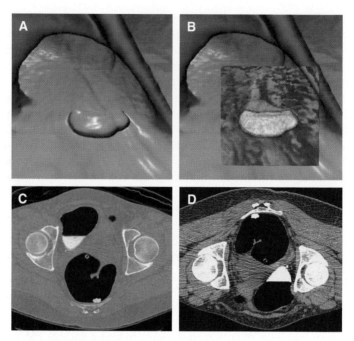

Fig. 1. (*A*) Volume-rendered intraluminal 3D view demonstrates a possible polyp at 6:00 o'clock. (*B*) 3D translucency rendering technique reveals high-attenuation internal density of polypoid structure, compatible with barium-tagged stool. (*C,D*) Axial images with different window/level settings allow user to recognize high internal density of small polypoid lesion, unequivocally identifying it as tagged stool. (Images courtesy of Dr. Perry Pickhardt, Madison, WI.)

conspicuous when dedicated primary 3D viewing technique is employed. CTC with primary 2D viewing can lead to excessive eye strain, especially when radiologists are performing serial evaluations, and has yielded disappointing results in multicenter trials of low-prevalence groups [23,25]. However, results in smaller studies with polyp-rich patient cohorts have been promising [45,46] as Pickhardt pointed out [32].

Novel image postprocessing

Novel image postprocessing methods under investigation provide "unwrapping" of the circular colon for ease of inspection. So-called "translucency rendering" may allow incorporated contrast visible in small wall-adherent feces, and help distinguish fecal material from polyps [47]. The term "electronic cleansing" describes automated removal of labeled stool by expert software before inspection by a radiologist [48–50]. However, this technique can produce significant artifacts by removing some of the polyps instead of feces and slow-down image analysis. Computer-aided detection software has been used to label suspicious areas before final inspection by the radiologist, but requires further development before mainstream clinical use [51–53]. Improved 3D postprocessing and routine incorporation of the latter methods into screening protocols may eventually improve the sensitivity of CTC.

Training—accreditation

There is a steep learning curve associated with the successful interpretation of CTC. Some authors have postulated that up to 50 cases should be interpreted under supervision of an experienced reader before the radiologist is competent to render high-quality interpretations [24,54]. Accreditation of facilities and certification of readers, analogous to mammographic accreditation, are being considered and the American College of Radiology is currently developing practice guidelines for CTC.

Summary

Currently, there is no consensus for the single best CTC technique. Statistically, the best results have been obtained with primary 3D viewing and 2D problem solving, after cathartic preparation and stool tagging. Ultimately, this technique may be the optimum strategy for CTC. Prone and supine imaging with adequate distention of the colon is crucial to yield the high-quality datasets necessary to perform both 3D and 2D analysis.

CT Colonography in symptomatic patients

Although the role of CTC in the asymptomatic screening population is a matter of ongoing investigation, there seems to be little disagreement about its use in the examination of patients with incomplete colonoscopies, detection of synchronous lesions in obstructing colon cancers, and superior localization of lesions before surgery, allowing for evaluation of extraluminal and remote findings [55–58]. Several studies found that between 10% and 13% of patients have significant extracolonic findings, often requiring further workup, additional or immediate therapy [59,60].

Magnetic resonance colonography

MRC has become more feasible secondary to technologic advancements in phased array coil technology and the development of faster image acquisition protocols. Potential uses include screening for, and staging of, colorectal pathology. Analogous to CTC, MRC is less invasive than conventional colonoscopy (CC), allows for evaluation of intra- as well as extraluminal disease, and is an opportunity for synchronous evaluation of distant sites, particularly the liver, for spread of disease. Soft tissue contrast resolution of MRC is superior to that of CTC, which aids in the assessment of local staging. The absence of ionizing radiation may represent an important advantage of MRC over CTC in the context of screening for colorectal cancer, because repeat CTC every 5 years exposes individuals to potentially significant cumulative radiation exposure.

Most MRC imaging protocols use a body coil for the abdomen and phased array coil for the pelvis. Phased array coils are capable of acquiring higher resolution datasets but allow only limited craniocaudal anatomic coverage. Similar to CTC, patients are imaged prone and supine, allowing for optimal distension while shifting residue and fluid in the colon.

Several imaging sequences have been developed, and can be classified into bright- or dark-lumen techniques. Bright-lumen techniques, such as a balanced steady state free-precession sequence (true FISP, FIESTA, balanced FFE), show colorectal masses as dark filling defects/areas of low signal on a background of bright-distended colon after a water enema. A dark-lumen technique can demonstrate enhancing lesions on a background of a dark distended colon. Most clinical studies on MRC use the dark-lumen technique. Lauenstein and colleagues [61] demonstrated better results with a dark-lumen compared with the bright-lumen technique in their study of 37 patients. The dark lumen was able to identify all polyps > 5 mm without any false positive findings. The overall sensitivity of dark- compared with bright-lumen MRC was 79% versus 69%, respectively. However, the bright-lumen technique (balanced steady state free-precession sequence) had better image quality and was less susceptible to motion; this may be preferred in patients unable to hold their breath or lay still sufficiently long.

As with CTC, distention of the colon is an essential prerequisite to correctly identify colorectal pathology. Multiple schemes have been developed including water, water with paramagnetic contrast, carbon dioxide, and barium enema, depending upon desired dark- or bright-lumen techniques on MRC. Recently, a study compared colonic distension with water versus carbon dioxide. The authors found similar accuracy for lesion detection; however, air provided better contrast-to-noise ratio and better distention [62]. Water combined with paramagnetic contrast and barium oral/rectal enema has been used for stool tagging. The use of paramagnetic contrast for bright-lumen MRC stool tagging is prohibitively expensive. However, oral and rectal barium administration will result in a good dark-lumen MRC [63]. Satisfactory fecal tagging may allow for a less cathartic bowel preparation and therefore enhance patient acceptance of MRC. This approach and its limitations have been further discussed in context with CTC. Past attempts to achieve stool tagging with diet modification have been unsuccessful [64].

An extensive meta-analysis comparing MRC and CC involving 563 patients demonstrated an overall MRC sensitivity and specificity of 75% and 96%, respectively [65]. MRC was able to identify synchronous lesions proximal to high-grade stenosing lesions that were not accessible by colonoscopy. The results of this study are encouraging, although limited by the inherent differences in employed techniques, as in the studies date from 1990 to 2004 [66]. Several studies have demonstrated high accuracy of MRC in detecting lesions greater than 10 mm [67–70]. In a study of 122 patients MRC was nearly 90% sensitive for lesions greater than 5 mm [67]. In a separate study of 100 patients, the sensitivity for lesions 6 to

9 mm was 85% [71]. MRC routinely missed lesions less than 5 mm and flat adenomas.

Most medical centers use CT rather than MRI for staging of colorectal carcinoma in accordance with recommendations by the radiology diagnostic oncology group II study [72]. Since its publication, technical advancements in MRC have shown improved accuracy in differentiating clinically favorable intramural (T1/T2) from unfavorable higher local stage tumor (T3/T4), especially in rectal cancer staging. Low and colleagues [73] were able to appropriately identify the TNM stage in 21 of 27 colon cancer patients, resulting in an overall accuracy of 78%, while the accuracy rate for rectal cancer was 95%, correctly staging 20 out of 21 cancers. Therefore, MRC was able to differentiate T1/2 from T3/4 stage cancers 95% of the time. Differentiating nodal metastatic disease from reactively enlarged lymph nodes has proven to be difficult solely based on size criteria. Accurate assessment of nodal status should also take in account the morphology of the perinodal tissue. Clinical research on lymph node imaging agents such as ultrasmall iron–oxide particles, as described in the rectal staging portion of this article, may improve accuracy of staging nodal involvement [74,75].

In summary, MRC may become an important tool in the screening for, and assessment of, known colorectal cancer. It uses no ionizing radiation and has powerful properties in determining local stage and evaluating for the presence of distant metastases. Performance of MRC is technically challenging, expensive, and requires significant patient cooperation, all of which represent barriers to broad implementation. Further refinement of the MRC technique is necessary. In addition, more prospective evaluations in comparison to existing modalities such as CC and CTC are required to fully understand its role in the preoperative evaluation of symptomatic patients and screening of the asymptomatic population.

Summary—what to choose?

Local practice pattern, available expertise in the involved medical/surgical subspecialties, and availability of the various imaging resources will have a great impact on preferences for total colon imaging. In our opinion, the sensitivity of an optimal CTC probably equals or exceeds that of DCBE in all but a few practices where highly skilled fluoroscopists are still available. After a gradual decline in performance of DCBE in both clinical practice and training, and considering its high examiner dependence, CTC will likely become the radiologic procedure of choice for colon cancer screening. The sensitivity of a carefully executed CTC in the asymptomatic screening population may be similar to that of Colonoscopy, although further investigation is needed. If equality can be demonstrated in rigorous trials, CTC could be added to the current reimbursable options available for colorectal carcinoma screening, which include fecal occult blood testing, sigmoidoscopy, DCBE examination, and colonoscopy.

At this point, most colon examination techniques require similar patient preparation. If cathartic preparation is not performed for patient comfort reasons, same-day polyp removal will not be feasible. Patients should probably be given the choice after explaining risks and benefits of the cathartic versus noncathartic prep.

To fully leverage the advantages of a less invasive technique (ie, decrease in number of complications per polyp detected), practices could attempt to stratify patients into primary invasive and noninvasive groups based on history and clinical parameters (age, prior studies, clinical risk profile). If immediate interpretation of CTC is feasible and established in a given practice, patients with positive findings who have been adequately prepped can proceed to diagnostic/therapeutic colonoscopy on the same day. Although this requires considerable interdisciplinary coordination, it would almost certainly result in high patient acceptance. Practices planning for new colon cancer screening facilities, or restructuring existing services, should keep this in mind. A combined CTC/colonoscopy approach may require a shift of resource allocation to free up dedicated CT scanning time in Radiology departments, or perhaps necessitate the installation of dedicated equipment in a screening facility and the acquisition of dedicated workstations. Close collaboration between colonoscopists and radiologists would be inevitable under such circumstances, and would likely result in higher quality patient care. Although most facilities have adequate scanner hardware to obtain sufficient source images, there is probably a lack of experienced interpreting radiologists in some areas. This shortfall may be overcome in the age of digital images as teleradiology technology makes remote interpretation by dedicated expert radiologists feasible.

Rectal cancer staging

Traditionally, the focus of preoperative radiologic evaluation of rectal cancer was stratification of patients into those receiving primary curative surgery alone and those who would benefit from preoperative neoadjuvant chemotherapy/radiation. Based on imaging criteria established by Hildebrandt and Feifel [76], the primary concern for endorectal ultrasound (EUS) became differentiating T2 from T3 disease. However, more recent advances in surgical techniques and neoadjuvant therapy for a subgroup of rectal cancer patients have significantly reduced cancer-related morbidity and mortality. Identifying optimum treatment parameters based on local staging, and precise differentiation of both superficial and locally invasive lesions, are of utmost importance in preoperative radiology evaluation.

Radical surgery for rectal cancer is associated with potential mortality as well as morbidity of poor bowel or sexual function, and possibly a stoma. Transanal excisions of superficial lesions (carcinoma in situ or ultrasound stage T1), and in particular, transanal endoscopic microsurgery, allow for improved functional outcome. Although their value as a curative cancer operation is seen as controversial by some [77], other studies found similar recurrence rates to more radical surgeries [78,79]. Preoperative chemoradiation followed by local excision of ultrasound stage T2, node-negative lesions, has also been advocated [78,80]. Thus, accurate discrimination of T1 from T2 disease is becoming crucial for preoperative staging.

Recent surgical management for T3/T4 lesions has focused on total mesorectal excision (TME). This incorporates the radical en bloc resection of tumor, local draining nodes, and surrounding mesorectal fat, including the thin mesorectal fascia. The success of TME surgery in preventing local recurrence has been linked to circumferential resection margin (CRM) and nodal status rather than T-staging [81]. The spatial relationship between tumor and mesorectal fascia is essential in determining the status of the CRM. Tumor found within 1 mm of the thin mesorectal fascia is an ominous prognostic indicator of a positive CRM and ultimately local recurrence.

Use of neoadjuvant radiation or chemotherapy within the past decade has had a major impact on treatment. The Swedish Rectal Cancer Trial showed that a short course of preoperative radiation therapy reduces the recurrence rate from 27% to 11% [82]. The Dutch TME trial stratified the patient population of locally advanced T3 or T4 stage lesions in whom neoadjuvant therapy is indicated [83]. Neoadjuvant radiation should be reserved for tumors with extramural spread or nodal metastasis [84]. Intensive and targeted preoperative therapy has rendered previously irresectable tumor resectable.

Staging techniques

The role of endorectal ultrasound in local staging of rectal cancer

EUS is the mainstay of local staging in many institutions across the United States. A metanalysis of the pertinent radiology literature comparing US/MR/CT published in 2004 [85] suggested that EUS is currently the modality of choice for local staging of all rectal carcinomas. Most practices use a 7.5 MHz or 10 MHz rigid US transducer with a saline-filled balloon tip, providing a 360-degree field of view. Accurate depiction of the five layers of the rectal wall is easily obtained. Tumor most commonly appears as a hypoechoic lesion invading or disrupting layers of the rectal wall. Those lesions invading just into the submucosa are ultrasound stage T1, those into but not beyond the muscularis propria are considered ultrasound stage T2 (Fig. 2), those lesions invading into the adjacent perirectal fat are ultrasound stage T3, and invasion into adjacent organs represent ultrasound stage T4.

Many consider EUS the imaging modality of choice for early T1/T2 rectal staging because of its superior depiction of tumor ingrowth into superficial layers of the rectal wall [86], with T staging accuracy ranging

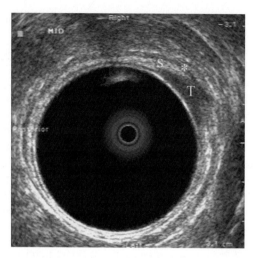

Fig. 2. EUS depicting an ultrasound Stage T2 lesion. Hypoechoic tumor (T) is invading through the echogenic submucosa (S), and up to, but not beyond, the muscularis propria (*).

from 69% to 97% [87]. In comparison, pelvic phased array coil MRI has been shown to be less accurate in differentiating T1 from T2 lesions [88]. It is important to note that EUS can only detect those lymph nodes within depth of range of the transducer resulting in potential understaging of disease. In the metanalysis performed by Bipat and colleagues [85], there was an overall sensitivity of 67% and specificity of 78% for lymph node involvement. Also, over staging of T2 tumors as T3 lesions is relatively common with EUS, because frequently peritumoral inflammatory changes have a similar appearance as primary tumor [89]. This possible overstaging may result in more radical therapy and expose patients to unnecessary chemoradiation.

Although some studies suggest that EUS is better suited for imaging of superficial lesions, its accuracy in locally advanced disease has recently been questioned, particularly in light of advancements in MRI [88]. In Bipat's meta-analysis, US had an overall sensitivity of 90% and specificity of 75% for perirectal fat invasion, better than CT or MRI [85]. However, it is important to note that their meta-analysis included studies performed over a 16-year time frame, and during that time, little has changed in EUS technique. During the same time interval significant technologic advancements have occurred in MRI rectal cancer staging, as discussed below.

EUS is limited in its assessment of advanced rectal cancer by its limited acoustic window, depth of penetration, and small field of view. Tumors beyond 13 cm superior to the dentate line are difficult to stage with the fixed-length rigid probe. Additional disadvantages of EUS are operator dependence, the need for a bowel prep, and occasionally proper positioning. Some patients are unable to tolerate the examination due to pain associated with highly stenotic lesions, which one may not be able to cross with the probe. In addition, recent studies have identified CRM, rather than traditional local T staging, as the more important preoperative indicator of local recurrence after surgery. EUS cannot accurately depict the relationship of the tumor to the mesorectal fascia.

3D endoluminal ultrasound and ultrasound miniprobe examinations are examples of recent advancements in endoluminal ultrasound technology. 3D endoluminal ultrasound allows the examiner to gain a different perspective on the lesion itself, particularly in regard to longitudinal extent and relationships to adjacent organs. Sequential transverse images are "stacked" upon one another, and using a separate workstation, the lesion can then be depicted in any plane. However, the scanning technique is identical to traditional EUS, with the same limitations in terms of depth of penetration and patient factors, as outlined previously. Miniprobe endoscopic ultrasound (m-EUS) uses an ulrathin probe (3–4 mm diameter) that can be used for local staging during routine colonoscopies. The advantages are a smaller and flexible probe, allowing for staging of higher rectal and colonic lesions, and the potential for crossing stenotic lesions. The use of m-EUS in the rectum may be limited, given that m-EUS has similar problems to traditional EUS in terms of depth of penetration, and in differentiating T3 from T4 lesions, which may be crucial in stenotic lesions [90]. The accuracy of m-EUS in determining lymph node status is approximately 80% [91]. Thus, its clinical use in the assessment of rectal lesions maybe limited. However, m-EUS does have a potential role in the local staging of colonic neoplasms, particularly in selected groups of patients, or in confirming superficial lesions in patients who may be poor candidates for an open surgical procedure [90].

The role of MRI in local staging of rectal cancer

A growing body of literature is supporting the use of pelvic phased array coil MRI (PA-MRI) over endorectal MRI, endoluminal ultrasound, CT, and digital rectal exam (DRE) for staging locally advanced extramural tumors. Early MRI studies were less encouraging because images were obtained with low-resolution body coils. However, the advent of high-resolution phased array coils in combination with improved imaging sequences has produced superior image quality to accurately assess tumor extent. In essence, a phased array coil has multiple surface coils that simultaneously detect signal, allowing for higher signal-to-noise ratios (SNRs), better spatial resolution, and faster imaging. High spatial resolution MRI can identify tumor features associated with poorer outcome, namely degree of extramural extension, venous invasion, nodal involvement, and peritoneal infiltration. State-of-the-art rectal MRI staging should be performed on a magnet with 1 or1.5 T field strength, phased array surface pelvic coil, and thin T2-weighted fast spin echo sequence (T2W-FSE) images. T2W-FSE provides superior discrimination between hyperintense mesorectal fat, intermediate tumor, hypointense rectal wall, and mesorectal fascia compared with other pulse sequences. Further technical details are discussed in an article by Brown and colleagues, in the *British Journal of Radiology* [92].

PA-MRI can be accurate in predicting T stage and CRM status. In 98 patients, Brown and colleagues [93] had 94% and 92% accuracy rate in predicting T-stage and CRM status, respectively. In addition, a study of 76 patients by Beets-Tan and colleagues [94] resulted in 83% accuracy rate in predicting CRM when examined by an experienced observer 1. Linear regression analysis of the study revealed that a distance from the tumor to the mesorectal resection plane of at least 2 mm could be predicted with 97% CI. A histologic distance of at least 1 mm can accurately was predicted with high confidence when the measured distance on MRI is at least 5 mm [94].

In 2002, the MERCURY Study (Magnetic Resonance Imaging and Rectal Cancer European Equivalence Study) was launched [95,96]. This study is assessing the equivalence of PA-MRI and histopathology, while evaluating the prediction of CRM positive tumors using MRI in 11 European centers [96]. Results of this study may eventually validate an MR-based preoperative staging system, stratifying patients into prognostic groups, and identifying patients who may benefit from neoadjuvant therapy [95]. At the time of writing of this article, the results have yet to be formally published, but the results presented at the RSNA in 2004 demonstrate an 82% accuracy in predicting involvement of the CRM, compared with histology, by using a 1-mm cutoff on MRI [96a].

Comparative analysis of modalities used for staging and histology of tumor prognostic favorability resulted in accuracy of 94% (MRI), 69% (EUS), and 65% (DRE) [88]. Clinical favorability was defined as T1, T2, and T3a lesions without lymph nodes metastasis. Borderline T3a lesions are considered prognostically favorable because they present with low risk of surgical failure, and neoadjuvant therapy would not be beneficial [97]. All 98 patients were able to tolerate the MRI examination. However, only 54 and 74 patients were able to undergo EUS and DRE, respectively. EUS and DRE were aborted for various reasons, including poor bowel prep, pain, and high tumor location out of reach.

MRI is limited in differentiating benign reactive lymph nodes (LN) from micrometastasis in small nodes. Of concern is the fact that greater than 50% of nodes containing metastases from rectal cancer are less than 5 mm in size [98]. Therefore, determination of LN involvement has been variable across all imaging modalities. When nodes of greater than 5 mm maximum short axis diameter are considered malignant, the nodal status accuracy rate of MRI ranges from 59% [97] to 85% [93]. Multiple small comparative studies between multiple modalities favor the use of PA-MRI, endorectal (ERC)-MRI, and EUS, in order of greatest accuracy [98,99]. One study of lymph nodes in 75 patients with rectal cancer demonstrated that nodes >4 mm had a higher rate of involvement, and nodes >8 mm were invariably affected by metastases [100]. However, the use of morphologic criteria to determine whether LNs are affected, such as spiculation, indistinctness, lobulation, and roundness, are similar to the use of a 5-mm size criteria. Additional characteristics that have a high correlation with LN involvement include mottled heterogenous post contrast-enhancement appearance, associated venous encasement, and dirty perirectal fat [100,101].

Early investigational studies of MRI using ultrasmall particles of iron oxide (USPIO) for LN detection in patients with rectal cancer have shown encouraging results. LNs are normally populated among other cells by macrophages, which will take up USPIO and result in signal loss (appear dark) on aT2* weighted sequence. Invasion of the lymph nodes with malignant cells displaces the macrophages, resulting in higher signal on USPIO-enhanced T2* imaging. Multiple uptake patterns can be visualized including uniform low, central low, eccentric high, and uniform high signal in order of increasing malignant potential. In a small study, Koh and colleagues [75] demonstrated 96% of benign LNs have a pattern of uniform or central low-signal intensity, while eccentric or uniform high signal is seen in those nodes containing metastases. Nodes containing metastatic foci smaller than 1 mm could not be recognized as containing tumor.

Multiple small studies have claimed that ERC-MRI and EUS have no statistical significant difference in T-staging accuracy [99,102,103]. In a study of 20 patients Akin and colleagues [104] claimed an accuracy of 85% for T staging when using ERC-MRI. The largest study of 89 patients showed that ERC-MRI and EUS had similar results, both of which were far superior to CT in the preoperative evaluation of rectal wall and adjacent organ invasion [105]. ERC-MRI uses an endorectal surface coil with balloon cover. Balloon insufflation is required for optimal contact with the affected bowel wall to maximize the inherent high SNRs; however, it may be impossible to cross stenotic lesions. The higher SNR with small field of view (FOV) in ERC-MR greatly increases image resolution, and rectal wall layers are clearly delineated. The limitation of ERC-MRI is the small field of view that is provided, with a very rapid drop in signal intensity beyond its immediate vicinity [95]. Therefore, adequate evaluation of CRM and mesorectal nodal status is difficult. ERC-MRI and EUS have similar technical advantages and disadvantages.

The role of CT in local staging of rectal cancer

Significant advances in CT technology allow high-resolution imaging of more anatomy in less time than ever before. However, its clinical use in local rectal cancer staging may be limited, particularly in light of the contemporaneous advancements in MR technology. A CT meta-analysis of 78 studies with 4897 patients revealed T-staging accuracy of only 73% [106]. The metanalysis of Bipat and colleagues [85] also demonstrated that

EUS was at least as good as CT in terms of local staging and lymph node status. A prospective blinded study published in 2002 demonstrated that EUS was superior to CT in local staging of rectal lesions [107]. Technical advancements in MRI, as previously described, have replaced conventional CT in assessing locally advanced tumors owing largely to its superior soft tissue resolution capability. Small comparative studies between MRI and CT demonstrated superior accuracy for MRI in predicting invasion into the bladder/uterus [108], pelvic wall, and subtle bone marrow involvement [109]. Although CT may not be able to depict the CRM as well as MRI due to its limitation in contrast resolution, it may represent an imaging alternative for patients with contraindications to MRI (implanted cardiac pacemaker, and so on).

Restaging after neoadjuvant therapy and detection of local recurrence

Despite improvements in therapy, a significant number of treated rectal cancers will recur. As discussed previously, the advent of local therapies has dramatically reduced the morbidity of those undergoing surgical treatment for rectal neoplasms. However, this decrease in morbidity must be weighed against a potential increased risk of local recurrence. There is a significant recurrence rate after local resection of superficial lesions [110], but those patients could undergo salvage surgery for cure if detected early. In addition, preoperative therapy may result in downstaging, potentially making local resection feasible in place of more radical therapy [80,111]. In this subgroup, accurate preoperative assessment, after neoadjuvant therapy, would be crucial to identify those patients who can undergo local excision for cure. Thus, accurate radiographic evaluation for local recurrence of rectal cancer, and accurate restaging after neoadjuvant therapy, both have a crucial impact on morbidity and long-term survival of these patients.

EUS was found to be accurate in detection of local recurrence in those patients who underwent local resection for superficial lesions [112]. In a study including 108 patients who underwent local excision for cure, 32 developed local recurrence. Twenty-six of these 32 patients were asymptomatic, and 10 of those who developed local recurrence (31%) were detected only by EUS [113]. These same authors, as well as others, believe that postoperative surveillance using EUS in those undergoing radical surgeries is also useful [113–117]. However, a normal postoperative EUS does not entirely exclude residual disease [118], and close postoperative surveillance of these patients is necessary.

Many studies exploring the role of EUS and MRI after neoadjuvant chemoradiation demonstrate poor accuracy in detecting local recurrence for both. EUS interpretation is limited by the inflammatory fibrotic reaction seen after neoadjuvant therapy [119]. Although some believe that EUS is valuable in evaluation of rectal lesions after chemoradiation [119], there are many reports of a dramatic decrease in accuracy after therapy, and

EUS alone in this clinical scenario may be of little use [120–122]. However, EUS-guided biopsy in combination with routine EUS surveillance is useful in the evaluation of suspicious postoperative lesions [123,124].

Recent results from restaging MRI in patients with locally advanced tumor after neoadjuvant chemoradiation therapy have been poor in accurately predicting both T and N stage [125,126]. MRI cannot reliably distinguish radiation fibrosis or postsurgical scarring from residual tumor, resulting in overstaging. In a study by Peschaud and colleagues [127], an MRI restaging study encountered overestimation errors particularly with tumors located in the low anterior rectum.

Fluoro-2-deoxy-D-glucose-positron emission tomography (FDG-PET), combined with CT, may offer the greatest advantage in detection of local recurrence. Although some regions of fibrosis can still have minor radiotracer uptake, recent studies have demonstrated high accuracy in detection of local recurrence after abdominal personal resections and anterior resections, even after chemoradiation exposure [128–130]. Combining the images with CT allows for simultaneous depiction of regional anatomy, decreasing the potential for false positive studies [128]. The study performed by Moore and colleagues [130], also demonstrated an increase in accuracy when performed 12 months after radiation, possible secondary to a decrease in inflammatory response related to radiation. FDG-PET also has the advantage of visualizing the rest of the body, detecting hepatic metastases, and evaluating a rising carcinoembryonic antigen level after a curative rectal cancer resection [131].

Summary

The advent of new surgical techniques and multimodality treatment paradigms aimed at improved functional outcomes in patients with rectal cancer has made preoperative staging of rectal carcinomas even more critical. Endoscipic ultrasound is currently the mainstay of local preoperative staging in most institutions. Although superficial lesions are best depicted with endoscopic ultrasound, there are limitations, and pelvic phase array coil MRI appears to be more accurate in visualization and depiction of advanced lesions. There is increasing reliance on assessment of the integrity of the CRM in regard to preoperative planning and use of neoadjuvant chemoradiation, and we suspect that more and more institutions will depend heavily on pelvic phase array coil MRI in the preoperative assessment of rectal cancer. The results of the MERCURY study could have a major impact on the utility of MRI in the preoperative staging of rectal lesions. Expect to see these results soon in the journal *Radiology*.

Endoscopic ultrasound, particularly when combined with guided biopsy, is valuable in the detection of local recurrence after initial therapies for rectal carcinoma. Although to date MRI has been disappointing in distinguishing posttherapeutic changes from local recurrence, FDG-PET is both sensitive and specific, especially when combined with CT, and perhaps MRI, and offers the additional advantage of a whole-body metastatic survey.

The role of positron emission tomography imaging in colorectal malignancy

PET, using fluoro-2-deoxy-D-glucose (18FDG), is impacting preoperative staging and evaluation for recurrence of colorectal cancer. It is the most sensitive and specific technique for in vivo imaging of metabolism and receptor ligand interactions in human tissue [132].

PET localization is based on abnormally increased tissue metabolism of cancer cells. In vivo imaging to detect increased glucose metabolism in cancer cells can be linked to increased expression of epithelial glucose transporter proteins and increased activity of the principle enzymes of the glycolytic pathway [132]. There is resulting intracellular accumulation, also known as "metabolic trapping," of 18FDG molecules. This mechanism is, in large part, responsible for the high sensitivity of FDG-PET, but also explains its limited specificity. Tracer may accumulate in any cells with hypermetabolism, such as leukocytes, macrophages, and other inflammatory cells.

Typically, a whole-body PET scan is obtained 60 minutes after administration of 10 mCi of 18FDG. The whole body is imaged in axial plane over 30 to 40 minutes with correction for variable soft tissue attenuation. Semi-quantitative index assessment of the radioactive uptake is determined by standardized uptake value (SUV). SUV is based on tumor radiotracer concentration (Q) normalized to the injected activity (Q_{inj}) and to the body weight (W). The (limited) spatial resolution of a current PET scanner is in the vicinity of 5 to 8 mm.

The utility of PET scanning alone is limited by poor spatial resolution and difficulty in exact anatomic localization of areas of abnormal radiotracer uptake. On the other hand, while much less sensitive, CT and MRI have inherent high spatial resolution that aids anatomic localization of lesions. Hybrid technology such as PET-CT has evolved, combining functional evaluation with anatomic localization and improved spatial resolution.

PET imaging has been available for staging of colorectal cancer since the 1980s using 18FDG; however, recently it has had more of an impact on staging and evaluation for recurrence. Other imaging modalities such as CT, MRI, and ultrasound (US) have traditionally been used for staging. However, the recurrence rate after initial treatment of colorectal malignancy has been reported to be as high as 30% to 40%, often within the first 2 years of treatment [133]. High recurrence rates so shortly after diagnosis suggest limitations in accuracy of the traditional staging tools.

The main applications of PET imaging in colorectal carcinoma are staging of disease at time of initial diagnosis, staging of recurrent disease, and assessment of response to therapy. Based on a study by Meta and colleagues [134], FDG-PET has a major impact on the management of colorectal cancer patients and contributed to changes in clinical stage and management decisions in >40% of the patients. In this study, PET had the highest sensitivity (95%) of all the modalities, which was confirmed by other studies. The sensitivity of PET was also dependent on histology, limited to 58% for detection of mucinous carcinoma versus 92% for nonmucinous carcinoma [135].

The sensitivity for detection of lymph node involvement was low (29%); however, the specificity and accuracy were higher: 88% and 75%, respectively. The sensitivity, accuracy, and specificity for detection of liver metastasis were similar comparing FDG-PET and CT. The sensitivity for detection of liver metastasis by PET was found to be 78% in the study by Meta and colleagues [134]. Other studies have cited higher sensitivity for detection of liver metastasis using PET [136–138]. However, study by Selzner [139] showed that hybrid PET/CT provided similar information regarding hepatic metastasis. PET/CT was superior to contrast-enhanced CT for detection of recurrent intrahepatic metastatic disease, extrahepatic metastases, and local recurrence at the initial surgical site [139] (Fig. 3).

One has to be aware of the information that can be obtained for different imaging modalities and how it may affect overall management in terms of initial staging and for evaluation of recurrent disease. Tzimas and colleagues [140] showed that the performance of different imaging modalities used for colon and rectal cancer staging including tumor depth, lymph node invasion, and metastasis does vary. PET has sensitivity of 87% to 100% and specificity of 43% to 100%. The positive predictive value (PPV) is relatively high, with 90% to 93% compared with CT, which has overall sensitivity of 48% to 97% in initial colorectal cancer staging. The specificity and PPV for CT was 57% to 100% and 100%, respectively. MRI had variable sensitivity and specificity based on the type of coil used such as external body coil or endorectal coil. The sensitivity was lower with external body coil with 22% to 89% versus 81% to 83% with endorectal coil. Specificity for staging was 43% to 100% for PET, 57% to 100% for CT, 71% to 100% external body coil MRI, and 42% to 100% for endoluminal rectal coil MRI, respectively [140].

The evaluation of the recurrent disease is limited by the postsurgical changes and fibrosis. There are also changes such as inflammation or fibrosis from chemotherapy and radiation (Fig. 4). PET imaging has been useful in differentiation of fibrotic or inflammatory changes from the recurrent disease. Thus, another major benefit of PET in evaluation of recurrent disease has been avoidance of inappropriate local therapies that may carry significant morbidity by documentation of widespread disease [141]. In the context of elevated carcinoembryogenic antigen (CEA), PET imaging is

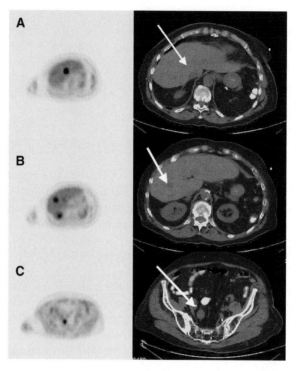

Fig. 3. (*A*) A focus of radiotracer uptake in the segment VIII of the right lobe of the liver corresponding to a hypodense lesion in the noncontrast-enhanced CT, probable focus of metastasis. (*B*) Another focus of FDG-PET uptake in the segment VI of the right lobe of the liver with corresponding hypodense lesion in the noncontrast-enhanced CT. (*C*) An 83-year-old female with a recent diagnosis of hepatic flexure colon cancer with increased uptake in the pelvis with a FDG-PET scan. This corresponds to the soft tissue mass noted in the right presacral space most likely a metastatic lymph node. (Images courtesy of Yamin Dou M.D, Methuen, MA.)

shown to have superior sensitivity in detection of recurrent disease. It has been shown by Selzner [139] that contrast-enhanced CT is not as sensitive as PET/CT for evaluation of local recurrence, with sensitivity of 20% versus 93%.

The use of PET has also been evaluated for recurrence of colorectal cancer and its effect on patient management. A meta-analysis by Huebner and colleagues [142] determined that the overall sensitivity and specificity of FDG-PET for detection of recurrent colorectal carcinoma is 97% and 76%, respectively. The overall change in the management of patient treatment based on the PET findings was 29%. Meta and colleagues [134] evaluated the impact of the use of FDG-PET from a referring physician's point of view, in terms of change in patient management. Changes in the management were classified as intramodality (eg, altered medical, surgical, or radiation treatment) or intermodality (eg, change from surgical to medical,

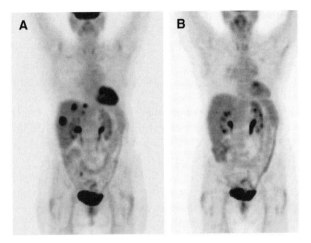

Fig. 4. (A) Initial full-body 18FDG-PET scan demonstrates four foci of increased uptake in the liver. There is normal uptake seen in the renal collecting system, bladder, ureters, cardiac muscle, with mild activity in the colon. (B) Postchemotherapy full-body PET scan performed 5 months after treatment shows excellent response to chemotherapy with complete resolution of the uptake in liver lesions. However, there is still normal expected uptake in the kidneys and bowel. Repeat CT at this time also demonstrates decrease in the size of the liver lesions. (Images courtesy of Yamin Dou M.D, Methuen, MA.)

surgical to radiation, medical to no treatment). Based on this study, FDG-PET had a significant impact on the management of patients and contributed to changes in treatment or staging in >40% of the patients. Based on this study, clinicians report changes in the staging in 42% of the patients. The colon cancer was upstaged in 80% and downstaged in 20% of the patients. The PET findings contributed to intermodality changes in 37%, intramodality changes in 18%, combination of management changes in 7%, and no change in 32% of the patients [134]. There are additional limitations to PET. One is the use of chemotherapy, which decreases the sensitivity of PET scan in detecting tumors. It was observed that the FDG uptake increases if imaging is performed at 4 to 5 weeks after treatment. It is postulated that there is a "flare" phenomenon based on increased macrophage infiltration with greater tumor cell kill [132]. FDG uptake is also limited in tumors less than 5 mm. Foci of inflammation and infection can result in false positive scans. In addition, high blood glucose levels and chemotherapy within 1 month of a study significantly decrease sensitivity [135,139].

The utility of combining CTC and whole-body FDG-PET has also been studied by Veit and colleagues [143]. Based on their study, although a small number of patient population, the integrated protocol may have substantial benefit in staging patients with suspected colorectal malignancy focusing on patients with incomplete colonoscopy and synchronous lesions. All but one of the lesions in the colon were detected. An additional polyp was identified as malignant. It also proved accurate in lymph node staging and detecting extracolonic tumor sites [143]. Combined contrast-enhanced CTC and PET is almost equivalent to having a routine staging CT; however, it is more sensitive in detection of small polyps in the colon, which may be other synchronous lesions, but may not be detected otherwise due to false positive uptake of FDG in the colon.

Based on the current evidence, FDG-PET has utility in the initial staging of colorectal cancer, and for evaluation of recurrent disease. Contrast-enhanced CT and FDG- PET imaging appear to increase the sensitivity, specificity, and accuracy for staging. Contrast-enhanced CT increases the spatial localization, while FDG-PET adds functional information. The future of tumor imaging is growing by new innovations in molecular imaging with tumor-specific agents for improved initial staging and evaluation for recurrence of colorectal carcinoma.

Acknowledgments

The authors thank Dr. Gina Brown, Consultant Radiologist and Honorary Senior Lecturer, Department of Radiology, The Royal Marsden Hospital NHS Trust, UK, for her insights into rectal cancer imaging, and, in particular, PA-MRI. Furthermore, we owe thanks to Drs. Perry Pickhardt, of Madison, WI, and Yamin Dou, of Methuen, MA, for some illustrative case material.

References

[1] Jemal A, Murray T, Samuels A, et al. Cancer statistics, 2003. CA Cancer J Clin 2003;53:5.

[2] Winawer S, Zauber A, Ho M. Prevention of colorectal cancer by colonoscopic polypectomy. The National Polyp Study Workgroup. N Engl J Med 1993;329:1977.

[3] Anderson LM, May DS. Has the use of cervical, breast, and colorectal cancer screening increased in the United States? Am J Public Health 1995;85:840.

[4] Fischer A. Fruehdiagnose des Dickdarmkrebses, insbesondere seine Differentialdiagnose gegen Tuberkulose mit Hilfe der kombinierten Luft- und Bariumfuellung des Dickdarms. Deutsch Ges Med 1923;35:86.

[5] Rubesin SE, Levine MS, Laufer I, et al. Double-contrast barium enema examination technique. Radiology 2000;215:642.

[6] Gazelle GS, McMahon PM, Scholz FJ. Screening for colorectal cancer. Radiology 2000; 215:327.

[7] Fork FT, Lindstrom C, Ekelund G. Double contrast examination in carcinoma of the colon and rectum. A prospective clinical series. Acta Radiol Diagn (Stockh) 1983;24:177.

[8] Johnson CD, Carlson HC, Taylor WF, et al. Barium enemas of carcinoma of the colon: sensitivity of double- and single-contrast studies. AJR Am J Roentgenol 1983;140:1143.

[9] Rex DK, Rahmani EY, Haseman JH, et al. Relative sensitivity of colonoscopy and barium enema for detection of colorectal cancer in clinical practice. Gastroenterology 1997; 112:17.

[10] Fork FT. Double contrast enema and colonoscopy in polyp detection. Gut 1981;22:971.

[11] Steine S, Stordahl A, Lunde OC, et al. Double-contrast barium enema versus colonoscopy in the diagnosis of neoplastic disorders: aspects of decision-making in general practice. Fam Pract 1993;10:288.

[12] Winawer SJ, Stewart ET, Zauber AG, et al. A comparison of colonoscopy and double-contrast barium enema for surveillance after polypectomy. National Polyp Study Work Group. N Engl J Med 2000;342:1766.

[13] Glick SN, Fibus T, Fister MR, et al. Comparison of colonoscopy and double-contrast barium enema. N Engl J Med 2000;343:1728.

[14] Anderson ML, Heigh RI, McCoy GA, et al. Accuracy of assessment of the extent of examination by experienced colonoscopists. Gastrointest Endosc 1992;38:560.

[15] Godreau CJ. Office-based colonoscopy in a family practice. Fam Pract Res J 1992;12: 313.

[16] Lieberman DA, Smith FW. Screening for colon malignancy with colonoscopy. Am J Gastroenterol 1991;86:946.

[17] Rex DK, Lehman GA, Hawes RH, et al. Screening colonoscopy in asymptomatic average-risk persons with negative fecal occult blood tests. Gastroenterology 1991;100:64.

[18] Laufer I, Smith NC, Mullens JE. The radiological demonstraction of colorectal polyps undetected by endoscopy. Gastroenterology 1976;70:167.

[19] Miller RE, Lehman G. Polypoid colonic lesions undetected by endoscopy. Radiology 1978; 129:295.

[20] Jentschura D, Raute M, Winter J, et al. Complications in endoscopy of the lower gastrointestinal tract. Therapy and prognosis. Surg Endosc 1994;8:672.

[21] Waye JD, Lewis BS, Yessayan S. Colonoscopy: a prospective report of complications. J Clin Gastroenterol 1992;15:347.

[22] Pickhardt PJ, Choi JR, Hwang I, et al. Computed tomographic virtual colonoscopy to screen for colorectal neoplasia in asymptomatic adults. N Engl J Med 2003;349:2191.

[23] Cotton PB, Durkalski VL, Pineau BC, et al. Computed tomographic colonography (virtual colonoscopy): a multicenter comparison with standard colonoscopy for detection of colorectal neoplasia. JAMA 2004;291:1713.

[24] Ferrucci JT. Colonoscopy: virtual and optical—another look, another view. Radiology 2005;235:13.

[25] Rockey DC, Paulson E, Niedzwiecki D, et al. Analysis of air contrast barium enema, computed tomographic colonography, and colonoscopy: prospective comparison. Lancet 2005; 365:305.

[26] Johnson CD, Harmsen WS, Wilson LA, et al. Prospective blinded evaluation of computed tomographic colonography for screen detection of colorectal polyps. Gastroenterology 2003;125:311.

[27] Pickhardt PJ. Differential diagnosis of polypoid lesions seen at CT colonography (virtual colonoscopy). Radiographics 2004;24:1535.

[28] Dachman AH. Diagnostic performance of virtual colonoscopy. Abdom Imaging 2002;27: 260.

[29] Halligan S, Altman DG, Taylor SA, et al. CT colonography in the detection of colorectal polyps and cancer: systematic review, meta-analysis, and proposed minimum data set for study level reporting. Radiology 2005;237:893.

[30] Ristvedt SL, McFarland EG, Weinstock LB, et al. Patient preferences for CT colonography, conventional colonoscopy, and bowel preparation. Am J Gastroenterol 2003;98: 578.

[31] Iannaccone R, Laghi A, Catalano C, et al. Computed tomographic colonography without cathartic preparation for the detection of colorectal polyps. Gastroenterology 2004;127: 1300.

[32] Pickhardt PJ. CT colonography without catharsis: the ultimate study or useful additional option? Gastroenterology 2005;128:521.

[33] Gluecker TM, Johnson CD, Harmsen WS, et al. Colorectal cancer screening with CT co-lonography, colonoscopy, and double-contrast barium enema examination: prospective assessment of patient perceptions and preferences. Radiology 2003;227:378.

[34] Fletcher JG, Johnson CD, MacCarty RL, et al. CT colonography: potential pitfalls and problem-solving techniques. AJR Am J Roentgenol 1999;172:1271.

[35] Macari M, Lavelle M, Pedrosa I, et al. Effect of different bowel preparations on residual fluid at CT colonography. Radiology 2001;218:274.

[36] Lefere PA, Gryspeerdt SS, Dewyspelaere J, et al. Dietary fecal tagging as a cleansing method before CT colonography: initial results polyp detection and patient acceptance. Radiology 2002;224:393.

[37] Ji H, Rolnick JA, Haker S, et al. Multislice CT colonography: current status and limitations. Eur J Radiol 2003;47:123.

[38] Barish MA, Soto JA, Ferrucci JT. Consensus on current clinical practice of virtual colonoscopy. AJR Am J Roentgenol 2005;184:786.

[39] Chen SC, Lu DS, Hecht JR, et al. CT colonography: value of scanning in both the supine and prone positions. AJR Am J Roentgenol 1999;172:595.

[40] Fletcher JG, Johnson CD, Welch TJ, et al. Optimization of CT colonography technique: prospective trial in 180 patients. Radiology 2000;216:704.

[41] Fletcher RH. The end of barium enemas? N Engl J Med 2000;342:1823.

[42] Laks S, Macari M, Bini EJ. Positional change in colon polyps at CT colonography. Radiology 2004;231:761.

[43] Morrin MM, Farrell RJ, Keogan MT, et al. CT colonography: colonic distention improved by dual positioning but not intravenous glucagon. Eur Radiol 2002;12:525.

[44] Wessling J, Fischbach R, Meier N, et al. CT colonography: protocol optimization with multi-detector row CT—study in an anthropomorphic colon phantom. Radiology 2003;228:753.

[45] Fenlon HM, Nunes DP, Schroy PC 3rd, et al. A comparison of virtual and conventional colonoscopy for the detection of colorectal polyps. N Engl J Med 1999;341:1496.

[46] Yee J, Akerkar GA, Hung RK, et al. Colorectal neoplasia: performance characteristics of CT colonography for detection in 300 patients. Radiology 2001;219:685.

[47] Pickhardt PJ. Translucency rendering in 3D endoluminal CT colonography: a useful tool for increasing polyp specificity and decreasing interpretation time. AJR Am J Roentgenol 2004;183:429.

[48] Pickhardt PJ, Choi JH. Electronic cleansing and stool tagging in CT colonography: advantages and pitfalls with primary three-dimensional evaluation. AJR Am J Roentgenol 2003;181:799.

[49] Zalis ME, Hahn PF. Digital subtraction bowel cleansing in CT colonography. AJR Am J Roentgenol 2001;176:646.

[50] Zalis ME, Perumpillichira J, Del Frate C, et al. CT colonography: digital subtraction bowel cleansing with mucosal reconstruction initial observations. Radiology 2003;226:911.

[51] Nicholson FB, Taylor S, Halligan S, et al. Recent developments in CT colonography. Clin Radiol 2005;60:1.

[52] Summers RM, Yao J, Johnson CD. CT colonography with computer-aided detection: automated recognition of ileocecal valve to reduce number of false-positive detections. Radiology 2004;233:266.

[53] Yoshida H, Masutani Y, MacEneaney P, et al. Computerized detection of colonic polyps at CT colonography on the basis of volumetric features: pilot study. Radiology 2002;222:327.

[54] Ferrucci J, Barish M, Choi R, et al. Virtual colonoscopy. JAMA 2004;292:431.

[55] Dachman AH, Kuniyoshi JK, Boyle CM, et al. CT colonography with three-dimensional problem solving for detection of colonic polyps. AJR Am J Roentgenol 1998;171:989.

[56] Fenlon HM, McAneny DB, Nunes DP, et al. Occlusive colon carcinoma: virtual colonoscopy in the preoperative evaluation of the proximal colon. Radiology 1999;210:423.

[57] Macari M, Berman P, Dicker M, et al. Usefulness of CT colonography in patients with incomplete colonoscopy. AJR Am J Roentgenol 1999;173:561.

[58] Morrin MM, Farrell RJ, Raptopoulos V, et al. Role of virtual computed tomographic colonography in patients with colorectal cancers and obstructing colorectal lesions. Dis Colon Rectum 2000;43:303.

[59] Hara AK, Johnson CD, MacCarty RL, et al. Incidental extracolonic findings at CT colonography. Radiology 2000;215:353.

[60] Morrin MM, Kruskal JB, Farrell RJ, et al. Endoluminal CT colonography after an incomplete endoscopic colonoscopy. AJR Am J Roentgenol 1999;172:913.

[61] Lauenstein TC, Ajaj W, Kuehle CA, et al. Magnetic resonance colonography: comparison of contrast-enhanced three-dimensional vibe with two-dimensional FISP sequences: preliminary experience. Invest Radiol 2005;40:89.

[62] Ajaj W, Lauenstein TC, Pelster G, et al. MR colonography: how does air compare to water for colonic distention? J Magn Reson Imaging 2004;19:216.

[63] Lauenstein TC, Goehde SC, Debatin JF. Fecal tagging: MR colonography without colonic cleansing. Abdom Imaging 2002;27:410.

[64] Goehde SC, Ajaj W, Lauenstein T, et al. Impact of diet on stool signal in dark lumen magnetic resonance colonography. J Magn Reson Imaging 2004;20:272.

[65] Purkayastha S, Tekkis PP, Athanasiou T, et al. Magnetic resonance colonography versus colonoscopy as a diagnostic investigation for colorectal cancer: a meta-analysis. Clin Radiol 2005;60:980.

[66] Villavicencio RT, Rex DK. Colonic adenomas: prevalence and incidence rates, growth rates, and miss rates at colonoscopy. Semin Gastrointest Dis 2000;11:185.

[67] Ajaj W, Pelster G, Treichel U, et al. Dark lumen magnetic resonance colonography: comparison with conventional colonoscopy for the detection of colorectal pathology. Gut 2003; 52:1738.

[68] Lauenstein TC, Debatin JF. Magnetic resonance colonography for colorectal cancer screening. Semin Ultrasound CT MR 2001;22:443.

[69] Luboldt W, Debatin JF. Virtual endoscopic colonography based on 3D MRI. Abdom Imaging 1998;23:568.

[70] Meier C, Wildermuth S. Feasibility and potential of MR-Colonography for evaluating colorectal cancer. Swiss Surg 2002;8:21.

[71] Hartmann D, Bassler B, Schilling D, et al. Colorectal polyps: detection with dark-lumen MR colonography versus conventional colonoscopy. Radiology 2005;238:143.

[72] Zerhouni EA, Rutter C, Hamilton SR, et al. CT and MR imaging in the staging of colorectal carcinoma: report of the Radiology Diagnostic Oncology Group II. Radiology 1996; 200:443.

[73] Low RN, McCue M, Barone R, et al. MR staging of primary colorectal carcinoma: comparison with surgical and histopathologic findings. Abdom Imaging 2003;28:784.

[74] Harisinghani MG, Saini S, Hahn PF, et al. MR imaging of lymph nodes in patients with primary abdominal and pelvic malignancies using ultrasmall superparamagnetic iron oxide (Combidex). Acad Radiol 1998;5(Suppl 1):S167.

[75] Koh DM, Brown G, Temple L, et al. Rectal cancer: mesorectal lymph nodes at MR imaging with USPIO versus histopathologic findings—initial observations. Radiology 2004;231:91.

[76] Hildebrandt U, Feifel G, Schwarz HP, et al. Endorectal ultrasound: instrumentation and clinical aspects. Int J Colorectal Dis 1986;1:203.

[77] Paty PB, Nash GM, Baron P, et al. Long-term results of local excision for rectal cancer. Ann Surg 2002;236:522.

[78] Stipa F, Burza A, Lucandri G, et al. Outcomes for early rectal cancer managed with transanal endoscopic microsurgery: a 5-year follow-up study. Surg Endosc 2006;20:541.

[79] Winde G, Nottberg H, Keller R, et al. Surgical cure for early rectal carcinomas (T1). Transanal endoscopic microsurgery vs. anterior resection. Dis Colon Rectum 1996;39: 969.

[80] Kim CJ, Yeatman TJ, Coppola D, et al. Local excision of T2 and T3 rectal cancers after downstaging chemoradiation. Ann Surg 2001;234:352.

[81] Nagtegaal ID, Marijnen CA, Kranenbarg EK, et al. Circumferential margin involvement is still an important predictor of local recurrence in rectal carcinoma: not one millimeter but two millimeters is the limit. Am J Surg Pathol 2002;26:350.

[82] Improved survival with preoperative radiotherapy in resectable rectal cancer. Swedish Rectal Cancer Trial. N Engl J Med 1997;336:980.

[83] Kapiteijn E, Marijnen CA, Nagtegaal ID, et al. Preoperative radiotherapy combined with total mesorectal excision for resectable rectal cancer. N Engl J Med 2001;345:638.

[84] Camma C, Giunta M, Fiorica F, et al. Preoperative radiotherapy for resectable rectal cancer: a meta-analysis. JAMA 2000;284:1008.

[85] Bipat S, Glas AS, Slors FJ, et al. Rectal cancer: local staging and assessment of lymph node involvement with endoluminal US, CT, and MR imaging—a meta-analysis. Radiology 2004;232:773.

[86] Akasu T, Kondo H, Moriya Y, et al. Endorectal ultrasonography and treatment of early stage rectal cancer. World J Surg 2000;24:1061.

[87] Beets-Tan RG, Beets GL. Rectal cancer: review with emphasis on MR imaging. Radiology 2004;232:335.

[88] Brown G, Davies S, Williams GT, et al. Effectiveness of preoperative staging in rectal cancer: digital rectal examination, endoluminal ultrasound or magnetic resonance imaging? Br J Cancer 2004;91:23.

[89] Heriot AG, Grundy A, Kumar D. Preoperative staging of rectal carcinoma. Br J Surg 1999; 86:17.

[90] Schulzke JD. Does miniprobe endoscopic ultrasound have a role in the diagnostic repertoire for colorectal cancer? Int J Colorectal Dis 2003;18:450.

[91] Stergiou N, Haji-Kermani N, Schneider C, et al. Staging of colonic neoplasms by colonoscopic miniprobe ultrasonography. Int J Colorectal Dis 2003;18:445.

[92] Brown G, Daniels IR, Richardson C, et al. Techniques and trouble-shooting in high spatial resolution thin slice MRI for rectal cancer. Br J Radiol 2005;78:245.

[93] Brown G, Radcliffe AG, Newcombe RG, et al. Preoperative assessment of prognostic factors in rectal cancer using high-resolution magnetic resonance imaging. Br J Surg 2003;90: 355.

[94] Beets-Tan RG, Beets GL, Vliegen RF, et al. Accuracy of magnetic resonance imaging in prediction of tumour-free resection margin in rectal cancer surgery. Lancet 2001;357: 497.

[95] Brown G, Daniels IR. Preoperative staging of rectal cancer: the MERCURY research project. Recent Results Cancer Res 2005;165:58.

[96] Strassburg J. Magnetic resonance imaging in rectal cancer: the MERCURY experience. Tech Coloproctol 2004;8(Suppl 1):s16.

[96a] Brown G, Daniels I, Norman A. MRI predicts surgical resection margin status in patients with rectal cancer: results from the Mercury Study Group. Abstract presented at the Radiological Society of North America Meeting 2004.

[97] Ferri M, Laghi A, Mingazzini P, et al. Pre-operative assessment of extramural invasion and sphincteral involvement in rectal cancer by magnetic resonance imaging with phased-array coil. Colorectal Dis 2005;7:387.

[98] Kotanagi H, Fukuoka T, Shibata Y, et al. The size of regional lymph nodes does not correlate with the presence or absence of metastasis in lymph nodes in rectal cancer. J Surg Oncol 1993;54:252.

[99] Maldjian C, Smith R, Kilger A, et al. Endorectal surface coil MR imaging as a staging technique for rectal carcinoma: a comparison study to rectal endosonography. Abdom Imaging 2000;25:75.

[100] Kim JH, Beets GL, Kim MJ, et al. High-resolution MR imaging for nodal staging in rectal cancer: are there any criteria in addition to the size? Eur J Radiol 2004;52:78.

[101] Oh YT, Kim MJ, Lim JS, et al. Assessment of the prognostic factors for a local recurrence of rectal cancer: the utility of preoperative MR imaging. Korean J Radiol 2005;6:8.

[102] Gualdi GF, Casciani E, Guadalaxara A, et al. Local staging of rectal cancer with transrectal ultrasound and endorectal magnetic resonance imaging: comparison with histologic findings. Dis Colon Rectum 2000;43:338.

[103] Hunerbein M, Pegios W, Rau B, et al. Prospective comparison of endorectal ultrasound, three-dimensional endorectal ultrasound, and endorectal MRI in the preoperative evaluation of rectal tumors. Preliminary results. Surg Endosc 2000;14:1005.

[104] Akin O, Nessar G, Agildere AM, et al. Preoperative local staging of rectal cancer with endorectal MR imaging: comparison with histopathologic findings. Clin Imaging 2004;28:432.

[105] Kim NK, Kim MJ, Yun SH, et al. Comparative study of transrectal ultrasonography, pelvic computerized tomography, and magnetic resonance imaging in preoperative staging of rectal cancer. Dis Colon Rectum 1999;42:770.

[106] Kwok H, Bissett IP, Hill GL. Preoperative staging of rectal cancer. Int J Colorectal Dis 2000;15:9.

[107] Harewood GC, Wiersema MJ, Nelson H, et al. A prospective, blinded assessment of the impact of preoperative staging on the management of rectal cancer. Gastroenterology 2002;123:24.

[108] Blomqvist L, Holm T, Nyren S, et al. MR imaging and computed tomography in patients with rectal tumours clinically judged as locally advanced. Clin Radiol 2002;57:211.

[109] Beets-Tan RG, Beets GL, Borstlap AC, et al. Preoperative assessment of local tumor extent in advanced rectal cancer: CT or high-resolution MRI? Abdom Imaging 2000;25:533.

[110] Madbouly KM, Remzi FH, Erkek BA, et al. Recurrence after transanal excision of T1 rectal cancer: should we be concerned? Dis Colon Rectum 2005;48:711.

[111] Mohiuddin M, Marks G, Bannon J. High-dose preoperative radiation and full thickness local excision: a new option for selected T3 distal rectal cancers. Int J Radiat Oncol Biol Phys 1994;30:845.

[112] Sengupta S, Tjandra JJ. Local excision of rectal cancer: what is the evidence? Dis Colon Rectum 2001;44:1345.

[113] de Anda EH, Lee SH, Finne CO, et al. Endorectal ultrasound in the follow-up of rectal cancer patients treated by local excision or radical surgery. Dis Colon Rectum 2004;47:818.

[114] Beynon J, Mortensen NJ, Foy DM, et al. The detection and evaluation of locally recurrent rectal cancer with rectal endosonography. Dis Colon Rectum 1989;32:509.

[115] Lohnert MS, Doniec JM, Henne-Bruns D. Effectiveness of endoluminal sonography in the identification of occult local rectal cancer recurrences. Dis Colon Rectum 2000;43:483.

[116] Makela JT, Laitinen SO, Kairaluoma MI. Five-year follow-up after radical surgery for colorectal cancer. Results of a prospective randomized trial. Arch Surg 1995;130:1062.

[117] Novell F, Pascual S, Viella P, et al. Endorectal ultrasonography in the follow-up of rectal cancer. Is it a better way to detect early local recurrence? Int J Colorectal Dis 1997;12:78.

[118] Garcia-Aguilar J, Hernandez de Anda E, Rothenberger DA, et al. Endorectal ultrasound in the management of patients with malignant rectal polyps. Dis Colon Rectum 2005;48:910.

[119] Barbaro B, Schulsinger A, Valentini V, et al. The accuracy of transrectal ultrasound in predicting the pathological stage of low-lying rectal cancer after preoperative chemoradiation therapy. Int J Radiat Oncol Biol Phys 1999;43:1043.

[120] Fleshman JW, Myerson RJ, Fry RD, et al. Accuracy of transrectal ultrasound in predicting pathologic stage of rectal cancer before and after preoperative radiation therapy. Dis Colon Rectum 1992;35:823.

[121] Napoleon B, Pujol B, Berger F, et al. Accuracy of endosonography in the staging of rectal cancer treated by radiotherapy. Br J Surg 1991;78:785.

[122] Rau B, Hunerbein M, Barth C, et al. Accuracy of endorectal ultrasound after preoperative radiochemotherapy in locally advanced rectal cancer. Surg Endosc 1999;13:980.

[123] Hunerbein M, Totkas S, Moesta KT, et al. The role of transrectal ultrasound-guided biopsy in the postoperative follow-up of patients with rectal cancer. Surgery 2001;129:164.

[124] Morken JJ, Baxter NN, Madoff RD, et al. Endorectal ultrasound-directed biopsy: a useful technique to detect local recurrence of rectal cancer. Int J Colorectal Dis 2006;21: 258.

[125] Kuo LJ, Chern MC, Tsou MH, et al. Interpretation of magnetic resonance imaging for locally advanced rectal carcinoma after preoperative chemoradiation therapy. Dis Colon Rectum 2005;48:23.

[126] Chen CC, Lee RC, Lin JK, et al. How accurate is magnetic resonance imaging in restaging rectal cancer in patients receiving preoperative combined chemoradiotherapy? Dis Colon Rectum 2005;48:722.

[127] Peschaud F, Cuenod CA, Benoist S, et al. Accuracy of magnetic resonance imaging in rectal cancer depends on location of the tumor. Dis Colon Rectum 2005;48:1603.

[128] Even-Sapir E, Parag Y, Lerman H, et al. Detection of recurrence in patients with rectal cancer: PET/CT after abdominoperineal or anterior resection. Radiology 2004;232:815.

[129] Fukunaga H, Sekimoto M, Ikeda M, et al. Fusion image of positron emission tomography and computed tomography for the diagnosis of local recurrence of rectal cancer. Ann Surg Oncol 2005;12:561.

[130] Moore HG, Akhurst T, Larson SM, et al. A case-controlled study of 18-fluorodeoxyglucose positron emission tomography in the detection of pelvic recurrence in previously irradiated rectal cancer patients. J Am Coll Surg 2003;197:22.

[131] Chessin DB, Kiran RP, Akhurst T, et al. The emerging role of 18F-fluorodeoxyglucose positron emission tomography in the management of primary and recurrent rectal cancer. J Am Coll Surg 2005;201:948.

[132] Flamen P. Positron emission tomography in colorectal cancer. Best Pract Res Clin Gastroenterol 2002;16:237.

[133] Arulampalam TH, Costa DC, Loizidou M, et al. Positron emission tomography and colorectal cancer. Br J Surg 2001;88:176.

[134] Meta J, Seltzer M, Schiepers C, et al. Impact of 18F-FDG PET on managing patients with colorectal cancer: the referring physician's perspective. J Nucl Med 2001; 42:586.

[135] Whiteford MH, Whiteford HM, Yee LF, et al. Usefulness of FDG-PET scan in the assessment of suspected metastatic or recurrent adenocarcinoma of the colon and rectum. Dis Colon Rectum 2000;43:759.

[136] Boykin KN, Zibari GB, Lilien DL, et al. The use of FDG-positron emission tomography for the evaluation of colorectal metastases of the liver. Am Surg 1999;65:1183.

[137] Topal B, Flamen P, Aerts R, et al. Clinical value of whole-body emission tomography in potentially curable colorectal liver metastases. Eur J Surg Oncol 2001;27:175.

[138] Zhuang H, Sinha P, Pourdehnad M, et al. The role of positron emission tomography with fluorine-18-deoxyglucose in identifying colorectal cancer metastases to liver. Nucl Med Commun 2000;21:793.

[139] Selzner M, Hany TF, Wildbrett P, et al. Does the novel PET/CT imaging modality impact on the treatment of patients with metastatic colorectal cancer of the liver? Ann Surg 2004; 240:1027.

[140] Tzimas GN, Koumanis DJ, Meterissian S. Positron emission tomography and colorectal carcinoma: an update. J Am Coll Surg 2004;198:645.

[141] Kalff V, Hicks RJ, Ware RE, et al. The clinical impact of (18)F-FDG PET in patients with suspected or confirmed recurrence of colorectal cancer: a prospective study. J Nucl Med 2002;43:492.

[142] Huebner RH, Park KC, Shepherd JE, et al. A meta-analysis of the literature for whole-body FDG PET detection of recurrent colorectal cancer. J Nucl Med 2000;41:1177.

[143] Veit P, Kuhle C, Beyer T, et al. Whole body positron emission tomography/computed tomography (PET/CT) tumour staging with integrated PET/CT colonography: technical feasibility and first experiences in patients with colorectal cancer. Gut 2006;55:68.

ELSEVIER
SAUNDERS

SURGICAL
CLINICS OF
NORTH AMERICA

Surg Clin N Am 86 (2006) 849–865

Advances in Gastrointestinal Endoscopic Techniques

David E. Beck, MD

Department of Colon and Rectal Surgery, Ochsner Clinic Foundation,
1514 Jefferson Highway, New Orleans, LA 70121, USA

Colonoscopy is a common and useful technique for the diagnosis and management of colorectal diseases. Improved understanding of disease processes and equipment advances has expanded the options that are available to experienced endoscopists. This article discusses several of these diagnostic and therapeutic techniques.

Advanced diagnostic maneuvers

Chromoscopy

Surface staining (or dye spraying) during colonoscopy is termed "chromoscopy," and involves the application of dyes to highlight surface features of the mucosa and suspected neoplasia [1]. Surface staining assists the endoscopist in identifying lesions or different types of epithelium and has the potential to allow better differentiation of normal from neoplastic or preneoplastic tissue, to improve screening of high-risk populations, and to ensure complete removal of neoplastic tissue by endoscopic means [2]. Several types of stains can be used; these include contrast stains (which highlight surface topography detail by pooling into crevices), absorptive (vital) stains (which enter the epithelial cells by absorption or diffusion), and reactive stains (which interact with specific types of epithelium to produce a chemically induced color change) (Table 1).

Indigo carmine (0.8% solution, American Regent Laboratories, Inc., Shirley, New York) is a blue contrast stain that highlights surface details. Indigo carmine can be ingested (mixed with an oral electrolyte lavage) or applied with a spray catheter as a 0.8% solution. The epithelium stains a dark blue, but tends to fade after a short period of time because of

E-mail address: dbeckmd@aol.com

doi:10.1016/j.suc.2006.05.003
surgical.theclinics.com

Table 1
Stains used for chromoendoscopy

Type of stain	Stain	Mechanism	Clinical use
Contrast	Indigo carmine	Pools in crypts/folds/ mucosal irregularities	Highlights small mucosal lesions
Absorptive	Lugol's solution	Absorbed by glycogen-containing epithelium	Outlines intestinal metaplasia
	Methylene blue	Absorbed by intestinal/colonic metaplasia	Intestinal metaplasia
	Toluidine blue	Absorbed by nucleic acid of malignant epithelium	Squamous cell cancer of esophagus
	Cresyl violet	Absorbed by colonic epithelium surrounding pits	Identification of pit pattern
Reactive	Congo red	Red at alkaline pH, blue/black at acid pH	Demonstrates areas of gastric secretion

dispersion of the contrast by gut secretion and motility. It also can be washed away easily with irrigation. Although indigo carmine is helpful to stain polyps, its short duration makes frequent applications necessary for large polyps. Indigo carmine has been reported to be helpful in the evaluation of Barrett's esophagitis, flat adenomas, gastric cancer, collagenous colitis, and malabsorption [1,3–6].

Absorptive stains, such as methylene blue, toluidine blue, cresyl violet, and Lugol's iodine, are absorbed actively into the mucosal cells. Methylene blue (1% solution, Hope Pharmaceuticals, Scottsdale, Arizona) is widely available and has been used to assist in identifying flat adenomas, ulcerative colitis, and aberrant crypt foci [7,8]. Methylene blue is applied in a 1% aqueous solution and absorbed into the epithelial cytoplasm. This absorption is facilitated by spraying a 10% acetylcysteine, which removes the mucus layer. The mucolytic effect of acetylcysteine takes several minutes to occur and can be assisted by collapsing the bowel. The pooled agent can be reaspirated into the catheter and reapplied to any missed areas. Toluidine blue is an aniline dye that fixes to nucleic acids, and, thus, stains tissue with increased mitotic activity [1]. A 1% to 2% solution has been used in the esophagus, but it will stain erosions, inflammation, or food particles false positively. Cresyl violet is absorbed by colonic epithelium surrounding pit openings. This defines the pit pattern that has been correlated with histologic examinations [7,9]. Lugol's solution contains potassium iodine and iodine (1%–5% solution) [1]. The iodine reacts with glycogen in nonkeratinized squamous epithelium and results in a deep green-brown staining of the normal mucosa. Dysplastic areas have less glycogen and do not stain. Lugol's solution may give rise to an allergic reaction in individuals who are allergic to iodine.

Some stains react with mucosa to produce a specific color. Congo red in a 0.3% bicarbonate solution combined with methylene blue has been used to demark the outline of polyps to aid excision [10]. Specific situations in which chromoscopy is being used include differentiating colon polyps (hyperplastic versus adenomas, or folds versus adenomas), screening/surveillance, neoplastic margins, and residual tissue [11].

Chromoscopy is cumbersome, time consuming, and can be messy. Few endoscopy units have these dyes readily available. Although mainly a research tool, these techniques merit further evaluation to define their roles in routine clinical practice.

Narrow band imaging

Narrow band imaging uses different light frequencies and filters. Special endoscopes and processors are required. Tissue has varied blood flow and varied light absorption. Adenomas tend to darken in the narrow band spectrum. Narrow band imaging is available on production endoscopes. It remains to be determined how useful clinicians will find this modality.

Magnification endoscopy

Optic or electronic magnification can enlarge images and improve visualization of normal and abnormal epithelium. High-resolution endoscopy is available and involves an increase in magnification up to 1.5×, an increase in pixels (eg, >400,000 versus 100,000 to 200,000 for earlier videoscopes), and a higher-speed electronic shutter [1]. These modifications usually are performed in the video chips and the video processors. Special processors and high-resolution monitors often are required to take full benefit of this technology.

These instruments allow the colonoscopist to recognize the honeycomb pit pattern and to discern nonspecific erythremia from mucosal hemorrhage and angiectasis [1]. High-resolution colonoscopy is especially suited for chromoscopy, because surface patterns are crisp and margins of sessile lesions are delineated well.

Magnification endoscopy is a technique that is used for the examination of subtle changes on the mucosa and colonic crypts [1,10,12]. Using scopes with a movable lens (similar to the lens of a microscope) to zoom, images can be magnified from 3× to 170× (most in the range of 10×–35×). The current scopes use dials, levers, or electronic foot pedals to move the lens. The distance between the tip of the scope and the mucosa, the presence or absence of fluid, and movement affect the viewing field and the quality of the image. These factors have hindered the value of endoscopic magnification in the proximal colon, but have allowed it to be useful in the rectum. Applications has been directed toward identification of aberrant crypt foci that are believed to be precursors of adenomas and cancer [12,13]. Aberrant crypt foci are enlarged colonic crypts that typically are grouped together. When viewed under magnification chromoscopy they appear as an elevated mound of markedly enlarged crypts [1]. These lesions may serve as intermediate markers and predictors for colorectal neoplasia [13,14].

Magnification is used frequently for anal cryptography and in the evaluation of Barrett's esophagitis, but remains a research tool for the colon. High-resolution endoscopes are now available commercially. Widespread availability will help to delineate the value of this technology.

Colonic marking

Unless a lesion is adjacent to the ileocecal valve or located in the rectum, it is difficult to localize its exact location in the colon accurately. Localization is important for small lesions or polyps that may not be palpable during open surgery, and if laparoscopic surgery or endoscopic follow-up is anticipated [15]. For lesions that are not confirmed with radiologic studies, such as barium enemas or CT scans, some type of colonic marking can be helpful.

Tattooing

Tattooing of the bowel has been performed with India ink, tattoo ink (Lasting Impressions Inc., Englewood, New Jersey), or carbon particles (SPOT, GI Supply, Camp Hill, Pennsylvania). The India ink is permanent, can be difficult to obtain, and lacks US Food and Drug Administration (FDA) approval [16]. The carbon particle solution is approved by the FDA and has been reported to last up to 38 months [17]. A list of commercially available agents is obtainable at the American Society of Gastrointestinal Endoscopy Web site [18].

The technique of tattooing is similar to other mucosal injection methods. The needle is exposed and passed at a tangential angle into the mucosa. Care is taken to maintain a superficial entry to avoid a transmural or intraperitoneal injection. A fluid bleb is produced by injection of 0.2 mL to 1 mL of solution (Fig. 1A). If a bleb is not apparent the needle is withdrawn and repositioned. The tattoos should be placed just distally to the lesion. If operative localization is desired, two or three additional tattoos should be placed in a circumferential location (Figs. 2 and 3).

Clipping

An alternative to tattooing is placement of endoscopic clips [7]. The clips can be identified by palpation in open operative procedures or with ultrasound in laparoscopic procedures. Because the clips are placed in the mucosa, their duration is short and they should be used for localization only if the surgery is planned shortly after the endoscopic procedure. Another option is to take an abdominal radiograph at the completion of the endoscopic procedure. The residual air in the colon provides an air contrast enema, and the clips can identify the segment of colon that contains the lesion (Figures 4 and 5). Two or three clips should be placed in

A

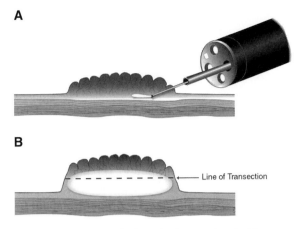

B

Line of Transection

Fig. 1. (*A–B*) Injection of submucosal material.

a circumferential manner a few centimeters distal to the lesion. The Quick-clip (Olympus America, Inc., Melville, New York) is a single-fire device. The Resolution clip device (Boston Scientific Corporation, Natick, Massachusetts) can be opened and closed before firing. Either device requires some familiarity with it before use.

Clips also have been used to close polypectomy sites that may be deeper than anticipated, to produce hemostasis at polypectomy sites or bleeding diverticulum, and to anchor feeding or decompression tubes [18,19].

The equipment for colonic marking should be available in all endoscopy units. The increasing use of minimally invasive surgery, along with marking indications that were described previously, support the increasing need for marking techniques.

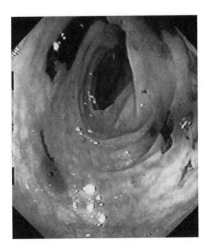

Fig. 2. Endoscopic view of colonic tattoo in three locations.

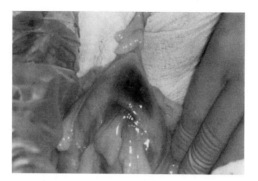

Fig. 3. Operative view of colonic tattoos.

Advanced therapeutic maneuvers

Dilatation

Endoscopic balloon dilatation of gastrointestinal obstruction developed from procedures for the treatment of achalasia. Balloon dilatation of colonic anastomotic strictures, Crohn's strictures, ischemic strictures, endometriotic strictures, and obstructing colorectal cancers has been described. The technique has been used as an alternative to surgery and to eliminate the need for a diverting colostomy before surgery.

In 1989, Aston and colleagues [20] reported their experience with nine patients who underwent balloon dilatation of colon and rectal anastomotic strictures. Six of the nine strictures resolved after a single dilatation. Also in 1989, Stone and Bloom [21] described balloon dilatation of obstructing colorectal cancer in three patients, which allowed elective one stage colon resection or neodymium:yttrium-aluminum-garnet (Nd:YAG) laser palliation in a clean field. In 1991, Williams and Palmer [22] reported the balloon dilatation of seven patients with obstructing symptoms secondary to

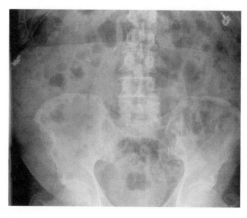

Fig. 4. Supine radiograph of abdomen demonstrating mucosal clips in transverse colon.

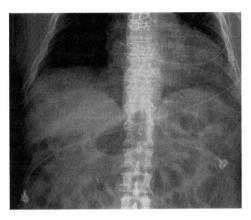

Fig. 5. Upright radiograph of abdomen demonstrating mucosal clips (same patient as in Fig. 4).

Crohn's strictures. Five patients had strictures at the site of a previous ileo-transverse colon anastomosis. They obtained a sustained improvement in five patients over a follow-up period of 18 to 24 months, but were unsuccessful in two patients. In a more recent, larger series, Dear and Hunter [23] reported balloon dilatation in 22 patients who had Crohn's strictures. Sixteen patients were dilated successfully, although one third of the patients required more than two dilatations. Six patients failed balloon treatment and required surgery. There were no complications after any of the 71 dilatations performed. Lastly, Miller and colleagues [24] reported successfully treating an endometriotic stricture of the sigmoid colon. Thus, balloon dilatation in selected patients seems to be safe and effective in eliminating the need for additional surgeries.

Intestinal strictures result from several conditions. Benign conditions, such as inflammation (inflammatory bowel disease) or postoperative anastomosis, often respond to dilatation. Several endoscopically guided balloons are available. For colonic use, the balloons range in size from 6 mm to 20 mm in diameter. The technique involves placing a guidewire across the stricture. The balloon catheter is advanced over the guidewire to the midpoint of the stricture and is inflated with a pressure- or volume-controlled handle.

Colonic stents

Intraluminal colonic stents are an extension of technology that initially was used for vascular, biliary, and esophageal obstructive pathology [25]. The main indication for their use is in the treatment of colonic obstruction: (1) in an attempt to obtain adequate mechanical bowel preparation before definitive resection (a bridge to surgery), and (2) for palliation in patients who are poor operative candidates because of comorbid disease or a limited life expectancy secondary to extensive metastases. Although most stents have been used in malignant disease, there are several reports of their use to manage fistulas and ischemic and anastomotic strictures.

Up to 30% of patients who have colorectal cancers present with obstruction. The operative morbidity and mortality for emergent surgery is higher than for elective colonic resections [25]. Right-sided obstructions have been managed with resection and ileocolic anastomosis, or, occasionally, an ileostomy. Left-sided colonic obstructions are managed most frequently with immediate resection without anastomosis (Hartmann's procedure), subtotal colectomy, primary resection with anastomosis (with or without on-table colonic irrigation), colonic stenting with delayed primary resection, and anastomosis [26]. Table 2 lists a comparison of the advantages and disadvantages of these procedures. All of these management options have the advantage of addressing the primary lesion early in the treatment course. Less commonly used operations include cecostomy and three-stage procedures (diversion, resection, stoma closure). Although colorectal adenocarcinomas account for most of the large bowel obstructions that are treated with intraluminal stents, obstruction from cancers of the prostate, ovaries, stomach, pancreas, and uterine cervix have been treated in this manner [27–30].

Colonic stenting for obstruction was described in the early 1990s [31,32]. Most reports on colonic stenting involve the use of uncovered esophageal-

Table 2
Advantages and disadvantages of procedures for managing chronic obstruction

Procedure	Advantages	Disadvantages
Resection without anastomosis	No anastomosis, time to optimize patient's nutritional status and comorbidities before anastomosis	Repeat operation, stoma (stoma closure never performed in 25%), combined mortality rate 6%–12%
Subtotal colectomy	No stoma, no bowel preparation needed	Lengthier operation, increased bowel frequency, liquid stool (especially an issue in older patients and for lesions in the distal sigmoid and rectum); mortality 3%–11%
Resection with on-table colonic irrigation primary anastomosis	No stoma, no additional operation required	Time consuming, risk for anastomosis (dilated, edematous colon; malnourished patient)
Colonic stenting, delayed resection, primary anastomosis	Opportunity to stage patient before surgery, opportunity to correct nutritional/comorbid factors	Risks for perforation, migration of stent, reobstruction

type stents. As of this writing, three uncovered, self-expandable, metal colonic stents have FDA approval. These include the Enteral Wallstent (Microvasive Corporation/Boston Scientific, Natick, Massachusetts), the colonic Z-stent (Wilson-Cook Medical, Winston-Salem, North Carolina), and the Precision Colonic Ultraflex (Microvasive Corporation/Boston Scientific). The stents are wire (stainless steel, Elgiloy, or Nitinol), have a predeployment diameter of 10 to 30 French and a postdeployment diameter of 20 mm to 25 mm. Contraindications to stent placement are existing perforation or distal rectal lesions in which the stent cannot be placed above the levator muscles. Stents can be placed radiographically, endoscopically, or using a combined technique.

Rectal, rectosigmoid, and distal sigmoid obstructions frequently are amenable to stent placement under fluoroscopic guidance [25]. The patient is sedated and appropriate monitoring of heart rate, blood pressure, and oxygenation is performed. A single dose of a broad-spectrum antibiotic is given intravenously. An angiography catheter is inserted by way of the anus and advanced to the level of obstruction. Water-soluble radiographic contrast is injected to demonstrate the obstruction, and a guidewire is placed through the catheter beyond the level of obstruction. The angiography catheter is removed and the stent delivery system is inserted over the guidewire. The length of the stent should be at least 4 cm longer than the obstruction to allow a 2-cm overlap at either end. The stent is deployed and contrast is injected to rule out perforation.

Most endoscopists prefer a combined endoscopic-fluoroscopic approach, whereas others use an endoscope-only technique. For the combined technique, sedation and monitoring are used as described previously. The endoscope is inserted until the distal portion of the obstruction is visualized. The length of the obstruction is determined by measurement with the endoscope. If the endoscope will not pass through the lesion, radiographic contrast is injected by way of a biliary or an angiography catheter placed through the scope. A guidewire is placed through the scope and beyond the level of the obstruction. If the stent is designed to fit through the colonoscope (Wallstent), it is inserted over the guidewire into position. Radiographic markers identify the location of the proximal portion of the stent. The stent is deployed under endoscopic visualization of its distal end with fluoroscopic confirmation. If the stent is not designed to fit through the endoscope, the endoscope is removed (leaving the guidewire in place), and the stent is inserted over the guidewire through the obstruction. The endoscope is reinserted to the distal portion of the obstruction and the stent is deployed under endoscopic visualization. Once the stent is deployed, contrast is injected to verify appropriate placement and detect colonic perforation. Several investigators have reported placement of two stents at the same procedure. This is necessary for long strictures or when the initial stent is not effective in resolving the obstruction because of malpositioning. Patients frequently pass stool through the stent immediately after successful deployment. Symptoms of obstruction should be relieved within the first 24 hours after deployment in most patients, but improvement over the first 72 hours can occur as the stent continues to expand. A plain film of the abdomen should be taken immediately following placement for comparison should concerns about stent migration arise.

As a bridge to surgery, technical success was obtained in 92% of 407 cases from a pooled analysis of 1198 patients from 54 case series that were reviewed by Sebastian and colleagues [33]. Clinical success, defined as the ability to perform a one-stage operation without creation of a stoma, was 72%. In 791 patients treated for palliation, technical success was achieved in 93%, and clinical success, defined by colonic decompression within 48 hours without other intervention, was 91%. Treatment success is higher in shorter lesions, distal lesions, and obstruction from colonic primaries. Inability to pass the guidewire or the stent catheter is the most common reason for technical failure. Laser treatment of a completely obstructing lesion may allow passage of a guidewire [34]. Balloon dilatation has been used before and after stent placement, but perforation has been reported [35–37]. Self-expanding stents should not need to be dilated, and, therefore, the risk for perforation seems unwarranted. Failure to relieve obstruction after successful deployment is rare, and usually is related to placing a stent that is too short relative to the length of the stenosis or failure to identify proximal obstruction in patients who have carcinomatosis and multiple-level obstruction [27,38]. No specific management is required after placement; however, most investigators recommend patients take a stool softener or product (eg, Miralax) to avoid fecal obstruction.

Complications of stent placement in the pooled analysis included perforation (3.8%), stent migration (11.8%), reobstruction (7.3%), rectal bleeding, anal pain, and tenesmus [33]. Perforation may occur during placement of the guidewire or stent carrier across the area of stenosis, during stent deployment or expansion, or remote from the procedure. Asymptomatic perforations that resulted from guidewire placement have been treated successfully with antibiotics [39,40]. Perforation that is related to stent deployment often is identified as increased pain following the procedure. Surgical treatment, most commonly with diversion, is required frequently in these situations. Delayed perforation, as late as 2 months after successful stenting, also has been reported [34,41]. Camunez and colleagues [35] found asymptomatic erosion of the colonic wall from the end of the stent in three patients in whom the stent was used as a bridge to surgery. Cumulative intervention-related mortality was 0.6% [33].

Stent migration may occur at any time, but is seen most frequently in the first several weeks following placement. It has been reported in 0% to 22% of cases. Most cases are detected within 5 days after placement; however, intervals up to 11 months have been reported [34,36]. Cases of delayed stent migration or expulsion are related to tumor response to chemotherapy or radiation [34,35,42]. Uncovered stents may be less likely to migrate than are covered ones, but tumor ingrowth leads to reobstruction. Covered stents have less tumor ingrowth but lack FDA approval [43]. Patients with normal mucosa, as is seen in obstruction secondary to extrinsic compression, also are at higher risk for stent migration. Stents typically migrate distally and have been expelled by way of the anus without complication. More commonly they are removed using endoscopic biopsy forceps or a snare.

In addition to large bowel obstruction from malignancy, colonic stenting has been applied to benign disease but with less success. Disease processes that are managed with stents include strictures from diverticular disease and intestinal fistulas [44,45]. Binkert and colleagues [39] performed a cost analysis of patients who were treated with colonic stents. Twelve of 13 patients were stented successfully, and 10 underwent subsequent operations for their tumor. They compared these patients with a control group of patients that was treated with initial surgery at the same hospital. Overall, an average cost reduction of 20% was demonstrated in the stented group. This group also had shorter hospitalization (6.1 days), fewer surgical procedures, and fewer ICU days. A second analysis by Targownik and colleagues [46] also showed that early colonic stent placement was less expensive than was emergency surgery for acute malignant obstruction because of the avoidance of a second operation to reestablish intestinal continuity.

In conclusion, colonic stenting is an effective and safe tool in the management of malignant, left-sided colorectal obstruction. It provides an opportunity for adequate bowel cleansing, medically optimizing the patient, and conversion of an emergent surgical problem into an elective one in which primary anastomosis is more likely to be performed. It also affords the treating surgeon the chance to stage the patient, and, thereby, to select out patients who would not benefit from further surgery while providing acceptable palliation of obstructive symptoms. Recurrent obstruction can be treated frequently with repeat stenting.

Lasers in colonoscopy

It is possible to transmit lasers fiber optically, and argon and Nd:YAG lasers are being used clinically. The Nd:YAG laser beam scatters more on impact and is not absorbed as readily by red-pigmented areas. It also penetrates deeper into tissue, which allows for greater destruction of large tumors [47,48]. The Nd:YAG laser has been used to destroy colon and rectal polyps; stop bleeding and relieve obstruction secondary to colorectal cancers; and control radiation proctitis, hereditary hemorrhagic telangiectasia, angiodysplasias, and photoablation of colorectal adenomas [49]. The laser also has been used in place of operative diversion in hopeless clinical situations, such as hemorrhage, obstruction, or prohibitive operative risk in patients who had advanced colorectal carcinoma.

The Nd:YAG laser and the argon plasma coagulator (which is not a laser) also have been used to control bleeding secondary to radiation proctitis [50].

Laser-induced fluorescence spectroscopy also has been used to differentiate adenomas from nonadenomas [51,52].

Advanced polypectomy techniques (endoscopic mucosal resection)

Endoscopic removal of lesions is an outgrowth of transanal techniques and a learned skill of wildly variable difficulty. Small lesions may be removed or destroyed with biopsy forceps, whereas larger lesions are suitable for cautery snare removal. Basic techniques for safe colonoscopic polypectomy are described below [53].

The endoscopist must be familiar with the electrosurgical unit and be able to develop a standard routine. Choose a combination of cutting and coagulation and check all of the connections, the plate position, and the electrosurgical unit setting before performing a polypectomy. Make sure that the foot pedal is in a comfortable position and have your foot positioned over the pedal, so that once the snare is around the polyp, you do not need to look away from the procedure. Premature cutting through the stalk of a polyp before adequate coagulation can result if the snare wire is too thin or if the snare handle is closed too completely or too forcibly. This can be avoided by placing a mark on the snare handle, which indicates the point at which the tip of the snare loop has closed to the end of the outer sheath. When a thick stalk is snared the mark gives a useful approximate measure of its size. The outer sheath of a closed snare also can be used to assess the base of the polyp and its fixity.

The view and position of the polyp should be at the 6 o'clock position for the best control of the snare. To achieve this view the patient may need to change position or the snare should be rotated to improve the view of the polyp. The colon lumen should not be distended excessively because this thins the wall and flattens the polyp. The colonoscope is advanced proximal to the lesion and the snare is passed fully through the biopsy channel. The snare is opened and the colonoscope is retracted until the polyp head comes into the field of view. The colonoscope is maneuvered to bring the polyp into the snare loop. Alternatively, the loop can be pushed proximally over a difficult polyp positioned to one side or the other of the polyp head, and then swung over it by appropriate movements of the instrument. When snaring a small- or average-sized polyp it usually is best to have the loop fully open, and then to maneuver the scope so that the snare loop is placed over the polyp head almost entirely by manipulation of the endoscope. Rotatable snares exist and can be useful for the difficult polyp.

Snare the polyp and push the snare sheath against the stalk; this ensures that the loop of the snare will tighten it exactly at the same point. If there is any doubt that the snare is positioned properly over the polyp head, try shaking the snare or opening and closing the loop repeatedly, so as to help it slip down around the stalk. Also try angling the colonoscope tip in the relevant direction. Close the snare loop gently, to the mark or by feel until it is snug, ideally near the top of the stalk at its narrowest part. Leave a short segment of normal tissue on the stalk to help pathologic interpretation. Initial snare closure should be gentle, because the loop may be positioned incorrectly. Once the wire has cut into polyp tissue it may be difficult to release and reposition it. With longer stalks, if there is a suspicion of malignancy, it may be possible and desirable to snare lower down on the stalk to increase the chance of resecting all invasive tissue in the stalk.

If the loop is stuck in the wrong position or it is apparent that the polyp cannot be transected safely, releasing the snare loop is made easier by lifting the snare up over the polyp head and pushing it into the colon, with the whole colonoscope if necessary. It is almost always possible to dismantle the snare or to sacrifice it by cutting it with the wire cutters, withdrawing the colonoscope and leaving the loop in situ. Either the polyp head will fall off and the snare will be expelled, or another attempt can be made with a second snare.

Electrocoagulate using a low-power current (15W or dial setting 2.5–3) with the snare loop kept gently closed against the neck of tissue to create favorable circumstances for electrocoagulation. Apply the current for 2 to 5 seconds at a time, watching for visible swelling or whitening. When the snared portion of the stalk or base is coagulating visibly, gently squeeze the handle more tightly while continuing electrocoagulation; transection will start.

Be certain to observe the polyp head as it falls off, because it can be lost. If a polyp is lost, try to identify the dependent portion of the bowel where the head is likely to be. If not visible, irrigate with some water by way of a syringe and watch where it flows; if the water just refluxes back over the lens, then the polyp also will be behind the instrument tip. The endoscope is withdrawn to find the specimen. Retrieval of the specimen may be with the snare, basket, or retrieval device, or by aspiration through the channel into a filtered suction trap. When numerous polyps are present it may be necessary to snare/transect some specimens of medium size to allow them to be aspirated and so save time.

Various other techniques for excising large polyps or flat lesions have been described as saline assisted polypectomy, strip biopsy, or endoscopic mucosal resection. Investigators have used submucosal injections of fluid or suction devices to elevate the lesion, and cautery snares or knives with single- or double-channel scopes [54–57]. Sessile lesions up to 5 cm in diameter have been removed; however, those that occupy more than one third of the colonic circumference or involve two haustral folds usually are too large for safe endoscopic removal. Similarly, the inability to elevate a colonic lesion adequately using submucosal injection indicates that endoscopic removal may not be possible [55]. If in doubt, it is better to perform piecemeal excision at different endoscopic sessions to lessen the risk for full-thickness bowel wall injury. This method also gains time for histologic assessment, which may help in case of a malignancy.

Saline-assisted polypectomy provides a safety cushion of engorged submucosal stroma that protects the bowel wall from dissipated heat and creates a "bloodless" excision. Solutions used include 1:10,000 adrenaline in 0.9% saline, which dissipates in 2 to 3 minutes, or hypertonic solutions (2N saline or 20% dextrose, with or without adrenaline, sodium hyaluronate), or autologous blood, which makes the injection bleb last longer [55–59]. To inject the solution, a 10-mL syringe and a sclerotherapy needle are used. The needle is angled tangentially into the mucosal surface under the polyp (Fig. 1A–B). A low-pressure injection is performed. If a bleb is not observed, the needle is withdrawn slightly until a submucosal bleb is noted. An injection of 1 to 3 mL is sufficient for most small polyps. For larger polyps, injection of fluid proximal to the polyp is performed first, followed by subsequent injection of fluid into the edge of the preceding bleb. This technique is particularly important for polyps that are hidden behind a fold or those that traverse a fold in a "clamshell" fashion. There is no hazard if the needle passes into the peritoneum and no contraindication to injecting through the substance of a shallow sessile polyp [55]. Additionally, based upon the experience gained from direct percutaneous needle aspiration of malignant lesions elsewhere in the body, the risk for seeding carcinoma cells is exceedingly rare and reported to be no more than 1 in 10,000 [54]. A confluent ring of injection that is sufficient to raise a 4- to 5-cm sessile polyp may need up to 30-mL total injection volume. A study by Karita and colleagues [57] examined the effectiveness of the saline injection strip biopsy technique. They found that all 71 colonic lesions that were resected by this technique, regardless of shape and size, could be removed completely and safely with this method. This study included lesions greater than 30 mm in size. Furthermore, there were no perforations; however, not all investigators have reported the same success rate. Yokota and colleagues [59], using the same technique, reported a success rate for complete excision of flat adenomas of 87%. In this study there were two perforations and one bleeding complication.

An endoscopic approach is desirable for patients who are of high risk because of comorbidity, but in a younger patient or in the presence of technical difficulties it may be wiser to proceed with surgery rather than to perform repeated aggressive endoscopy. This is especially true in the era of laparoscopic surgery [60].

Control of bleeding

Endoscopic bleeding is prevented best by using the techniques that were described previously. When it does occur several techniques are available. These include irrigation or injection of epinephrine solutions, fulguration or cautery, clipping, or resnaring. Another option is a preassembled single-use endoscopic ligating device (PolyLoop, Olympus America, Inc.,

Melville, New York). This device, which can be passed through the biopsy port of a colonoscope, has a detachable nylon loop that can ligate a polyp stalk securely. The device can be used on a bleeding polyp stalk or placed on the stalk proximal to a planned snare site.

Summary

An increasing number of techniques for endoscopic diagnosis and treatment is being described. Endoscopic surgeons should be familiar with these techniques. Although many of the diagnostic techniques, other than marking, do not have widespread clinical application, the therapeutic techniques that were described in this article are being used successfully in increasing numbers of appropriately selected patients. Additional experience and technologic advances will refine the endoscopic therapy that is available to patients with colorectal diseases.

References

[1] Sorbi D, Gostout CJ. Polyp identification and marking: chromoscopy: resolution and high-magnification endoscopy, tattooing, and clipping. Tech Gastrointest Endoscopy 2000;2:2–8.
[2] Eisen GM. Chromoendoscopy of the colon. Gastrointest Endosc Clin N Am 2004;14: 453–60.
[3] Mitooka H, Fujimori T, Maeda S, et al. Minute flat depressed neoplastic lesions of the colon detected by contrast chromoscopy using an indigo carmine capsule. Gastrointest Endosc 1995;41:453–9.
[4] Mitooka H, Fujimori T, Ohno S, et al. Chromoscopy of the colon using indigo carmine dye with electrolyte lavage solution. Gastrointest Endosc 1992;38:373–4.
[5] Sato S, Benoni C, Toth E, et al. Chromoendoscopic appearance of collagenous colitis—a case report using indigo carmine. Endoscopy 1998;30:S80–1.
[6] Saitoh Y, Obara T, Watari J, et al. Invasion depth diagnosis of depressed type early colorectal cancers by combined use of videoendoscopy and chromoendoscopy. Gastrointest Endosc 1998;48:362–70.
[7] Fleischer DE. Chromoendoscopy and magnification endoscopy in the colon. Gastrointest Endosc 1999;49:S45–9.
[8] Matsumoto T, Kuroki F, Mizuno M, et al. Application of magnifying chromoscopy for the assessment of severity in patients with mild to moderate ulcerative colitis. Gastrointest Endosc 1997;46:400–5.
[9] Iida M, Iwashita A, Yao T, et al. Endoscopic features of villous tumors of the colon: correlation with histological findings. Hepatogastroenterology 1990;37:342–4.
[10] Iishi H, Tatsuta M, Okuda S, et al. Diagnosis of colorectal tumors by the endoscopic Congo red-methylene blue test. Surg Endosc 1994;8:1308–11.
[11] Rutter MD, Saunders BP, Schofield G, et al. Pancolonic indigo carmine dye spraying for the detection of dysplasia in ulcerative colitis. Gut 2004;53:256–60.
[12] Dolara P, Caderni G, Lancioni L, et al. Aberrant crypt foci in human colon carcinogenesis. Cancer Detect Prev 1997;21:135–40.
[13] Takayama T, Katsuki S, Takahashi Y, et al. Aberrant crypt foci of the colon as precursors of adenoma and cancer. N Engl J Med 1998;339:1277–84.
[14] Dashwood RH. Early detection and prevention of colorectal cancer (review). Oncol Rep 1999;6:277–81.

[15] Ellis KK, Fennerty MB. Marking and identifying colon lesions. Tattoos, clips, and radiology in imaging the colon. Gastrointest Endosc Clin N Am 1997;7:401–11.

[16] Lane KL, Vallera R, Washington K, et al. Endoscopic tattoo agents in the colon. Tissue responses and clinical implications. Am J Surg Pathol 1996;20:1266–70.

[17] Naveau S, Bonhomme L, Preaux N, et al. A pure charcoal suspension for colonoscopic tattoo. Gastrointest Endosc 1991;37:624–5.

[18] American Society of Gastrointestinal Endoscopy. Available at http://www.asge.org. Accessed February 1, 2006.

[19] Kudo H. Endoscopic clipping hemostasis for diverticular bleeding of the colon: report of three cases. Endoscopic Forum for Digestive Disease 2003;19:63–6.

[20] Aston NO, Owen WJ, Irving JD. Endoscopic balloon dilatation of colonic anastomotic strictures. Br J Surg 1989;76:780–2.

[21] Stone JM, Bloom RJ. Transendoscopic balloon dilatation of complete colonic obstruction: an adjunct in the treatment of colorectal cancer: report of three cases. Dis Colon Rectum 1989;32:429–31.

[22] Williams AJ, Palmer KR. Endoscopic balloon dilatation as a therapeutic option in the management of intestinal strictures resulting from Crohn's disease. Br J Surg 1991;78:453–4.

[23] Dear KL, Hunter JO. Colonoscopic hydrostatic balloon dilatation of Crohn's strictures. J Clin Gastroenterol 2001;33:315–8.

[24] Miller ES, Barnett RM, Williams RB. Sigmoid endometriotic stricture treated with endoscopic balloon dilatation: case report and literature review. Md Med J 1990;39:1081–4.

[25] Whitlow CB, Timmcke AE. New techniques in colonoscopy. Clin Colon Rectal Surg 2003;16:163–72.

[26] Deans GT, Krukowski ZH, Irwin ST. Malignant obstruction of the left colon. Br J Surg 1994;81:1270–6.

[27] Carter J, Valmadre S, Dalrymple C, et al. Management of large bowel obstruction in advanced ovarian cancer with intraluminal stents. Gynecol Oncol 2002;84:176–9.

[28] Friedland S, Hallenbeck J, Soetikno RM. Stenting the sigmoid colon in a terminally ill patient with prostate cancer. J Palliat Med 2001;4:153–6.

[29] Dauphine CE, Tan P, Beart RW Jr, et al. Placement of self-expanding metal stents for acute malignant large-bowel obstruction: a collective review. Ann Surg Oncol 2002;9:574–9.

[30] Law WL, Chu KW, Ho JWC, et al. Self-expanding metallic stent in the treatment of colonic obstruction caused by advanced malignancies. Dis Colon Rectum 2000;43:1522–7.

[31] Itabashi M, Hamano K, Kameoka S, et al. Self-expanding stainless steel stent application in rectosigmoid stricture. Dis Colon Rectum 1993;36:508–11.

[32] Baron TH. Colonic stenting: technique, technology, and outcomes for malignant and benign disease. Gastrointest Endosc Clin N Am 2005;15:757–71.

[33] Sebastian S, Johnston S, Geoghegan T, et al. Pooled analysis of the efficacy and safety of self-expanding metal stenting in malignant colorectal obstruction. Am J Gastroenterol 2004;99:2051–7.

[34] Baron TH, Dean PA, Yates MR III, et al. Expandable metal stents for the treatment of colonic obstruction: techniques and outcomes. Gastrointest Endosc 1998;47:277–86.

[35] Camunez F, Echenagusia A, Simo G, et al. Malignant colorectal obstruction treated by means of self-expanding metallic stents: effectiveness before surgery and in palliation. Radiology 2000;216:492–7.

[36] Tamim WZ, Ghellai A, Counihan TC, et al. Experience with endoluminal colonic wall stents for the management of large bowel obstruction for benign and malignant disease. Arch Surg 2000;135:434–8.

[37] Canon CL, Baron TH, Morgan DE, et al. Treatment of colonic obstruction with expandable metal stents: radiologic features. AJR Am J Roentgenol 1997;168:199–205.

[38] Adamsen S, Holm J, Meisner S, et al. Endoscopic placement of self-expanding metal stents for treatment of colorectal obstruction with long-term follow-up. Dan Med Bull 2000;47:225–7.

[39] Binkert CA, Ledermann H, Jost R, et al. Acute colonic obstruction: clinical aspects and cost-effectiveness of preoperative and palliative treatment with self-expanding metallic stents: a preliminary report. Radiology 1998;206:199–204.

[40] Aviv RI, Shyamalan G, Watkinson A, et al. Radiological palliation of malignant colonic obstruction. Clin Radiol 2002;57:347–51.

[41] Han YM, Lee JM, Lee TH. Delayed colon perforation after palliative treatment for rectal carcinoma with bare rectal stent: a case report. Korean J Radiol 2000;1:169–71.

[42] Spinelli P, Mancini A. Use of self-expanding metal stents for palliation of rectosigmoid cancer. Gastrointest Endosc 2001;53:203–6.

[43] Repici A, Reggio D, De Angelis C, et al. Covered metal stents for management of inoperable malignant colorectal strictures. Gastrointest Endosc 2000;52:735–40.

[44] Paul L, Pinto I, Gomez H, et al. Metallic stents in the treatment of benign diseases of the colon: preliminary experience in 10 cases. Radiology 2002;223:715–22.

[45] Jeyarajah AR, Shepherd JH, Fairclough PD, et al. Effective palliation of a colovaginal fistula using a self-expanding metal stent. Gastrointest Endosc 1997;46:367–9.

[46] Targownik LE, Spiegel BM, Sack J, et al. Colonic stent vs. emergency surgery for management of acute left-sided malignant colonic obstruction: a decision analysis. Gastrointest Endosc 2004;60:865–74.

[47] Ball KA, editor. Lasers: the perioperative challenge. St. Louis (MO): CV Mosby; 1990.

[48] Nishioka NS. Applications of lasers in gastroenterology. In: Puliafito CA, editor. Laser surgery and medicine: principles and practice. New York: Wiley-Liss; 1996.

[49] Mathus-Vliegen EM, Tytgat GN. The potential and limitations of laser photoablation of colorectal adenomas. Gastrointest Endosc 1991;37:9–17.

[50] Kaassis M, Oberti E, Burtin P, et al. Argon plasma coagulation for the treatment of hemorrhagic radiation proctitis. Endoscopy 2000;32:673–6.

[51] Cothren RM, Sivak MV Jr, Van Dam J, et al. Detection of dysplasia at colonoscopy using laser-induced fluorescence: a blinded study. Gastrointest Endosc 1996;44:168–76.

[52] Mycek MA, Schomacker KT, Nishioka NS. Colonic polyp differentiation using time-resolved autofluorescence spectroscopy. Gastrointest Endosc 1998;48:390–4.

[53] Waye J. Colonoscopic polypectomy. Tech Gastrointest Endosc 2000;2:9–17.

[54] Waye JD. New methods of polypectomy. Gastrointest Endosc Clin N Am 1997;7(3):413–22.

[55] Waye JD. Saline injection colonoscopic polypectomy. Am J Gastroenterol 1994;89:305–6.

[56] Muto T, Kamiya J, Sawada T, et al. Small "flat adenoma" of the large bowel with special reference to its clinicopathologic features. Dis Colon Rectum 1985;28:847–51.

[57] Karita M, Tada M, Okita K, et al. Endoscopic therapy for early colon cancer: the strip biopsy resection technique. Gastrointest Endosc 1991;37:128–32.

[58] Shirai M, Nakamura T, Matsuura A, et al. Safer colonoscopic polypectomy with local submucosal injection of hypertonic saline-epinephrine solution. Am J Gastroenterol 1994; 89(3):334–8.

[59] Yokota T, Sugihara K, Yoshida S. Endoscopic mucosal resection for colorectal neoplastic lesions. Dis Colon Rectum 1994;37:1108–11.

[60] Eijsbouts QA, Heuff G, Sietses C, et al. Laparoscopic surgery in the treatment of colonic polyps. Br J Surg 1999;86(4):505–8.

ELSEVIER
SAUNDERS

Surg Clin N Am 86 (2006) 867–897

SURGICAL
CLINICS OF
NORTH AMERICA

Laparoscopic Colon Surgery: Past, Present and Future

Guillaume Martel, MD, CM,
Robin P. Boushey, BSc, MD, PhD, CIP, FRCSC*

*Division of General Surgery, Minimally Invasive Surgery Research Group,
University of Ottawa, The Ottawa Hospital—General Campus, 501 Smyth Road,
Ottawa, ON K1H 8L6, Canada*

In September 1985, Eric Mühe performed the first human laparoscopic cholecystectomy [1]. As is often the case, this revolutionary technique was not readily embraced by the surgical community; however, by 1989, Reddick and Olsen [2] had reported their own experience with the procedure, which would soon become the standard of care for patients with cholelithiasis. By 1992, the early success of minimally invasive surgery of the gallbladder had spread to include a number of first publications on laparoscopic splenectomy, Nissen fundoplication, adrenalectomy, nephrectomy, and appendectomy. Similarly, reports of laparoscopic colon surgery were published in 1991 [3,4], introducing a promising technique for the management of some of the most common abdominal pathologies. Nevertheless, minimally invasive surgical techniques for the colon have not enjoyed as rapid a rise in popularity as many other laparoscopic procedures have throughout the 1990s. Several factors account for this difference, including a steep learning curve for the surgeon, the need for laparoscopic intra-abdominal vascular control, the time required to perform the procedure, the need for larger incisions to retrieve specimens, and concerns over the oncologic safety of the procedure in malignant disease [5]. In this article, we review the current state of laparoscopic colon surgery, focusing on the evidence surrounding its use in malignant and benign disease, and addressing advantages, disadvantages, and common controversies. Finally, we explore several recent technological advances facilitating laparoscopic colon surgery, including hand-assist technologies, hemostatic devices, and new laparoscopic imaging systems.

---

* Corresponding author.
E-mail address: rboushey@ottawahospital.on.ca (R.P. Boushey).

0039-6109/06/$ - see front matter © 2006 Elsevier Inc. All rights reserved.
doi:10.1016/j.suc.2006.05.006   *surgical.theclinics.com*

Laparoscopic surgery for malignant disease

Port site metastases

In 1993, Alexander and colleagues [6] reported a case of wound recurrence at 3 months following a laparoscopically-assisted right hemicolectomy in a 67-year-old woman who had Dukes' C adenocarcinoma. In a similar fashion, O'Rourke and coworkers [7] described port site recurrences merely 10 weeks following resection of a Dukes' B adenocarcinoma with intent to cure. Overall, greater than 35 cases of port site metastases associated with laparoscopic colon cancer resection were published within a 2-year span of this initial report, including both limited and advanced primary lesions [8]. The true incidence of port site recurrences was unknown at the time, leading Wexner and Cohen [9] to report a series incidence of 6.3% (range 1.5%–21%) among all published cases up to 1995. These data stand in sharp contrast with rates of wound recurrences in colon resections performed via traditional laparotomy. Indeed, a retrospective series by Hughes and colleagues [10] found a rate of 0.81% (CI 0.43%–1.38%) among 1603 patients undergoing traditional open resection between 1950 and 1980, whereas Reilly and coworkers [11] found only 11 cases among 1711 reviewed patients (0.64%, CI 0.32%–1.15%) from 1986 to 1989. Thus, when compared with rates of wound metastases in open resections, early data did seem to indicate that laparoscopic management of colon malignancies compromised oncologic safety, despite the poor quality of the evidence available at the time.

In response to these concerns, the American Society of Colon and Rectal Surgeons recommended that laparoscopic colon resections for malignant disease be limited to formal prospective data collection [12]. The data obtained from these studies were most helpful in determining the true incidence of port site recurrences in minimally invasive colon surgery. In a critical review of the literature from 2001, Zmora and colleagues [8] analyzed a total of 16 series of laparoscopic colorectal resections for carcinoma published between 1993 and 2000, each comprising greater than 50 patients, and found an incidence of port site metastases of less than 1% among 1737 patients. Using a similar methodology, Allardyce [13] found an incidence of 0.85% (CI 0.14%–1.18%) among 1769 patients. More recently, data from well-designed, randomized controlled trials have provided definitive evidence against a higher incidence of port site metastases in laparoscopic colon surgery compared with traditional resection (Table 1). The Clinical Outcomes of Surgical Therapy (COST) study [14], in which 872 patients were randomized to laparoscopically assisted or open colectomy for cancer, reported only two such patients (0.5%) who had wound recurrences within the laparoscopic arm, compared with one for the open arm (0.2%, $P = 0.50$) after a median follow-up of 4.4 years. Similarly, Lacy and colleagues [15] found a single case of port site recurrence within their laparoscopic surgery group (n = 106) and none within their open group (n = 102) after a median follow-up of

Table 1
Major randomized controlled trials comparing laparoscopic and open surgery for colon cancer

Authors/studies	Year	No. patients (lap/open)	No. centers	Disease site	Conversion rate	Port site metastases	Outcomes	Follow-up
COLOR [22,38]	2005	627/621	Multi (29)	C	19%	-	Short-term, costs	-
Guillou et al [23]	2005	526/268	Multi (27)	C, R	29%	-	Short-term, QoL	-
COST [14,33,55]	2004	435/437	Multi (48)	C	21%	0.5%	Short-term, long-term, QoL, costs	4.4 years
Leung et al [50]	2004	203/200	Single	R, S	23%	0%	Short-term, long-term, costs	4.4 years
Kaiser et al [18]	2004	29/20	Single	C	45%	0%	Short-term, long-term	2.9 years
Hasegawa et al [32]	2003	29/30	Single	C, R	17%	0%	Short-term, immunology	1.7 year
Lacy et al [15]	2002	111/108	Single	C	11%	0.94%	Short-term, long-term	3.6 years
Braga et al [122]	2002	136/133	Single	C, R	5%	0%	Short-term, costs, immunology	1.0 year
Tang et al [123]	2001	118/118	Single	C, R	13%	-	Immunology	-
Curet et al [17]	2000	25/18	Single	C, R	28%	0%	Short-term, long-term	4.9 years
Milsom et al [16]	1998	55/54	Single	C, R	-	0%	Short-term	1.5 years
Schwenk et al [27,31]	1998	30/30	Single	C, R	-	-	Short-term	-
Stage et al [29]	1997	18/16	Single	C	17%	0%	Short-term, immunology	1.2 years

Abbreviations: C, colon, excluding transverse; Multi, multi-center trial; QoL, quality of life; R, rectum; S, sigmoid colon; Single, single-center trial.

43 months. Three additional smaller prospective trials comprising a total of 201 patients randomized between laparoscopic-assisted and open resection for colon cancer found no additional case of port site or wound tumor recurrence [16–18]. As such, the evidence to date indicates that patients undergoing laparoscopic resection of colon malignancies are at no increased risk of port site metastases compared with those undergoing open surgery. It appears that early reports of high rates of port site recurrences were in fact related to surgeon inexperience, and inappropriate handling of the tumor laparoscopically [19].

Adequacy of oncologic resection

The goals of laparoscopic colectomy performed in the setting of colon cancer are the same as for open surgery. Those involve appropriate vessel ligation, adequate resection with 5 cm proximal and distal resection margins, and radical mesenteric lymphadenectomy. In addition, a thorough inspection of the abdominal cavity and liver surface is expected, together with the creation of a reliable anastomosis. Many of these elements have been evaluated in the context of clinical trials. Perhaps the most extensively studied factors have been the number of recovered lymph nodes within surgical specimens and the adequacy of resection margins. A recent meta-analysis [20] reviewed five randomized controlled trials reporting specifically on these issues, and found no significant difference between laparoscopic and open resection groups. Similarly, a Cochrane Collaboration review of 7 trials comprising 688 patients [21] found no difference in the total number of retrieved lymph nodes between the two groups ($P = 0.86$). Recent pathological data from large-scale, randomized controlled clinical studies further support these conclusions. Indeed, the European Colon Cancer Laparoscopic or Open Resection (COLOR) Study Group found identical rates of positive resection margins of 2% between their two groups ($P = 1.0$) [22], whereas the UK Medical Research Council trial of Conventional versus Laparoscopic-Assisted Surgery in Colorectal Cancer (MRC CLASICC) reported nonsignificant positive circumferential resection margins of 7% and 5% ($P = 0.45$) in laparoscopic-assisted and open resections, respectively [23]. In the COST study [14], the median number of recovered lymph nodes was 12 in both study arms, whereas longitudinal resection margins of less than 5 cm were present in only 5% and 6% of laparoscopic and open colectomies, respectively ($P = 0.52$). Despite the lack of good data on other elements of adequate oncologic surgery mentioned earlier, there appears to be no appreciable difference in the oncologic outcomes between laparoscopic and open colectomies for cancer.

Short-term outcomes

Much like other minimally invasive surgical procedures, laparoscopic colon surgery offers numerous short-term benefits, including reduced postoperative pain, potentially improved quality of life, shorter length of stay in hospital, quicker recovery of bowel function, and potentially, costs savings (see Table 1). These factors can be extremely advantageous for the patient, but must nonetheless be balanced against increased operating time required to perform these procedures. Although the mean increase in operating time seems to approach 1 hour in the literature [24], this value does appear to decrease significantly with surgeon experience [25].

Faster recovery of bowel function is one of the important potential benefits of laparoscopic colon surgery, because this often impacts on the duration of the postoperative hospital stay. Schwenk and colleagues [21] found that first passage of flatus was typically 1.0 day earlier in the laparoscopic colectomy group ($P<0.0001$), whereas passage of first bowel movement was 0.9 days earlier ($P<0.0001$). More recent randomized controlled trials also demonstrated a shorter recovery in bowel function, namely a report by Kaiser and coworkers [18], as well as the recent COLOR trial [22], both of which showed a significant decrease in time to first stool after laparoscopic colectomy. The major criticism associated with these studies is that examiners were not blinded with respect to the procedure performed, thus potentially allowing a positive discriminating bias in favor of patients treated laparoscopically. In addition, several studies failed to standardize the postoperative diet regimen, although Lacy and colleagues [15] used a strict protocol and demonstrated faster initiation of peristalsis and oral intake in patients undergoing laparoscopic colectomy. Despite these limitations inherent to nonblinded trials, objective evidence of improved peristalsis favoring laparoscopic colectomy has been published in the form of animal experiments [26], as well as clinical motility studies involving radio-opaque markers [27] and manometric recordings at the splenic flexure [28]. Thus, high-level evidence indicates that laparoscopic colectomy offers faster bowel function recovery than open surgery.

Numerous randomized controlled trials have demonstrated a significant reduction in pain or analgesic requirements in the immediate postoperative period [14,16,18,22,29–32]. In fact, data from the Cochrane Collaboration meta-analysis by Schwenk and colleagues [21] supports a difference in pain perception limited to the first ($P<0.0001$) and third ($P = 0.0002$) postoperative days, with no statistically significant difference found on postoperative day 2 ($P = 0.16$). In another meta-analysis, Abraham and coworkers [20] found significant advantages for the laparoscopic colectomy group in pain levels at rest and during coughing, from 6 to 8 hours until 3 days postoperatively. More recently, data from the COST study [14] showed that patients treated with laparoscopic colectomy required on average fewer days of both parenteral narcotics (3 versus 4 days, $P<0.001$) and oral analgesics (1 versus 2 days, $P = 0.02$), when compared with open resection. Similarly, short-term outcomes from the COLOR trial [22] showed a lower need for opioid analgesia on postoperative days 2 and 3, as well as a lower need for nonopioid analgesia on postoperative day 1 within the laparoscopy group. When compared with postoperative pain indices, results from quality of life surveys have been less impressive in demonstrating a difference between patients treated by laparoscopic versus open colon resection. In an interim analysis of the COST trial, Weeks and colleagues [33] administered three different quality of life assessment scales to patients randomized to either laparoscopic-assisted (n = 228) or open colectomy (n = 221). Although the authors did show a significant difference in the number of days of oral and parenteral analgesia requirements, they did not find any significant differences in quality of life indices at 2 days, 2 weeks, and 2 months postoperatively, except for the global rating scale at 2 weeks in favor of the laparoscopic group. Similarly, the authors of the MRC CLASICC trial [23] administered the QLQ-C30 and QLQ-CR38 quality of life questionnaires to patients randomized to laparoscopic-assisted (n = 526) or open surgery (n = 268) for colon cancer. They found very little difference between the two treatment arms at 2 weeks and 3 months follow-up, with most instruments showing equally worse quality of life at 2 weeks, with a return to baseline at 3 months. Despite these disappointing results, it should be noted that the quality of life instruments used in the COST and MRC CLASICC trials were not designed to assess acute to subacute postoperative patients who have potentially curable cancers. Although convenient because of their established validity, all but one of the questionnaires used were taken from the oncology literature, focusing heavily on chronic pain issues. Thus it is possible that meaningful quality of life differences between the two groups may have been missed because of the lack of a more sensitive and appropriate instrument. Therefore, based on the literature available thus far, the superiority of laparoscopic surgery in reducing immediate postoperative pain following colon resection seems evident. On the other hand, short- to medium-term quality of life indices assessed in two randomized controlled trials do not appear to improve with laparoscopic surgery, warranting further investigation using quality of life instruments dedicated for colon cancer surgery.

Length of hospital stay following colorectal surgery is often dependent upon bowel function recovery and the severity of postoperative pain. With the exception of one study [16], all reported randomized studies thus far have shown a shorter length of stay in hospital with laparoscopic colon resection compared with open surgery, with a wide variability in total length of stay between centers [14,15,17,18,22,23,29,31–33]. Although none of these studies were blinded to the treating surgical team, it is unlikely that this overwhelming trend in the literature is the result of an early discharge selection bias in favor of patients treated laparoscopically. A more recent meta-analysis [21] found that the length of stay in hospital was indeed 1.5 days shorter in the laparoscopic group (CI -1.94 to -1.12, $P < 0.0001$). It should be noted that patients whose laparoscopic procedure was converted to open had in fact a longer length of stay than those who had conventional open resections, highlighting the importance of identifying this subgroup of patients preoperatively [23]. Nevertheless, there is high-level evidence indicating that laparoscopy for colon cancer is associated with a shorter stay in hospital compared with laparotomy.

Costs

Direct costs following laparoscopic surgery for colon cancer are generally assumed to be higher than those incurred with equivalent open procedures; however, certain authors have argued that total costs to society may actually be lower for patients receiving laparoscopic surgery, given the improved short-term and potential long-term outcomes associated with the minimally invasive approach. A number of early publications limited to malignant disease have found conflicting data, with all papers reporting higher or similar costs associated with laparoscopic colon resection [34–36]. One of these studies by Philipson and colleagues [35] retrospectively assessed 61 consecutive patients who had undergone either laparoscopic-assisted (n = 28) or open (n = 33) right hemicolectomy for adenocarcinoma. By breaking down total incurred expenditures into direct (operating room, recovery, ward, intensive care unit) and indirect (hospital overhead) costs, but excluding any preoperative or postdischarge expenses, the authors reported a total of $9064 for laparoscopic-assisted procedures versus $7881 for open hemicolectomy ($P<0.001$). It is important to note that this study has significant limitations, including its retrospective nature and the lack of data regarding postdischarge societal costs, which one would predict to be lower in the laparoscopic surgery group. In addition, this report is one of only a handful that failed to show a shorter length of stay in hospital with a laparoscopic approach, a fact which could have substantially increased the hospital costs associated with this group. On the other hand, another retrospective study by Khalili and colleagues [36] reported no significant difference in total costs between the procedures ($P = 0.48$), despite higher operating room costs in the laparoscopic group. More recently, data from a case-controlled series of 150 laparoscopic and 150 open colorectal procedures [37] demonstrated higher operating room expenses associated with laparoscopy. The total direct costs were significantly lower in this same group, however, owing to shorter stay in hospital and lower pharmacy, laboratory, and nursing expenditures. The only costs data available from high-quality, randomized controlled trials have recently been reported in two separate studies. The first one [38], an interim analysis of the European COLOR study, compared 98 cases of laparoscopic colectomy for cancer compared with 112 open cases. In the context of a significantly longer operating room time in the laparoscopic group and a similar length of stay in hospital, Janson and co-workers found significantly higher total primary operation costs (€3493 versus €2322, $P<0.001$) and total cost of first admission (€6931 versus €5375, $P = 0.015$) in the laparoscopic colectomy group compared with the open group; however, productivity loss was greater in the open group (€2579 versus €2181), yielding no statistically significant difference in total costs between the two groups (€11,660 versus €9814, $P = 0.104$) [38]. On the other hand, the second major trial [39] assessed 512 patients randomized to laparoscopic versus open colectomy for colorectal cancer. The authors reported net extra costs per patient of €125 within the laparoscopic group, related to €1171 in additional operating costs, and savings of €1046 in postoperative complications [39]. Therefore, the data available in the literature do not provide adequate evidence on whether total costs significantly differ between laparoscopy and conventional open surgery in the treatment of colonic malignancy. It appears that costs may differ significantly, depending on health care systems and local practices.

Long-term outcomes

Long-term outcomes following laparoscopic resection for colon cancer—namely tumor recurrence, disease-free survival, and overall survival—are much more challenging to assess than short-term outcomes. Since the inception of minimally invasive techniques for resecting colon cancer, a number of prospective and retrospective case series [40–46], cohort studies [47–49], and randomized controlled trials [18,50] have provided low- to moderate-quality evidence regarding the equivalency of laparoscopic and open colonic resections. The vast majority of comparative studies published thus far have found no significant difference in long-term outcomes between laparoscopic and open resections, and case series have found recurrence and survival data that measure up favorably with accepted rates for traditional colon resections.

In 2002, Lacy and colleagues [15] published one of the first landmark randomized controlled trials comparing laparoscopic-assisted (n = 105) and open resection (n = 101) for colon cancer. The study authors reported tumor recurrence rates of 17% and 27% respectively, with a nonsignificant trend favoring laparoscopic resection ($P = 0.07$). Similarly, based on an intention-to-treat analysis, the overall mortality rates were not significantly different between the laparoscopic and open resection groups (18% versus 26%, $P = 0.14$), but the rates of cancer-related mortality favored the laparoscopic group (9% versus 21%, $P = 0.03$). When analyzed by procedure actually performed, the differences in rates of tumor recurrence, overall mortality, and cancer-related mortality, all became strongly statistically significant in favor of the laparoscopic approach. Interestingly, by analyzing patients based on cancer staging, the Lacy group demonstrated that the overall advantages found with the laparoscopic approach were attributable to a subgroup of patients who had locally-advanced Stage III disease [15]. Indeed, these data by Lacy and coworkers seem to suggest that laparoscopic resections may provide a potential survival advantage for Stage III colon cancer. The mechanism behind these data is speculative at best, but may be related to alterations in immune function with laparoscopy. At least one other large case series has described a similar survival advantage in locally-advanced disease [51]. Although very interesting and provocative, these results have yet to be replicated in other large-scale randomized studies.

Despite Lacy's report, laparoscopic surgery for malignant disease of the colon has only recently become an acceptable routine procedure, following the publication of long-term outcomes data from the COST study [14]. As stated earlier, this multicenter trial randomized 435 patients to laparoscopic-assisted colectomy and 428 patients to undergo traditional open colectomy. The surgeons participating in this study were required to meet strict adherence criteria, providing video evidence of proficiency in laparoscopic colon surgery. Despite this safeguard mechanism, the conversion rate in this study was 21%. After a median follow-up of 4.4 years, the study authors reported tumor recurrence in 76 and 84 patients ($P = 0.32$) within the laparoscopic and open groups, respectively, with no significant difference noted for time to recurrence and at different stages of disease. Similarly, the 3-year survival rate was 86% for the laparoscopic-assisted group and 85% for the open group ($P = 0.51$), with comparable disease-free survival rates ($P = 0.70$). It is fair to say that the COST study group demonstrated that laparoscopic colectomy for curable cancer is safe and at least equivalent to open resection in experienced hands [14]. The implications of the COST trial results have been far-reaching, including endorsement by American Society of Colon & Rectal Surgeons in a recent position statement [52]. It should be noted that long-term outcomes data from the European COLOR and MRC CLASICC trials had yet to be published at the time of manuscript preparation.

Finally, the issue of conversion to open surgery after attempting laparoscopic resection for colon cancer should be discussed briefly. Indeed, data exist in the literature indicating that patients undergoing attempted laparoscopic resection who are subsequently converted to traditional laparotomy fare substantially worse than either open procedures or laparoscopic resections, both with respect to short- and long-term outcomes. A recent report by Moloo and colleagues [53] reviewing 377 consecutive cases of laparoscopic resections for colorectal cancer described a significantly lower overall 2-year survival rate among converted patients who had curable Stage I through III malignancies, compared with those who had their colectomy completed laparoscopically (75.7% versus 87.2%, $P = 0.0201$). Similarly, recently published short-term data from the multicenter MRC CLASICC trial [23] revealed that converted patients had significantly higher postoperative complication rates, in-hospital mortality, transfusion requirements, and proportion of Dukes' C2 cancers than did completed patients. It is unclear whether these surprising outcomes were the result of an active learning curve documented by the authors throughout this study, or whether this represents a true unexpected outcome. Adverse outcomes associated with conversion have been examined by several additional groups, including a recent report by Casillas and coworkers [54], who used a case-control strategy to evaluate 51 such converted cases. The authors of this report found no significant short-term outcome differences between their groups of converted and open control patients. Similarly, a recent post-hoc analysis by the COST trial study group [55] reported no significant difference in oncologic outcome after conversion to open surgery, both in terms of overall survival and disease-free survival at 3 years. Thus, although there appear to be conflicting results regarding short-term outcomes, long-term data from one important multicenter randomized trial do not appear to demonstrate any adverse oncologic outcome with conversion to open surgery [55]. Short- and long-term follow-up results from the COLOR and MRC CLASICC trials will have to be released before one can make any further conclusions.

Laparoscopic surgery for benign disease

Inflammatory bowel disease

It is known that patients suffering from inflammatory bowel diseases (IBD) have a high lifetime likelihood of requiring surgery. Specifically, patients who have Crohn's disease (CD) have an 80% overall chance, whereas patients suffering from ulcerative colitis (UC) have a 30% to 40% probability of requiring a colectomy [56]. Given their proportionally younger age and the risk of requiring multiple procedures, patients are increasingly seeking care from specialized colorectal centers offering laparoscopic treatment of IBD. Several short-term benefits similar to those described in colon cancer have been associated with laparoscopic surgery for IBD. In addition, theoretical long-term advantages include fewer adhesions formation, decreased rates of bowel obstruction, decreased likelihood of chronic pain, and decreased incidence of infertility or wound hernias [56,57].

In Crohn's disease involving the colon, the presence of inflammatory changes, thickened mesentery, skip lesions, and fistulas and abscesses makes the laparoscopic approach to surgery particularly challenging. Nevertheless, the indications for surgery remain the same as with open techniques. According to one review [57], up to three different minimally invasive procedures can be performed, including diagnostic laparoscopy, diversion procedures, and bowel resections, which can be approached using pure laparoscopic methods or hand-assisted techniques. Two randomized controlled trials have been published to date [58,59], with numerous small comparative case series [60–66], making it very difficult to assess the superiority of laparoscopic techniques when compared with conventional open outcomes (Table 2). In the first study, Milsom and colleagues [58] randomized 60 patients to elective laparoscopic-assisted (n = 31) or open (n = 29) ileocolic resection for CD. They reported a decreased incidence of minor complications favoring the laparoscopic group (four versus eight, $P < 0.05$), with a significantly faster return to preoperative pulmonary function within this same group (2.5 versus 3.5 days, $P = 0.03$). Interestingly, total morphine requirements and recovery of bowel function were not significantly different between the two groups, whereas operative time was significantly shorter within the open group (140 ± 45 versus 85 ± 21 minutes, $P<0.0001$). As expected, incision length was substantially shorter within the laparoscopic group (5.3 ± 1.6 versus 12.7 ± 5.5 cm, $P<0.0001$). Recently, a second trial by Maartense and coworkers [59] used a similar comparative strategy with 60 patients who had CD. They reported shorter hospital stays (5 versus 7 days, $P = 0.008$), lower 30-day postoperative morbidity rates (10% versus 30%, $P = 0.028$), and lower total costs over 3 months (€6412 versus €8196, $P = 0.042$) within the laparoscopic resection group. Interestingly, no significant quality of life difference was found between the two groups using the SF-36 Health Survey and the Gastro-Intestinal Quality of Life Index. Based on the data obtained from these two randomized controlled trials, it appears that laparoscopic ileocolic resection for CD is advantageous over open approaches, in addition to providing an apparent cosmetic benefit [67]. It should be noted that the short-term benefits of laparoscopic surgery for CD have also been supported by a recent meta-analysis on the topic [68]. Finally, long-term outcomes following laparoscopic ileocolic resection for CD have simply not been addressed in prospective trials. As such, proposed long-term benefits associated with the laparoscopic approach remain hypothetical, and should not form the basis for choosing this method over a traditional open approach.

The surgical management of UC by minimally invasive methods is complex, and has thus far been limited to highly experienced laparoscopic surgeons working in specialized centers. The three procedures currently performed are laparoscopic subtotal colectomy, total proctocolectomy, and restorative proctocolectomy [69]. As is the case in open surgery, these procedures require the mobilization of the entire colon, as well as the taking of several important vascular pedicles. This area of laparoscopic colon surgery has paralleled the development of operative experience within specialized colorectal centers, and has been facilitated by the evolution of laparoscopic technologies. Many early publications on the topic described significantly worse postoperative outcomes among UC patients treated laparoscopically compared with those receiving traditional open procedures [70], in addition to longer operative times of up to 8 hours [71]. More recently, however, data from case-controlled studies have demonstrated that patients undergoing laparoscopic surgery for UC had no worse outcomes than those receiving open procedures [72], despite operative times that have remained significantly longer in most series (see Table 2). In fact, many groups have documented shorter postoperative stays in hospital by approximately 1 day within their laparoscopic groups [72–74], in addition to superior body image data, and equivalent functional outcomes [74,75]. Larson and colleagues [75] have recently reported comparable functional outcomes at a median follow-up of 13 months, among patients who had undergone laparoscopic (n = 33) and open (n = 33) ileal pouch-anal

Table 2

Major studies of laparoscopic colon resection for benign disease

Authors	Year	Study type	No. patients (lap/open)	Disease site	Conversion rate	Comparative outcomes*
Crohn's disease						
Maartense et al [59]	2006	RCT	30/30	IC	10%	↑ OR time, ↓ hospital stay, ↓ morbidity, ↓ costs
Huilgol et al [66]	2004	CC	21/19	IC	5%	↓ time PO intake, ↓ bowel time, ↓ hospital stay
Msika et al [61]	2001	PNS	20/26	SB, IC, C	0%	↑ OR time, ↓ bowel time, ↓ hospital stay, ↓ complications, ↓ costs
Milsom et al [58]	2001	RCT	31/29	IC	6%	↑ OR time, ↓ pulmonary recovery time, ↓ complications
Ulcerative colitis						
Larson et al [75]	2005	CC	33/33	C	–	No difference in morbidity or functional outcomes
Dunker et al [74]	2001	CC	16/19	C	0%	↑ OR time, ↓ hospital stay, ↓ bowel time, ↑ body image
Hashimoto et al [73]	2001	RCS	11/13	C	0%	↑ OR time, ↓ blood loss, ↓ pain, ↓ hospital stay, ↑ cosmesis
Araki et al [124]	2001	RCS	21/11	C	–	↓ time PO intake, ↓ bowel time, ↑ cosmesis
Marcello et al [72]	2000	CC	20/20	C	0%	↑ OR time, ↓ bowel time, ↓ hospital stay

Diverticular disease						
Alves et al [80]	2005	PNS	163/169	15%	S	↑ OR time, ↓ blood loss, ↓ hospital stay, ↓ morbidity
Lawrence et al [79]	2003	RCS	56/215	7%	S	↑ OR time, ↓ hospital stay, ↓ complications, ↓ costs
Dwivedi et al [78]	2002	RCS	66/88	20%	S	↑ OR time, ↓ blood loss, ↓ hospital stay, ↓ time PO intake, ↓ costs
Senagore et al [77]	2002	PNS	61/71	7%	S	↓ hospital stay, ↓ complications, ↓ costs

Abbreviations: CC, case controlled study; IC, ileocolic; OR, operating room; PNS, prospective non-randomized study; RCS, retrospective case series; RCT, randomized controlled trial; SB, small bowel; ↑, increased; ↓, decreased.

* Outcome results are pertaining to the laparoscopic group, relative to the comparison group; non-statistically significant results are omitted.

anastomosis for UC or familial adenomatous polyposis. Despite numerous reports highlighting the safety and feasibility of laparoscopic surgery for UC among expert hands, no comparative randomized trial with open surgery has yet been completed. The current level of evidence in the literature is thus insufficient to conclude the superiority of one approach over another. Nevertheless, it is likely that the minimally invasive approach will continue to gain in popularity among expert laparoscopists, given its clear cosmetic advantages and potentially improved short-term outcomes.

Diverticular disease

In recent years, laparoscopic resection methods have been successfully applied to diverticulitis of the sigmoid colon [76]. Good data exist from a number of nonrandomized studies highlighting the advantages of laparoscopic sigmoid resection in uncomplicated diverticular disease (see Table 2). These benefits include most of the advantageous short-term outcomes associated with laparoscopic colon surgery, and also include decreased postoperative wound and pulmonary complications, as well as lower direct costs [77–79]. Recently, Alves and coworkers [80] published the results of a prospective national study involving 332 consecutive patients undergoing laparoscopic (n = 163) or open (n = 169) elective sigmoid resection for diverticular disease. They reported significantly higher overall morbidity rates within the open group (16.0% versus 31.4%, $P<0.001$), including higher wound complications, abscesses, and fistulas, as well as significantly longer lengths of stay in hospital within this same group. Although this study suffered from a significant patient selection bias associated with its lack of randomization, the study authors did determine that open colectomy was an independent risk factor for morbidity, using a multiple logistic regression analysis model. Therefore, despite the lack of large randomized trials comparing open and laparoscopic sigmoid colectomy for diverticulitis, good evidence exists supporting the use of laparoscopy for elective resections, based on improved short-term outcomes [76]. One should keep in mind, however, that this conclusion does not necessarily hold true for complicated diverticular disease. Some groups have shown significant increases in morbidity and conversion rates associated with laparoscopic resection of complicated diverticulitis [81]. It is recommended that such resections be performed by experienced laparoscopists.

Emerging techniques and technologies

Since the early days of laparoscopic colon surgery, techniques and technologies have evolved to render this procedure more amenable to routine use by general surgeons. Putting aside issues of oncologic safety and outcome equivalency between laparoscopic and open colorectal procedures, it remains that laparoscopic-assisted colectomy is a difficult technique to adopt for surgeons without advanced minimally invasive surgical training. Conversion rates as high as 29% have been described [23], highlighting the steep learning curve associated with this procedure. Many new techniques and technologies have emerged in an attempt to flatten this learning curve, in part by relying upon skills surgeons have acquired in open surgery.

Hand-assist devices

Simply stated, hand-assisted laparoscopic surgery (HALS) involves the insertion of a hand inside the abdomen during a laparoscopic procedure, while maintaining pneumoperitoneum, to facilitate the procedure. The potential clinical benefits of hand-assist technology in laparoscopic colon surgery are significant. They include the restoration of tactile sensation and proprioception, the ability to perform blunt dissection, the ability to retract organs atraumatically, the ability to apply immediate hemostatic pressure, and a potential reduction in the total number of ports required during surgery. In cases of resection for malignancy, hand-assist devices restore the surgeon's ability to palpate the tumor. In short, hand-assist devices have the potential to provide the operating surgeon with many of the technical advantages of open surgery, while maintaining the short-term benefits of minimally invasive surgery.

Since the early days of laparoscopic colon resections, attempts have been made at inserting a hand inside the abdomen to help with the procedure. The evolution of hand-assisted laparoscopic surgery has paralleled the evolution of technologies to maintain pneumoperitoneum, while allowing for convenient access to the abdomen by a hand or laparoscopic instruments [82]. In 1995, Ou [83] first reported his experience with the hand-assisted technique, whereby he inserted his hand in the peritoneal cavity using a 5 to 6 cm incision and maintained pneumoperitoneum with two stay stitches to tighten the fascia around his hand. Comparing two cohorts of 12 patients each undergoing hand-assisted laparoscopic or open colectomy, Ou reported shorter lengths of stay in hospital for the hand-assisted group (5.6 versus 8.3 days), despite slightly longer total operating time (135 versus 100 minutes). Other groups have also reported their own uncontrolled case series, emphasizing short stays in hospital and the lack of conversion to open resection [84,85].

Based on these early results, a number of hand-access devices have been marketed to facilitate hand-assistance in minimally invasive surgery. So-called "first generation devices" were all built in a similar fashion, including a type of sleeve secured between the abdominal wall and the surgeon's forearm to prevent leakage of carbon dioxide, as well as a circular base designed to adapt to the contour of the abdominal wound [82]. These devices include the Dexterity Pneumo Sleeve (Dexterity Surgical, San Antonio, Texas), Intromit (Applied Medical, Rancho Santa Margarita, California), Handport (Smith & Nephew Endoscopy, Andover, Massachusetts), and Omniport (Advanced Surgical Concepts, Bray, Ireland). These initial designs all suffered from similar problems, including hand fatigue for the operating surgeon and regular leakage of pneumoperitoneum in as many as 41% to 48% of cases [86,87]. The latter problem specifically resulted in conversion to open surgery in 14% of reported cases in one series [86]. More recently, sleeveless hand-port technology has been introduced on the market, including the Gelport (Applied Medical, Rancho Santa Margarita, California) and LapDisc (Ethicon Endosurgery, Cincinnati, Ohio) devices. These second-generation designs include a wound-contouring system that maintains the system in place, in addition to a reliable lock-on gel or disclike cover top that seals the device shut [82]. Effectively, the self-sealing nature of these new constructs provides a functional "port" into the abdomen, allowing the surgeon to insert or withdraw a hand at will. In addition, this property permits the use of laparoscopy trocars, cameras, or instruments, thus maximizing the utility of this port and minimizing the need for additional port sites on the abdominal wall.

Data regarding the validity of HALS in colon surgery now exists in the form of several case series, as well as an increasing number of randomized controlled trials (Table 3). In 1999, the Southern Surgeons' Club Study Group [86] published results of their multicenter prospective study involving 58 patients who underwent HALS, of whom 22 had mixed colon procedures. The average operating time for this subgroup was 157 minutes (94–240 minutes), with a mean length of stay in hospital of 6.4 days. Both figures compare favorably with previously published data from large trials of laparoscopic colectomy [14,22]. In another randomized controlled trial comparing hand-assisted (n = 22) versus standard laparoscopic (n = 18) colorectal resections for a variety of benign conditions and incurable malignancy, the HALS Study Group reported slightly shorter, albeit nonsignificant, operative time for the laparoscopic surgery group (152 ± 66 versus 141 ± 54 minutes, $P = 0.58$) [87]. After removing seven cases of conversion to open surgery from the analysis, operative time became somewhat more favorable for the hand-assisted group (144 versus 152 minutes, $P = 0.70$). Lengths of incision, number of cases converted to open, and stay in hospital were all similar between the two study groups. In another study, Targarona and colleagues [88] randomized 54 patients who had diagnoses of cancer, polyps, or volvulus to hand-assisted or laparoscopic colectomy. Although this group reported similar total anesthetic times, it did find higher conversion rates among laparoscopic patients (7% versus 22%), leading surgeons to find a clear subjective advantage for the hand-assisted procedure in 13 of 54 cases. The authors of this study found no significant difference in length of stay in hospital, requirements for analgesia, overall morbidity rate, oncological features, or costs of the procedures. Although not performed on an intention-to-treat basis, an analysis of interleukin-6 and C-reactive protein inflammatory markers revealed a significantly higher postoperative increase in the hand-assisted colectomy group, highlighting the greater tissue trauma generated by this procedure compared with simple laparoscopy [88].

Table 3
Major studies of hand-assisted laparoscopic surgery in colonic resections

Authors/studies	Year	Study type	Comparison groups	No. patients	Diseases	Comparative outcomes*
Segmental resections						
Chang et al [89]	2005	PNS	HALS versus LAP	66/85	B, M, P	↓ OR time ($P = 0.07$), ↑ incision, ↓ conversion
Kang et al [90]	2004	RCT	HALS versus OPS	30/30	B, M, P	↓ incision, ↓ analgesia, ↓ blood loss, ↓ bowel time
Targarona et al [88]	2002	RCT	HALS versus LAP	27/27	B, M, P	↓ conversion, ↑ inflammation
HALS Study Group [87]	2000	RCT	HALS versus LAP	22/18	B, I, P	Comparable results
Southern Surgeons' Club [86]	1999	PNS	HALS	24	B, M, P	N/A
Total abdominal colectomy/total proctocolectomy						
Maartense et al [94]	2004	RCT	HALS versus OPS	30/30	B	↑ OR time
Rivadeneira et al [92]	2004	RCT	HALS versus LAP	10/13	B	↓ OR time, ↓ bowel time
Nakajima et al [93]	2004	RCS	HALS versus LAP	12/11	B	↓ OR time, ↓ number of trocars

Abbreviations: B, benign; HALS, hand-assisted laparoscopic surgery; I, incurable malignant; LAP, laparoscopic surgery; M, malignant; OPS, open surgery; P, polyps; PNS, prospective non-randomized study.
* Outcome results are pertaining to HALS, relative to the comparison group; non-statistically significant results are omitted.

Though interesting, these data did not appear to influence the immediate postoperative clinical outcome.

More recently, Chang and coworkers [89] reported the results of a larger cohort study in which they compared 66 patients undergoing hand-assisted segmental resections with 85 undergoing standard laparoscopic colectomy. Both groups were well-matched in terms of demographics and diagnosis. The authors found a trend toward shorter average operative time in the hand-assisted group (189 versus 205 minutes, $P = 0.07$), with a significantly decreased need for conversion to open surgery in this same group (0% versus 13%, $P<0.01$). No differences were noted in any of the standard postoperative variables. Interestingly, the authors noted that despite the advantageous conversion data and equivalent postoperative results, proportionally more hand-assisted resections were performed by surgeons with limited minimally invasive surgery experience compared with the laparoscopic colectomy group (27% versus 16%, $P<0.05$), highlighting the potential value of this technology in training laparoscopic surgeons. In another recent study, Kang and colleagues [90] randomized 60 patients to undergo either hand-assisted laparoscopic colectomies or traditional open resections. To the authors' knowledge, this report is the only randomized-controlled trial to date comparing HALS and open surgery for segmental colon resections. Whereas reported operating times were similar between the two groups, the study authors reported significantly less blood loss (193 ± 85 cc versus 343 ± 143 cc, $P<0.001$), and shorter incision length (7.17 ± 0.38 cm versus 13.73 ± 1.87 cm, $P<0.001$) with the HALS procedure compared with open resections. They commented that the favorable operative time obtained in the hand-assisted group may have been related to the use of new dissection technologies. Similarly, time to oral intake, time to passage of flatus and stool, use of analgesia, and length of hospital stay were all significantly better in the hand-assisted group compared with the laparotomy group. Finally, pain scores were significantly lower on postoperative days 1, 3, and 14, but were equivalent on day 30 [90]. Overall, the data presented by Chang and colleagues and by Kang and coworkers indicate that hand-assisted laparoscopic techniques may be equivalent to standard laparoscopy for segmental resections of the colon in terms of short-term outcomes. Data from larger randomized-controlled trials will be necessary to confirm this statement. Given that most general surgeons perform only a few colon resections each year [91], it is likely that modern sleeveless handport devices will be helpful in flattening the learning curve associated with laparoscopic colon surgery, and will help in bridging the transition between the purely open and minimally invasive approaches.

Hand-assisted technologies were also recently studied in the context of highly complex colorectal procedures, such as total proctocolectomy with ileal pouch-anal anastomosis or total abdominal colectomy. Given the extent of the colonic and rectal dissections involved in these cases, it is logical to consider these procedures separately from simple segmental resections of the colon. Rivadeneira and colleagues [92] compared two series of patients who had undergone hand-assisted (n = 10) or standard laparoscopic (n = 13) restorative proctocolectomy for UC or familiar adenomatous polyposis using a prospective database. Interestingly, the study authors found no difference in incision size or length of stay in hospital between the two approaches, but did appreciate a small difference in operative time favoring the hand-assisted group (247 [210–390] versus 300 [240–400] minutes, $P<0.01$). In another retrospective study, Nakajima and coworkers [93] reported similar results, including shorter operative time in hand-assisted total colectomy, but otherwise equivalent intra- and postoperative courses. Although these two studies seem to indicate that total colectomy is easier to perform using hand-assist devices than standard laparoscopy, both suffer from very small sample sizes and retrospective methodologies. As such, a recent randomized controlled trial performed by Maartense and colleagues [94] is particularly interesting. In this study, the authors compared patients undergoing hand-assisted laparoscopic (n = 30) versus open (n = 30) total proctocolectomy with ileal pouch anal anastomosis. They found no difference in postoperative pain, morphine requirements, time to recovery of bowel function, length of stay in hospital, or quality of life between the two groups. The only significant results were related to increased operative time and costs associated with the hand-assisted laparoscopic procedure. It should be noted that the authors used relatively rigid postoperative care protocols, which may have skewed the results in favor of the open approach.

New dissection technologies

Obtaining reliable hemostatic control in mesocolic or mesorectal dissection is not always straightforward, particularly when inflammatory processes such as diverticulitis, or inflammatory bowel disease are present [95]. As such, a number of different methods have been used for hemostatic control, including monopolar and bipolar coagulation, clips, staples, sutures, and ultrasonic dissection. In this section, we review the use and role of two such relatively novel technologies: the high-frequency ultrasonic scalpel and the electrothermal bipolar vessel sealer.

The ultrasonic scalpel was first introduced for laparoscopic use by Amaral in 1994 [96]. Today, three different models of ultrasonically-activated scalpels exist on the market: Harmonic Scalpel/UltraCision (Ethicon Endosurgery, Cincinnati, Ohio), AutoSonix (United States Surgical, Norwalk, Connecticut), and SonoSurg (Olympus Surgical, Orangeburg, New York). These instruments consist of laparoscopic shears that are induced to vibrate at a frequency of 23.5 to 55.5 kHz using a piezoelectric transducer over a 80 to 200 μm arc at the functional tip. This high-frequency vibration is said to achieve hemostasis at low temperatures (50°C–100°C) by denaturing proteins, thus producing a sticky coagulum that effectively seals blood vessels up to 5 mm in diameter [97]. It should be noted that this proposed mechanism of action was challenged in a recent experimental study by Foschi and colleagues [98]. In contrast to ultrasonic dissection, traditional electrosurgery uses much higher temperatures ($150°C$–$400°C$) to rapidly desiccate and char tissues, resulting in eschar formation that seals the bleeding area. Based on these differences, several advantages favoring ultrasonic technology have been proposed, including the ability to coagulate in close proximity to other structures, given the theoretical lack of thermal damage to adjacent tissues, the absence of charring, the absence of smoke, and the ability to use the ultrasonic scalpel for dissection, cutting, grasping, and tissue coagulation, thus saving valuable operative time [97]. Potential limitations of this technology include high costs, the limited availability of reusable shears (both Harmonic Scalpel and AutoSonix are disposable), possible coagulation failure caused by inadequate power application or grip strength, and the creation of a vapor mist that has the potential to contain viable cells [97].

Despite the theoretical benefits of ultrasonic dissection, care must be taken given the data obtained by Emam and Cuschieri in a porcine model [99]. Indeed, they demonstrated histologically that despite the lack of macroscopic damage, ultrasonic dissection of the colon at power level 5 for more than 10 seconds caused partial- to full-thickness injury to the adjacent ureters, in the context of a large zone of significant hyperthermia surrounding the instrument. Nevertheless, the study authors found nonsignificant changes surrounding the dissection when they limited their use of the ultrasonic scalpel to 5 second bursts at a power level of 3. Emam and Cuschieri thus recommend the use of level 4 power in short bursts of 5 seconds or less for routine dissection, and level 3 power in the presence of important surrounding structures [99]. The cost of this technology is another important issue. It has been addressed in two studies of laparoscopic hysterectomy and Nissen fundoplication, comparing the use of ultrasonic shears with endoscopic staplers and clip applicators, respectively [100,101]. In both instances, the study authors reported lower costs associated with ultrasonic dissection, given the need for additional stapler cartridges or clip applicators. Finally, the issue of potentially viable cellular debris within the vapor mist created by ultrasonic dissection should be addressed, because it is directly relevant to the routine use of this technology in colon cancer. In an experimental rat tumor model, Nduka and colleagues [102] demonstrated that despite the release of airborne cellular debris from ultrasonic dissection, no viable cells were present and no subsequent growth occurred in vitro.

Only limited clinical data exists regarding the safety and efficacy of ultrasonic dissection in laparoscopic colon resection. In one such study, Heili and coworkers [103] reviewed 85 patients undergoing laparoscopic-assisted right hemicolectomy or sigmoid resection using either traditional instruments or ultrasonic shears. They reported favorable operative times ($P = 0.1989$) and lengths of stay in hospital ($P = 0.0018$) for the ultrasonic dissection group. Similarly, a recent prospective series of 34 colorectal resections by Msika and colleagues [104] demonstrated the short-term safety of this instrument, with no reported bleeding complications. Moreover, they also argued in favor of a cost advantage for ultrasonic dissection in this setting, when compared with the use of an average 2.5 clip applicators in laparoscopic colorectal resections. The only randomized controlled trial available to date was published recently, comparing ultrasonic versus monopolar electric dissection in laparoscopic colorectal surgery [105]. In this study, 146 patients were randomized to ultrasonic dissection (n = 74) or monopolar electrosurgery (n = 72), with bipolar cautery used in both groups at the discretion of the operating surgeon. The study authors reported equivalent operative times, except for low anterior resections, for which ultrasonic dissection was significantly shorter (95.4 versus 115.6 minutes, $P = 0.01$), and reported significantly reduced overall intraoperative blood loss (140.79 versus 182.58 mL, $P = 0.032$). All other studied parameters were found to be equivalent between the two study groups, including operative complications, conversion rates, time to recovery of bowel function, stay in hospital, and postoperative complications. Nevertheless, the authors did report a very significant rate of conversion to ultrasonic dissection (20.8% or 15/72 patients) within the standard electrosurgery group. This conversion was based on the operating surgeon's judgment that ultrasonic dissection was essential to the safe completion of the procedure laparoscopically, and was more frequent during right hemicolectomy (26%) and low anterior resection (26%) [105]. Despite concerns raised by the authors of that report regarding the high costs of the technology, ultrasonic dissection appears to be valuable in complex laparoscopic colorectal resections, perhaps more so when issues of learning curves are taken into consideration. Further studies will be required to ascertain the true effectiveness of the ultrasonic scalpel over other hemostatic devices.

The electrothermal bipolar vessel sealer (LigaSure, Valleylab, Boulder, Colorado) is another relatively new hemostatic device in laparoscopic surgery. Its mechanism of action is entirely different from that of the ultrasonic scalpel, relying on high current (4 amps) and low voltage (<200 volts) to denature the collagen and elastin within vessel walls [106]. This reaction, combined with the high compression pressure of the instrument, effectively seals vessels up to 7 mm in diameter by rearranging the collagen and elastin across the collapsed vessel wall. Clinically, this process yields a translucent band of tissue that can then be cut using a second instrument, or using the internal blade of the laparoscopic LigaSure Atlas variant. In theory, this technology is thus particularly well-suited for laparoscopic colon resections, because it allows the operating surgeon to obtain hemostatic control over most if not all large arteries encountered during this procedure. This fact was confirmed in ex vivo experimental protocols using isolated abattoir porcine veins and arteries ranging in diameter from 1.0 to 7.0 mm [107]. In this study, the authors recorded acute burst pressures of 761 ± 221 mmHg for arteries 3.1 to 5.0 mm in diameter, and of 654 ± 227 mmHg for arteries of 5.1 to 7.0 mm in diameter. Despite three of eight failed seals within the 5.1 to 7.0 mm category, the overall probability of burst strengths being less than 400 mmHg for the electrothermal sealer was only 0.04 (0.00–0.13), compared with 0.95 (0.82–1.00) for the ultrasonic coagulator. In another experimental study by Harold and colleagues [108], the superiority of the electrothermal bipolar vessel sealer over the ultrasonic shears was specifically addressed using small-, medium-, and large-sized arteries harvested from freshly euthanized pigs. Although the recorded burst pressures were statistically comparable for vessels of 2 to 3 mm, the electrothermal bipolar sealer had significantly higher burst pressures for both vessels of 4 to 5 mm (601 versus 205 mmHg, $P<0.0001$) and 6 to 7 mm diameter (442 versus 174 mmHg, $P<0.0001$). Finally, the study authors reported no significant difference in histological thermal injury between the two dissection technologies, although the mean reported spread using the ultrasonic shears (2.18 mm) is almost one order of magnitude smaller than that published recently by Emam and Cuschieri [99]. This discrepancy is difficult to explain at this time, but it may be related to differences in methodology between these two studies.

To our knowledge, only five clinical studies have assessed the electrothermal bipolar vessel sealer in laparoscopic colon surgery [106,109–112]. An initial study by Heniford and colleagues comprising 18 cases of laparoscopic colon and small bowel resections among 98 major operations yielded a hemostatic failure rate of only 0.3% for vessels of 2 to 7 mm diameter, demonstrating the safety and effectiveness of this new technology for vascular pedicles of large sizes [106]. Three of the five studies mentioned above were retrospective in nature, and compared small series of restorative proctocolectomies [109], hand-assisted total colectomies [110], and sigmoid and transverse colectomies [111] done using either the electrothermal bipolar sealer or the ultrasonic dissector. In all three series, the electrothermal bipolar sealer was found to be slightly superior to the ultrasonic dissector in terms of decreased mean total operating time [109,110], decreased intraoperative blood loss [110], decreased costs [109], fewer episodes of rebleeding [111], and decreased time to dissect the mesocolon [111]. Finally, Marcello and colleagues [112] reported recently published data from the only prospective randomized clinical trial comparing the electrothermal bipolar sealer (n = 52) to conventional staplers and clips (n = 48) during elective laparoscopic right, left, and total colectomies. In their study, the authors reported a non-statistically significant reduction in mean operative time of 11 minutes in the electrothermal bipolar sealer group ($P = 0.44$), in addition to a difference in vascular pedicle ligation failure rate that was significantly higher in the clips and staples group (3% versus 9.2%, $P = 0.02$). Blood loss associated with device failure was somewhat lower within the clips and staples group, because a single case of major hemorrhage associated with inadequate sealing of the inferior mesenteric vein occurred within the electrothermal bipolar sealing group. Interestingly, the study authors also reported significantly lower operative costs associated with the use of the LigaSure Atlas device over laparoscopic clips and staples ($317 ± 0 versus $400 ± $112, $P<0.001$) [112]. As expected, this difference was more pronounced for total colectomies, for which six to nine major vascular pedicles must be divided using multiple stapler reloads and clip applicators. It should be kept in mind that purchase prices for such proprietary devices vary enormously across the United States, Canada, and Europe, thus altering the validity of cost-benefit calculations presented above based on practice location. In addition, the calculation would have easily favored the traditional approach had the authors decided to compare the device to laparoscopic clips, instead of clips and staples. That being said, the electrothermal bipolar vessel sealer represents an exciting new tool in laparoscopic colon surgery.

Advances in camera technologies

Improvements in laparoscopic cameras and video imaging systems have paralleled the development of minimally invasive surgery. Recently, important advances in laparoscopic camera technologies have dramatically improved the ease with which surgeons can perform advanced laparoscopic surgery, including colonic resections. One such innovation has been the introduction of charged coupled device (CCD) chip cameras [113], which have essentially replaced traditional tube laparoscopes. Simply put, CCD chips work by acquiring optical or analog images, and converting them into electronic or digital information, which can then be displayed on a monitor for the surgeon to see. The image resolution provided by CCD chips is directly related to a vertical and horizontal grid of sensor elements known as pixels situated on the chip, which provide resolutions of 450 to 600 horizontal lines [114]. Three-chip cameras have also been developed, which function by separating the image signal into red, blue, and green components, thus providing an improved resolution of 700 horizontal lines. These cameras tend to be slightly heavier and to lose their alignment over time due to repeated handling and sterilization, however; hence the potential for deterioration in resolution [114]. More recently, new "chip-on-a-stick" video laparoscopes have been introduced [113,114]. These new designs of laparoscopic cameras involve the placement of a single CCD chip at the tip (patient's side) of the laparoscope, immediately behind the lens. This system allows the immediate processing of the image by the chip, and in doing so, eliminates the bulky fiber-optic apparatus traditionally located within the shaft of the laparoscope. By transmitting the image via cables from the CCD chip at the tip of the laparoscope to a camera now located on the endoscopic cart, this system has several advantages, including improved image quality and resolution, reduced possibility of inadvertent camera damage, less cumbersome video cables, and potentially smaller laparoscope shaft diameter.

The traditional rigid surgical laparoscope is based upon the Hopkins rod-lens system. It is currently available in 0° forward-viewing and 30° forward-oblique-viewing designs [115]. Although the 0° scope provides greater direct illumination on the field of vision, the 30° scope is particularly well-suited for advanced laparoscopic surgery, because it allows the operator to visualize an object from all directions by rotating the shaft of the laparoscope. It should be noted though, that the 30° scope requires somewhat more user experience than its 0° counterpart, but this additional requirement is easily offset by the improved field of vision provided by this laparoscope. Given its clear advantages and similar costs, the 30° scope is used routinely at the authors' center for laparoscopic colon surgery, because it is most valuable for difficult pelvic dissections requiring different points of view. Nevertheless, the need for even greater control and improved visualization over the surgical field has also led to the introduction of flexible-tip laparoscopes [116]. These novel devices provide an observation range of 14 to 120 mm, a vertical motion ability of 100°, and a horizontal motion ability of 60° to 90°, depending on the manufacturer. As such, these laparoscopes allow for a field of view of 80° to 90°, compared with 75° for the 30° scope. In a recent study by Perrone and coworkers [117], two models of flexible-tip laparoscopes (Fujinon EL2-R310 and Olympus LTF-V3) were compared with 30° and 0° models in performing three experimental tasks. Although the study authors did show a significant difference in procedure time, accuracy, and subjective difficulty between the 0° and all three other types of laparoscopes, they did not find a significant improvement when comparing the 30° scope and flexible-tip laparoscopes. Although surprising, these data may be attributable to the simplicity of the in-vitro model used in this study. Indeed, it is likely that the flexible laparoscope would perform much better in the setting of complex colorectal dissections. Based on the current data, however, it appears that the 30° laparoscope provides excellent surgical field visualization at a lesser cost than the novel flexible-tip laparoscopes. Further head-to-head clinical studies will be required to ascertain the true value of these new technologies in colorectal surgery.

Another recent advancement in camera technology is the development of three-dimensional (3D) video imaging systems for minimally invasive surgery [118]. It is well known that the lack of depth perception in laparoscopic surgery has a direct influence on the steep learning curve associated with learning new laparoscopic skills, whether basic ones for the novice surgeon, or advanced ones for the more experienced laparoscopist. Indeed, experimental data have demonstrated that specific tasks such as laparoscopic suturing or knot tying can be performed faster and more accurately using a 3D video imaging system [119]. This system relies upon a stereoendoscope, which acquires the surgical image from two separate side-by-side lenses, yielding two offset images that can be visualized into a single 3D image using simple shutter glasses. Experimental data obtained using early 3D laparoscopes was not very promising, revealing that 3D imaging was both tiring and awkward to use for the surgeon, and provided no benefit over standard 2D laparoscopy [120]. Nevertheless, more recent data obtained from new second-generation 3D laparoscopes are much more encouraging. Taffinder and colleagues [121] showed that 3D imaging reduced the handicap associated with traditional 2D laparoscopy by as much as 41% to 53% for a variety of experimental tasks, both for novice and experienced laparoscopists. Although not currently widely used, this system may have the potential to reintroduce 3D vision and depth perception to minimally invasive surgery, which would be most useful in colonic resections. Further clinical data will be required before this experimental system can become more widely used in surgical practice.

Summary

Since its first described case in 1991, laparoscopic colon surgery has lagged behind minimally invasive surgical methods for solid intra-abdominal organs in terms of acceptability, dissemination, and ease of learning. In colon cancer, initial concerns over port site metastases and adequacy of oncologic resection have considerably dampened early enthusiasm for this procedure. Only recently, with the publication of several large, randomized controlled trials [14,15,22,23], has the incidence of port site metastases been shown to be equivalent to that of open resection. Laparoscopic surgery for colon cancer has also been demonstrated to be at least equivalent to traditional laparotomy in terms of adequacy of oncologic resection, disease recurrence, and long-term survival. In addition, numerous reports have validated short-term benefits following laparoscopic resection for cancer, including shorter hospital stay, shorter time to recovery of bowel function, and decreased analgesic requirements, as well as other postoperative variables. In benign colonic disease, much less high-quality literature exists supporting the use of laparoscopic methods. Two recent randomized controlled trials have demonstrated some short-term benefits to laparoscopic ileocolic resection for CD [58,59], in addition to evident cosmetic advantages. On the other hand, the current evidence on laparoscopic surgery for UC does not support its routine use among nonexpert surgeons outside of specialized centers. Laparoscopic colonic resection for diverticular disease appears to provide several short-term benefits, although these advantages may not translate to cases of complicated diverticulitis.

Despite the increasing acceptability of minimally invasive methods for the management of benign and malignant colonic pathologies, laparoscopic colon resection remains a prohibitively difficult technique to master. Numerous technological innovations have been introduced onto the market in an effort to decrease the steep learning curve associated with laparoscopic colon surgery. Good evidence exists supporting the use of second-generation, sleeveless, hand-assist devices in this context. Similarly, new hemostatic devices such as the ultrasonic scalpel and the electrothermal bipolar vessel sealer may be particularly helpful for extensive colonic mobilizations, in which several vascular pedicles must be taken. The precise role of these hemostatic technologies has yet to be established, particularly in comparison with stapling devices and significantly cheaper laparoscopic clips. Finally, recent advances in camera systems are promising to improve the ease with which difficult colonic dissections can be performed.

References

[1] Mühe E. Die erste: Cholecystecktomie durch das Laparoskop [The first laparoscopic cholecystectomy]. Langenbecks Arch Surg 1986;369:804.
[2] Reddick EJ, Olsen DO. Laparoscopic laser cholecystectomy: a comparison with mini-lap cholecystectomy. Surg Endosc 1989;3:131–3.
[3] Fowler DL, White A. Laparoscopy-assisted sigmoid resection. Surg Laparosc Endosc 1991;1:183–8.
[4] Jacobs M, Verdeja JC, Goldstein HS. Minimally invasive colon resection (laparoscopic colectomy). Surg Laparosc Endosc 1991;1:144–50.
[5] Lacy A. Colon cancer: laparoscopic resection. Ann Oncol 2005;16(Suppl 2):ii88–95.
[6] Alexander RJ, Jaques BC, Mitchell KG. Laparoscopically assisted colectomy and wound recurrence. Lancet 1993;341:249–50.
[7] O'Rourke N, Price PM, Kelly S, et al. Tumour inoculation during laparoscopy. Lancet 1993;342:368.
[8] Zmora O, Gervaz P, Wexner SD. Trocar site recurrence in laparoscopic surgery for colorectal cancer: myth or real concern? Surg Endosc 2001;15:788–93.
[9] Wexner SD, Cohen SM. Port site recurrence after laparoscopic colorectal surgery for cure of malignancy. Br J Surg 1995;82:295–8.
[10] Hughes ESR, McDermott FT, Polglase AL, et al. Tumor recurrence in the abdominal wall scar tissue after large bowel cancer surgery. Dis Colon Rectum 1983;26:571–2.
[11] Reilly WT, Nelson H, Schroeder G, et al. Wound recurrence following conventional treatment of colorectal cancer: a rare but perhaps underestimated problem. Dis Colon Rectum 1996;39:200–7.
[12] American Society of Colon and Rectal Surgeons. Position statement on laparoscopic colectomy. Dis Colon Rectum 1992;35:5A.
[13] Allardyce RA. Is the port site really at risk? Biology, mechanisms and prevention: a critical review. Aust N Z J Surg 1999;69:479–85.
[14] The Clinical Outcomes of Surgical Therapy Study Group. A comparison of laparoscopically assisted and open colectomy for colon cancer. N Engl J Med 2004;350:2050–9.
[15] Lacy AM, García-Valdecasas JC, Delgado S, et al. Laparoscopy-assisted colectomy versus open colectomy for treatment of non-metastatic colon cancer: a randomized trial. Lancet 2002;359:2224–9.
[16] Milsom JW, Böhm B, Hammerhofer KA, et al. A prospective, randomized trial comparing laparoscopic versus conventional techniques in colorectal cancer surgery: a preliminary report. J Am Coll Surg 1998;187:46–57.
[17] Curet MJ, Putrakul K, Pitcher DE, et al. Laparoscopically assisted colon resection for colon carcinoma: perioperative results and long-term outcome. Surg Endosc 2000;14:1062–6.
[18] Kaiser AM, Kang JC, Chan LS, et al. Laparoscopic-assisted versus open colectomy for colon cancer: a prospective randomized trial. J Laparoendosc Adv Surg Tech A 2004;14:329–34.
[19] Schlachta CM, Mamazza J, Seshadri PA, et al. Defining a learning curve for laparoscopic colorectal resections. Dis Colon Rectum 2001;44:217–22.

[20] Abraham NS, Young JM, Solomon MJ. Meta-analysis of short-term outcomes after laparoscopic resection for colorectal cancer. Br J Surg 2004;91:1111–24.

[21] Schwenk W, Haase O, Neudecker J, et al. Short term benefits of laparoscopic colorectal resection. Cochrane Database Syst Rev 2005;(3):CD003145.

[22] The Colon Cancer Laparoscopic or Open Resection Study Group. Laparoscopic surgery versus open surgery for colon cancer: short-term outcomes of a randomized trial. Lancet Oncol 2005;6:477–84.

[23] Guillou PJ, Quirke P, Thorpe H, et al. Short-term endpoints of conventional versus laparoscopic-assisted surgery in patients with colorectal cancer (MRC CLASICC trial): multicentre, randomized controlled trial. Lancet 2005;365:1718–26.

[24] Chapman AE, Levitt MD, Hewett P, et al. Laparoscopic-assisted resection of colorectal malignancies: a systematic review. Ann Surg 2001;234:590–606.

[25] Lezoche E, Feliciotti F, Paganini AM, et al. Laparoscopic vs open hemicolectomy for colon cancer. Surg Endosc 2002;16:596–602.

[26] Tittel A, Schippers E, Anurov M, et al. Shorter postoperative atony after laparoscopic-assisted colonic resection? An animal study. Surg Endosc 2001;15:508–12.

[27] Schwenk W, Böhm B, Haase O, et al. Laparoscopic versus conventional colorectal resection: a prospective randomised study of postoperative ileus and early postoperative feeding. Langenbecks Arch Surg 1998;383:49–55.

[28] Kasparek MS, Muller MH, Glatzle J, et al. Postoperative colonic motility in patients following laparoscopic-assisted and open sigmoid colectomy. J Gastrointest Surg 2003;7: 1073–81.

[29] Stage JG, Schulze S, Moller P, et al. Prospective randomized study of laparoscopic versus open colonic resection for adenocarcinoma. Br J Surg 1997;84:391–6.

[30] Hewitt PM, Ip SM, Kwok SP, et al. Laparoscopic-assisted versus open surgery for colorectal cancer: comparative study of immune effects. Dis Colon Rectum 1998;41:901–9.

[31] Schwenk W, Böhm B, Müller JM. Postoperative pain and fatigue after laparoscopic or conventional colorectal resections: a prospective randomized trial. Surg Endosc 1998;12: 1131–6.

[32] Hasegawa H, Kabeshima Y, Watanabe M, et al. Randomized controlled trial of laparoscopic versus open colectomy for advanced colorectal cancer. Surg Endosc 2003;17: 636–40.

[33] Weeks JC, Nelson H, Gelber S, et al. Short-term quality-of-life outcomes following laparoscopically-assisted colectomy vs open colectomy for colon cancer: a randomized trial. JAMA 2002;287:321–8.

[34] Bokey EL, Moore JW, Chapuis PH, et al. Morbidity and mortality following laparoscopic-assisted right hemicolectomy for cancer. Dis Colon Rectum 1996;39(Suppl):S24–8.

[35] Philipson BM, Bokey EL, Moore JWE, et al. Cost of open versus laparoscopically assisted right hemicolectomy for cancer. World J Surg 1997;21:214–7.

[36] Khalili TM, Fleshner PR, Hiatt JR, et al. Colorectal cancer: comparison of laparoscopic with open approaches. Dis Colon Rectum 1998;41:832–8.

[37] Delaney CP, Kiran RP, Senagore AJ, et al. Case-matched comparison of clinical and financial outcome after laparoscopic or open colorectal surgery. Ann Surg 2003;238:67–72.

[38] Janson M, Björholt I, Carlsson P, et al. Randomized clinical trial of the costs of open and laparoscopic surgery for colon cancer. Br J Surg 2004;91:409–17.

[39] Braga M, Vignali A, Zuliani W, et al. Laparoscopic versus open colorectal surgery: cost-benefit analysis in a single-center randomized trial. Ann Surg 2005;242:890–6.

[40] Anderson CA, Kennedy FR, Potter M, et al. Results of laparoscopically assisted colon resection for carcinoma: the first 100 patients. Surg Endosc 2002;16:607–10.

[41] Lechaux D, Trebuchet G, Le Calve JL. Five-year results of 206 laparoscopic left colectomies for cancer. Surg Endosc 2002;16:1409–12.

[42] Lumley J, Stitz R, Stevenson A, et al. Laparoscopic colorectal surgery for cancer: intermediate to long-term outcomes. Dis Colon Rectum 2002;45:867–74.

[43] Scheidbach H, Schneider C, Hügel O, et al. Oncological quality and preliminary long-term results in laparoscopic colorectal surgery. Surg Endosc 2003;17:903–10.

[44] Baća I, Perko Z, Bokan I, et al. Technique and survival after laparoscopically assisted right hemicolectomy. Surg Endosc 2005;15:650–5.

[45] Jacob BP, Salky B. Laparoscopic colectomy for colon adenocarcinoma: an 11-year retrospective review with 5-year survival rates. Surg Endosc 2005;19:643–9.

[46] Sample CB, Watson M, Okrainec A, et al. Long-term outcomes of laparoscopic surgery for colorectal cancer. Surg Endosc 2006;20:30–4.

[47] Franklin ME Jr, Rosenthal D, Abrego-Medina D, et al. Prospective comparison of open versus laparoscopic colon surgery for carcinoma: five-year results. Dis Colon Rectum 1996;39(Suppl 10):S35–46.

[48] Patenkar SK, Larach SW, Ferrara A, et al. Prospective comparison of laparoscopic versus open resections for colorectal adenocarcinoma over a ten-year period. Dis Colon Rectum 2003;46:601–11.

[49] Zheng MH, Feng B, Lu AG, et al. Laparoscopic versus open right hemicolectomy with curative intent for colon carcinoma. World J Gastroenterol 2005;11:323–6.

[50] Leung LK, Kwok SPY, Lam SCW, et al. Laparoscopic resection of rectosigmoid carcinoma: prospective randomized trial. Lancet 2004;363:1187–92.

[51] Poulin EC, Mamazza J, Schlachta CM, et al. Laparoscopic resection does not adversely affect early survival curves in patients undergoing surgery for colorectal adenocarcinoma. Ann Surg 1999;229:487–92.

[52] American Society of Colon & Rectal Surgeons. Position statement: laparoscopic colectomy for curable cancer. Available at: http://www.fascrs.org/displaycommon.cfm?an=1&subarticlenbr=319. Accessed December 27, 2005.

[53] Moloo H, Mamazza J, Poulin EC, et al. Laparoscopic resections for colorectal cancer: does conversion affect survival? Surg Endosc 2004;18:732–5.

[54] Casillas S, Delaney CP, Senagore AJ, et al. Does conversion of a laparoscopic colectomy adversely affect patient outcome? Dis Colon Rectum 2004;47:1680–5.

[55] Young-Fadok TM, Sargent DJ, Nelson H, et al. Conversion does not adversely affect oncologic outcomes after laparoscopic colectomy for colon cancer: results from a multicenter prospective randomized trial. American Society of Colon and Rectal Surgeons Annual Meeting; 2005 April 30–May 3; Philadelphia, PA. S65. Available at: http://www.vioworks.com/clients/ascrs2005/presentations.asp. Accessed June 27, 2006.

[56] Bemelman WA, Dunker MS, Slors JFM, et al. Laparoscopic surgery for inflammatory bowel disease: current concepts. Scand J Gastroenterol 2002;37(Suppl 236):54–9.

[57] Milsom JW. Laparoscopic surgery in the treatment of Crohn's disease. Surg Clin N Am 2005;85:25–34.

[58] Milsom JW, Hammerhofer KA, Böhm B, et al. Prospective, randomized trial comparing laparoscopic versus conventional surgery for refractory ileocolic Crohn's disease. Dis Colon Rectum 2001;44:1–8.

[59] Maartense S, Dunker MS, Slors JFM, et al. Laparoscopic-assisted versus open ileocolic resection for Crohn's disease: a randomized trial. Ann Surg 2006;243:143–9.

[60] Luan X, Gross E. Laparoscopic assisted surgery for Crohn's disease: an initial experience and results. J Tongji Med Univ 2000;20:332–5.

[61] Msika S, Iannelli A, Deroide G, et al. Can laparoscopy reduce hospital stay in the treatment of Crohn's disease? Dis Colon Rectum 2001;44:1661–6.

[62] Dueprее HJ, Senagore AJ, Delaney CP, et al. Advantages of laparoscopic resection for ileocecal Crohn's disease. Dis Colon Rectum 2002;45:605–10.

[63] Benoist S, Panis Y, Beaufour A, et al. Laparoscopic ileocecal resection in Crohn's disease: a case-matched comparison with open resection. Surg Endosc 2003;17:814–8.

[64] Bergamaschi R, Pessaux P, Arnaud JP. Comparison of conventional and laparoscopic ileocolic resection for Crohn's disease. Dis Colon Rectum 2003;46:1129–33.

[65] Shore G, Gonzalez QH, Bondora A, et al. Laparoscopic vs conventional ileocolectomy for primary Crohn's disease. Arch Surg 2003;138:76–9.
[66] Huilgol RL, Wright CM, Solomon MJ. Laparoscopic versus open ileocolic resection for Crohn's disease. J Laparoendosc Adv Surg Tech A 2004;14:61–5.
[67] Dunker MS, Stiggelbout AM, van Hogezand RA, et al. Cosmesis and body image after laparoscopic-assisted and open ileocolic resection for Crohn's disease. Surg Endosc 1998;12:1334–40.
[68] Rosman AS, Melis M, Fichera A. Metaanalysis of trials comparing laparoscopic and open surgery for Crohn's disease. Surg Endosc 2005;19:1549–55.
[69] Wexner SD, Cera SM. Laparoscopic surgery for ulcerative colitis. Surg Clin N Am 2005;85:35–47.
[70] Schmitt SL, Cohen SM, Wexner SD, et al. Does laparoscopic-assisted ileal pouch anal anastomosis reduce the length of hospitalization? Int J Colorectal Dis 1994;9:134–7.
[71] Liu CD, Rolandelli R, Ashley SW, et al. Laparoscopic surgery for inflammatory bowel disease. Am Surg 1995;61:1054–6.
[72] Marcello PW, Milsom JW, Wong SK, et al. Laparoscopic restorative proctocolectomy: case-matched comparative study with open restorative proctocolectomy. Dis Colon Rectum 2000;43:604–8.
[73] Hashimoto A, Funayama Y, Naito H, et al. Laparoscope-assisted versus conventional restorative proctocolectomy with rectal mucosectomy. Surg Today 2001;31:210–4.
[74] Dunker MS, Bemelman WA, Slors JF, et al. Functional outcome, quality of life, body image, and cosmesis in patients after laparoscopic-assisted and conventional restorative proctocolectomy: a comparative study. Dis Colon Rectum 2001;44:1800–7.
[75] Larson DW, Dozois EJ, Piotrowicz K, et al. Laparoscopic-assisted versus open ileal pouch-anal anastomosis: functional outcome in a case-matched series. Dis Colon Rectum 2005;48:1845–50.
[76] Senagore AJ. Laparoscopic sigmoid colectomy for diverticular disease. Surg Clin N Am 2005;85:19–24.
[77] Senagore AJ, Duepree HJ, Delaney CP, et al. Cost structure of laparoscopic and open sigmoid colectomy for diverticular disease: similarities and differences. Dis Colon Rectum 2002;45:485–90.
[78] Dwivedi A, Chahin F, Agrawal S, et al. Laparoscopic colectomy versus open colectomy for sigmoid diverticular disease. Dis Colon Rectum 2002;45:1309–14.
[79] Lawrence DM, Pasquale MD, Wasser TE. Laparoscopic versus open sigmoid colectomy for diverticulitis. Am Surg 2003;69:499–503.
[80] Alves A, Panis Y, Slim K, et al. French multicentre prospective observational study of laparoscopic versus open colectomy for sigmoid diverticular disease. Br J Surg 2005;92:1520–5.
[81] Kockerling F, Schneider C, Reymond MA, et al. Laparoscopic resection of sigmoid diverticulitis: results of a multicenter study. Surg Endosc 1999;13:567–71.
[82] Ballantyne GH, Leahy PF. Hand-assisted laparoscopic colectomy: evolution to a clinically useful technique. Dis Colon Rectum 2004;47:753–65.
[83] Ou H. Laparoscopic-assisted mini laparotomy with colectomy. Dis Colon Rectum 1995;38:324–6.
[84] O'Reilly MJ, Saye WB, Mullins SG, et al. Technique of hand-assisted laparoscopic surgery. J Laparoendosc Surg 1996;6:239–44.
[85] Mooney MJ, Elliott PL, Galapon DB, et al. Hand-assisted laparoscopic sigmoidectomy for diverticulitis. Dis Colon Rectum 1998;41:630–5.
[86] Southern Surgeons' Club Study Group. Handoscopic surgery: a prospective multicenter trial of a minimally invasive technique for complex abdominal surgery. Arch Surg 1999;134:477–85.

[87] HALS Study Group. Hand-assisted laparoscopic surgery vs standard laparoscopic surgery for colorectal disease: a prospective randomized trial. Surg Endosc 2000;14: 896–901.

[88] Targarona EM, Gracia E, Garriga J, et al. Prospective randomized trial comparing conventional laparoscopic colectomy with hand-assisted laparoscopic colectomy: applicability, immediate clinical outcome, inflammatory response, and cost. Surg Endosc 2002;16:234–9.

[89] Chang YJ, Marcello PW, Rusin LC, et al. Hand-assisted laparoscopic sigmoid colectomy: helping hand or hindrance? Surg Endosc 2005;19:656–61.

[90] Kang JC, Chung MH, Chao PC, et al. Hand-assisted laparoscopic colectomy vs open colectomy: a prospective randomized study. Surg Endosc 2004;18:577–81.

[91] Hyman N. How much colorectal surgery do general surgeons do? J Am Coll Surg 2002;194: 37–9.

[92] Rivadeneira DE, Marcello PW, Roberts PL, et al. Benefits of hand-assisted laparoscopic restorative proctocolectomy: a comparative study. Dis Colon Rectum 2004;47:1371–6.

[93] Nakajima K, Lee SW, Cocilovo C, et al. Laparoscopic total colectomy: hand-assisted vs standard technique. Surg Endosc 2004;18:582–6.

[94] Maartense S, Dunker MS, Slors JF, et al. Hand-assisted laparoscopic versus open restorative proctocolectomy with ileal pouch anal anastomosis: a randomized trial. Ann Surg 2004;240:984–92.

[95] Sardinha TC, Wexner SD. Laparoscopy for inflammatory bowel disease: pros and cons. World J Surg 1998;22:370–4.

[96] Amaral JF. The experimental development of an ultrasonically activated scalpel for laparoscopic use. Surg Laparosc Endosc 1994;4:92–9.

[97] Gossot D, Buess G, Cuschieri A, et al. Ultrasonic dissection for endoscopic surgery. Surg Endosc 1999;13:412–7.

[98] Foschi D, Cellerino P, Corsi F, et al. The mechanism of blood vessel closure in humans by the application of ultrasonic energy. Surg Endosc 2002;16:814–9.

[99] Emam TA, Cuschieri A. How safe is high-power ultrasonic dissection? Ann Surg 2003;237: 186–91.

[100] Richards SR, Simpkins SS. Comparison of the harmonic scissors and endostapler in laparoscopic supracervical hysterectomy. J Am Assoc Gynecol Laparosc 1995;3:87–90.

[101] Laycock WS, Trus TL, Hunter JG. New technology for the division of short gastric vessels during laparoscopic Nissen fundoplication: a prospective randomized trial. Surg Endosc 1996;10:71–3.

[102] Nduka CC, Poland N, Kennedy M, et al. Does the ultrasonically activated scalpel release viable airborne cancer cell? Surg Endosc 1998;12:1031–4.

[103] Heili MJ, Flowers SA, Fowler DL. Laparoscopic-assisted colectomy: a comparison of dissection techniques. JSLS 1999;3:27–31.

[104] Msika S, Deroide G, Kianmanesh R, et al. Harmonic scalpel in laparoscopic colorectal surgery. Dis Colon Rectum 2001;44:432–6.

[105] Morino M, Rimonda R, Allaix ME, et al. Ultrasonic versus standard electric dissection in laparoscopic colorectal surgery: a prospective randomized clinical trial. Ann Surg 2005;242: 897–901.

[106] Heniford BT, Matthews BD, Sing RF, et al. Initial results with an electrothermal bipolar vessel sealer. Surg Endosc 2001;15:799–801.

[107] Kennedy JS, Stranahan PL, Taylor KD, et al. High-burst-strength, feedback-controlled bipolar vessel sealing. Surg Endosc 1998;12:876–8.

[108] Harold KL, Pollinger H, Matthews BD, et al. Comparison of ultrasonic energy, bipolar thermal energy, and vascular clips for the hemostasis of small-, medium-, and large-sized arteries. Surg Endosc 2003;17:1228–30.

[109] Hasegawa H, Watanabe M, Nishibori H, et al. Clipless laparoscopic restorative proctocolectomy using an electrothermal bipolar vessel sealer. Digestive Endoscopy 2003;15:320–2.

[110] Araki Y, Noake T, Kanazawa M, et al. Clipless hand-assisted laparoscopic total colectomy using LigaSure Atlas. Kurume Med J 2004;51:105–8.
[111] Takada M, Ichihara T, Kuroda Y. Comparative study of electrothermal bipolar vessel sealer and ultrasonic coagulating shears in laparoscopic colectomy. Surg Endosc 2005; 19:226–8.
[112] Marcello PW, Roberts PL, Rusin LC, et al. Vascular pedicle ligation techniques during laparoscopic colectomy: a prospective randomized trial. Surg Endosc 2006;20:263–9.
[113] Kourambas J, Preminger GM. Advances in camera, video, and imaging technologies in laparoscopy. Urol Clin North Am 2001;28:5–14.
[114] Berber E, Siperstein AE. Understanding and optimizing laparoscopic videosystems. Surg Endosc 2001;15:781–7.
[115] Cuschieri A. Technology for minimal access surgery. BMJ 1999;319:1304–10.
[116] Amory SE, Forde KA, Tsai JL. A new flexible videoendoscope for minimal access surgery. Surg Endosc 1993;7:200–2.
[117] Perrone JM, Ames CD, Yan Y, et al. Evaluation of surgical performance with standard rigid and flexible-tip laparoscopes. Surg Endosc 2005;19:1325–8.
[118] Birkett DH, Josephs LG, Este-McDonald J. A new 3-D laparoscope in gastrointestinal surgery. Surg Endosc 1994;8:1448–51.
[119] Babayan RK, Chiu AW, Este-McDonald J, et al. The comparision between 2-dimensional and 3-dimensional laparoscopic video systems in a pelvic trainer. J Endourol 1993;7:S195.
[120] Chan ACW, Chung SCS, Yim APC, et al. Comparison of two-dimensional vs three-dimensional camera systems in laparoscopic surgery. Surg Endosc 1997;11:438–40.
[121] Tafffinder N, Smith SGT, Huber J, et al. The effect of a second-generation 3D endoscope on the laparoscopic precision of novices and experienced surgeons. Surg Endosc 1999;13: 1087–92.
[122] Braga M, Vignali A, Gianotti L, et al. Laparoscopic versus open colorectal surgery: a randomized trial on short-term outcome. Ann Surg 2002;236:759–67.
[123] Tang CL, Eu KW, Tai BC, et al. Randomized clinical trial of the effect of open versus laparoscopically assisted colectomy on systemic immunity in patients with colorectal cancer. Br J Surg 2001;88:801–7.
[124] Araki Y, Ishibashi N, Ogata Y, et al. The usefulness of restorative laparoscopic-assisted total colectomy for ulcerative colitis. Kurume Med J 2001;48:99–103.

SURGICAL
CLINICS OF
NORTH AMERICA

Surg Clin N Am 86 (2006) 899–914

Laparoscopic Rectal Surgery: Rectal Cancer, Pelvic Pouch Surgery, and Rectal Prolapse

Robert P. Akbari, MD[a,b], Thomas E. Read, MD[a,b,*]

[a]*Division of Colon and Rectal Surgery, Western Pennsylvania Hospital,
4800 Friendship Avenue, Pittsburgh, PA 15224, USA*
[b]*Department of Surgery, Temple University School of Medicine,
Western Pennsylvania Hospital, 4800 Friendship Avenue, Pittsburgh, PA 15224, USA*

Laparoscopy for rectal cancer

The adoption of laparoscopic proctectomy for rectal cancer has been slow, primarily because of the technical difficulty of the procedure. The wide surgeon-to-surgeon variability in disease-free survival and local pelvic recurrence after open proctectomy probably is due to differences in surgical technique. These differences are likely to be magnified when the challenge of laparoscopy is added to the procedure. Oncologic and functional outcomes data are limited. Although the adoption of laparoscopic techniques to perform curative proctectomy likely will expand as technical challenges are overcome and experience and training improve, the results of prospective multicenter trials are necessary to ensure that the procedures provide equivalent oncologic and functional outcome to conventional surgery.

Technical aspects of laparoscopic proctectomy

The technical aspects of proctectomy for adenocarcinoma of the rectum have received considerable attention in recent years because of wide surgeon-to-surgeon variability in local pelvic recurrence and survival rates following curative resection [1–4]. The two most commonly identified surgeon-specific factors that are associated with good outcome have been specialty training and high case volume. The technique of mesorectal mobilization and resection has been demonstrated to have prognostic significance,

---

* Corresponding author. Department of Surgery 4600N, Western Pennsylvania Hospital, 4800 Friendship Avenue, Pittsburgh, PA 15224.

E-mail address: tread@wpahs.org (T.E. Read).

0039-6109/06/$ - see front matter
doi:10.1016/j.suc.2006.05.002 *surgical.theclinics.com*

even when combined with neoadjuvant radiotherapy [1]. Likewise, data from the Dutch Colorectal Cancer Group rectal cancer trial indicate that the benefits of meticulous surgical technique and preoperative radiotherapy are additive, not compensatory [5].

Thus, the technique of proctectomy is of critical importance, in terms of disease-free survival and local pelvic recurrence. Although performing an oncologically sound proctectomy for an upper rectal cancer in a thin woman may be straightforward, proctectomy for a distal rectal tumor in an obese man with a narrow pelvis may be difficult. Adding the technical challenges of laparoscopy to such an operation has led some surgeons to express skepticism as to the relative appropriateness of attempting laparoscopic proctectomy for rectal cancer. As is true of the evolution of many technically involved procedures, however, advances in instrumentation, combined with greater experience and better training, will allow surgeons to perform laparoscopic proctectomy for cancer and achieve excellent results.

In the past decade, there has been a rapid evolution of laparoscopic techniques to treat colorectal disease, as surgeons have sought to make laparoscopic colectomy and proctectomy more routine. In addition to advances in laparoscopic instrumentation and energy delivery, improvements in hand-assist technology have allowed surgeons to approach laparoscopic proctectomy with better tools [6].

The most appealing operation early on in the laparoscopic proctectomy experience was abdominoperineal resection (APR) [7]. APR does not require division of the distal rectum or mesorectum, nor does it require an abdominal extraction excision or anastomosis. Thus, the full benefits of the laparoscopic approach theoretically can be realized. Patients who require APR typically have tumors abutting the anal sphincter complex, so dissection in the immediate vicinity of the tumor is performed primarily from a perineal approach, as one would during an open operation. Fears of tumor dissemination due to pneumoperitoneum were minimized because of the position of the tumor.

Many patients who undergo open APR do not require mobilization of the splenic flexure because it is not necessary to bring the descending colon into the deep pelvis to create an anastomosis. As a consequence, open APR often can be completed by means of an infraumbilical incision, which makes the relative benefits of laparoscopic APR less obvious. Some surgeons use a small Pfannenstiel's incision to assist with laparoscopic proctectomy, and may place a hand-assist device through this incision. The difference, then, between an infraumbilical midline incision and a Pfannenstiel's incision to assist with laparoscopic APR in terms of short-term outcomes (pain, disability, immune suppression) in a thin patient may not be striking. If laparoscopic APR is performed without an abdominal incision, other than for ports and colostomy, there may be substantial benefit.

One of the concerns regarding laparoscopic proctectomy is the ability of the surgeon to mobilize the distal rectum and mesorectum, especially in the setting of a bulky rectal tumor (Fig. 1). If retraction is difficult in the deep pelvis and visualization is limited, the surgeon may have a natural tendency to perform more of the dissection from the perineal approach. Although not intrinsically dangerous, the same pelvic morphology that would lead to lesser transabdominal mobilization may make extensive perineal dissection more difficult. If complete resection of the tumor and mesorectum at risk for tumor spread is jeopardized by these technical issues, then the surgeon has done a great disservice to his or her patient by performing APR by way of a laparoscopic approach. Alternatively, if the rectum and mesorectum can be mobilized in the same planes as would be performed during open APR, oncologic outcomes should be equivalent.

Anterior resection with colorectal or coloanal anastomosis differs from APR in several fundamental ways. Excluding from the discussion those surgeons who perform transanal or transvaginal specimen extraction [8], most surgeons use an abdominal incision to extract the specimen. Additionally, an anastomosis is performed, and more extensive proximal mobilization of the colon is necessary to allow for a tension-free anastomosis. Surgeons have learned to use the extraction incision to facilitate mobilization, rectal transaction, and anastomosis. The ability to mobilize the splenic flexure completely, divide the inferior mesenteric artery at the aorta, and divide the inferior mesenteric vein adjacent to the ligament of Treitz without making a supraumbilical incision may prove to be the greatest benefit of laparoscopic proctectomy in the short term.

Some surgeons use a left lower quadrant or periumbilical incision to extract the specimen for any left-sided colorectal resectional procedure. Although tolerated well by the patient, such a technique requires closure of the wound and recreation of pneumoperitoneum to perform the anastomosis. Any anastomotic problems must be addressed laparoscopically. An

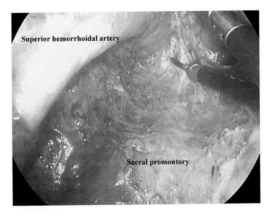

Fig. 1. Laparoscopic posterior mobilization of the rectum and mesorectum during laparoscopic abdominoperineal resection. (*From* Read TE. Laparoscopic treatment of rectal adenocarcinoma. Semin Colon Rectal Surg 2004;14(3):149; with permission.)

alternative is to use a Pfannenstiel's or lower midline incision to perform specimen extraction and anastomosis. This incision also can be used to assist with rectosigmoid mobilization directly, and allows for a hand-assist device to be placed at the start of the operation (Fig. 2). Because the incision is immediately over the pelvic inlet, anastomotic problems, difficult mobilization issues, or bleeding problems can be addressed directly. Transection of the rectum and mesorectum, one of the most difficult aspects of laparoscopic proctectomy, can be performed through this incision. Additionally, the Pfannenstiel's incision is cosmetically appealing to many patients, especially women.

As with laparoscopic restorative proctocolectomy, some surgeons are performing what has been termed a "hybrid" technique, using laparoscopic techniques to mobilize the proximal colon and performing much of the pelvic dissection and anastomosis through a small Pfannenstiel's or low vertical midline incision [9]. Although semantic purists may argue that this is not truly a completely laparoscopic method, the benefits of laparoscopy may be preserved. Because an incision is necessary for anterior resection with anastomosis regardless of method, the debate over what is laparoscopic and what is not seems somewhat specious. Prospective trials are necessary to determine if there are any differences in postoperative immune suppression [10], pain, ileus, or other short-term outcomes between the various techniques of laparoscopic proctectomy.

As surgeons have come to a better appreciation of the anatomy of the mesorectum and patterns of spread of rectal adenocarcinoma, there has been increasing enthusiasm for anal sphincter preservation and restoration of intestinal continuity. By extension, there has been an increasing need to divide the rectum and mesorectum in the deep pelvis. Transection of the mid or distal rectum and mesorectum can be difficult laparoscopically,

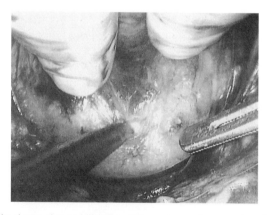

Fig. 2. Hand-assisted posterior mobilization of the rectum and mesorectum during anterior resection of the rectosigmoid. (*From* Read TE. Laparoscopic treatment of rectal adenocarcinoma. Semin Colon Rectal Surg 2004;14(3):149; with permission.)

although the use of articulating linear staplers and hand-assist technology has made this task easier (Figs. 3 and 4). An alternative to dividing the mesorectum with vascular staplers is the use of energy, either by harmonic scalpel or Ligasure (Valleylab, Tyco Health care Group, Boulder, Colorado). Retraction of the deep pelvic tissues, especially the prostate in a man, can be challenging laparoscopically as well. Placement of standard open retractors through a Pfannenstiel's incision often is helpful.

Because of the small numbers of patients who undergo laparoscopic proctectomy for rectal cancer reported in the literature, and the paucity of randomized, prospective trials, true comparisons of functional outcomes and perioperative morbidity between laparoscopic and open proctectomy are lacking. The anastomotic leak rates in some series of laparoscopic anterior resection have been 9% to 20% [11–14], which suggests that surgeons are still on steep portions of their learning curves. Alternatively, because many leaks are due to inadequate proximal blood supply and tension, it may suggest that surgeons are not enthusiastic about rigorous (and potentially time-consuming) mobilization of the splenic flexure and proximal mesentery when faced with the task of laparoscopic mobilization of the rectum and mesorectum.

Oncologic issues

Given the wide variability in oncologic outcomes following open proctectomy, and the technical challenges of laparoscopic proctectomy, it is logical to assume that the differences in outcome between surgeons will be magnified after laparoscopic proctectomy for rectal cancer. One of the major concerns regarding laparoscopic rectal resection is accidental tumor spillage that is caused by grasping and manipulating the rectum and mesorectum in a narrow pelvis. The prevalence of intraoperative tumor cell dissemination

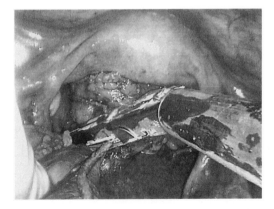

Fig. 3. Laparoscopic transaction of the rectum using a reticulating linear cutting stapler. (*From* Read TE. Laparoscopic treatment of rectal adenocarcinoma. Semin Colon Rectal Surg 2004;14(3):151; with permission.)

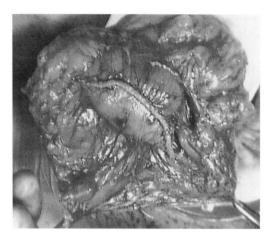

Fig. 4. Divided rectum and mesorectum. Note that the mesorectum has been divided at the level of rectal transaction. (*From* Read TE. Laparoscopic treatment of rectal adenocarcinoma. Semin Colon Rectal Surg 2004;14(3):151; with permission.)

that is caused by iatrogenic tumor perforation or transaction during laparoscopic APR has been reported to be as high as 5% [15]. Although large randomized, prospective trials may show that experienced laparoscopic colectomists can achieve good outcomes for patients who have curable intraperitoneal colon adenocarcinoma, these results cannot be extrapolated immediately to patients who have rectal cancer. Thus, it is critical to evaluate immediate pathologic and long-term oncologic results of laparoscopic proctectomy prospectively before recommending the technique for mass consumption.

There have been few reports of oncologic outcomes following laparoscopic proctectomy for rectal cancer [10,11,16–27]. There have been only a handful of published series with greater than 50 patients and greater than 3-year follow-up [21]. Although the German and Austrian Laparoscopic Colorectal Surgery Study Group recently reported results from 380 patients who underwent laparoscopic proctectomy, follow-up was short (24 months). In addition to the problems of small numbers and short follow-up, some investigators fail to perform time-to-event (actuarial, Kaplan-Meier) analysis of disease-free survival and local pelvic recurrence, which makes any conclusions regarding oncologic outcome difficult [27]. Many series report results for selected patients who have early-stage tumors, which is reasonable given the technical issues of laparoscopic manipulation of tumor; however, such reports are not useful in making generalizations as to the appropriateness of the technique for all patients who have rectal cancer. In two series of patients who underwent laparoscopic proctectomy for more advanced tumors [17,24], local pelvic recurrence rates were 19% and 25%, although exactly matched by the local pelvic recurrence rate in the comparison groups of patients who underwent open proctectomy in each study. Therefore, the reasons for the local recurrences probably are not a function of the laparoscopic technique *per se.*

The only data about the learning curve for rectal cancer come from the conventional versus laparoscopic-assisted surgery in patients with colorectal cancer (CLASICC) trial [28]. In this trial, which included colon and rectal resection, 242 laparoscopic rectal resections were performed. Experienced laparoscopic surgeons, who had done at least 20 laparoscopic colon resections before the trial began, performed the procedures. The conversion rate for colon resection was 25% and decreased over the course of the study. For rectal resection, the rate of conversion was higher (34%) and the conversion rate remained high throughout the course of the study. Tumor fixation and uncertainty of margins were the two most common reasons for conversion. This suggests that even in experienced hands, laparoscopic proctectomy is more technically demanding. The rates of positive margins were not statistically different when comparing laparoscopic with open proctectomy, although there was trend toward a higher positive margin rate for laparoscopic restorative procedures as compared with open techniques (12% versus 6%; $P = .19$).

Prospective analysis of outcomes by expert laparoscopic proctectomists will be the first step toward determining whether patients should undergo laparoscopic proctectomy for rectal cancer. Unfortunately, even the positive results of such a trial will not prove that nonexpert surgeons can achieve similar results. Surgeons with specialty training and high-volume practices achieve better results when treating patients who have rectal cancer by open techniques [1], which should not be surprising. Recent data from the American Board of Surgery suggests that the average general surgeon in the United States performs only one or two proctectomies per year for any reason [29,30]. This paucity of practice experience is compounded by the small number of patients who have rectal cancer that is encountered during a general surgical residency. Data from the Residency Review Committee and the American Board of Surgery indicate that the average colorectal surgery resident performs more colectomies and APRs in a single year of training than the average general surgical resident performs in 5 years of residency [31,32]. The number of laparoscopic proctectomies that is performed by general and colorectal surgeons undoubtedly will be much less than the number of open proctectomies. Therefore, the initial adoption of laparoscopic proctectomy as treatment for curable rectal cancer will be by well-trained surgeons who perform a high volume of laparoscopic colectomy and open proctectomy for cancer, and who are willing to invest the time and effort to build a successful operative team.

Costs and quality of life

The financial aspects of laparoscopic proctectomy for cancer have not been studied well. Data regarding the costs of laparoscopic versus open colorectal surgery, in general, are conflicting [33,34]. In general, the short-term costs of laparoscopy are higher because of equipment expense and increased operating time. Long-term costs are more difficult to assess, but shorter length of hospital stay, quicker return to work, and reduction in the rate of adhesive bowel obstruction [35] ultimately may make laparoscopic proctectomy financially equivalent or superior to open proctectomy.

Quality of life after laparoscopic versus open colorectal resections was assessed in the CLASICC trial [28]. Using the European Organization for Research and Treatment of Cancer-C30 questionnaire and the Quality of Life Questionnaire-CR38, there was no significant difference found in general or colorectal quality of life between the two groups at baseline, 2 weeks, or at 3 months; however, it should be emphasized that the proctectomy subgroups were not analyzed separately. As with other procedures, it will be difficult to determine conclusively whether laparoscopic proctectomy for rectal cancer results in improved "quality of life," because socioeconomic and cultural issues make rigorous comparisons virtually impossible.

Laparoscopic colostomy for obstructing rectal cancer

Laparoscopic creation of diverting colostomy has great usefulness in the management of patients who present with locally advanced obstructing or near-obstructing rectal cancer [36]. Laparoscopic exploration of the abdomen allows for evaluation of the liver (with or without laparoscopic ultrasound), pelvis, and peritoneum to look for occult metastatic disease that may change management. Recovery time is minimized to allow for the near-immediate institution of neoadjuvant radiotherapy or chemoradiotherapy. Laparoscopic colostomy can be accomplished using only two 5-mm ports and a port at the stoma extraction site, which limits the postoperative morbidity. Because of the virtual absence of postoperative adhesions, there is reduced risk for small bowel injury during radiotherapy, and proctectomy is easier to perform than after laparotomy and colostomy. The obvious benefits of this technique obviate the performance of a randomized, prospective trial to evaluate the differences between open and laparoscopic colostomy.

Laparoscopic pelvic pouch surgery (restorative proctocolectomy)

Indications for laparoscopic restorative proctocolectomy (proctocolectomy with ileal-pouch anal anastomosis) are, in general, the same as for open restorative proctocolectomy. Patients who have ulcerative colitis or familial adenomatous polyposis who have good anal sphincter function and who will tolerate a major laparoscopic abdominal operation are candidates for the procedure. Because laparoscopic restorative proctocolectomy remains a lengthy and taxing operation, even in experienced hands, patient selection may help to improve outcome. The best candidates for the laparoscopic approach tend to be thin and without a multitude of previous laparotomies. The benefits of laparoscopic restorative proctocolectomy have been more difficult to demonstrate than with other colorectal procedures, likely because of the magnitude of the operation, the removal of the organ that causes debilitation (in patients suffering from ulcerative colitis), and the construction of a temporary diverting ileostomy.

Technical aspects of laparoscopic restorative proctocolectomy

Techniques of laparoscopic restorative proctocolectomy vary [37–39]. The colonic portion of the operation essentially is a total abdominal colectomy, and can be performed totally laparoscopically or with the use of a hand-assist device. Mobilization of the transverse colon tends to be the most taxing for the surgeon. The proctectomy can be performed completely laparoscopically, using a laparoscopic stapler to divide the distal rectum at the pelvic floor, or by completing the proctectomy from a transanal approach and extracting the specimen through the anus. With either approach, an abdominal incision usually is required to exteriorize the ileum and construct the pouch. This incision usually is made in the midline at the umbilicus, in the lower midline, or as a Pfannenstiel's incision. The advantages of a lower midline or Pfannenstiel's incision are similar to what was outlined above in the discussion of laparoscopic proctectomy for rectal cancer. Following the proctectomy, the anastomosis is performed and a loop ileostomy may be constructed.

An alternative approach is to use a Pfannenstiel's or lower midline incision from the beginning of the operation, and place a hand-assist device through this incision. Current hand-assist technology allows the surgeon to perform the proctectomy by way of the open incision, laparoscopically with a hand in the abdomen to facilitate retraction, or purely laparoscopically with the cap of the device closed. Rivadeneira and colleagues [40] compared hand-assisted with "conventional" laparoscopic restorative proctocolectomy, and found no difference in outcome, except for a significant reduction in operative time. Given that these procedures are labor- and time-intensive, any method that shortens the operation and reduces surgeon stress and fatigue is a welcome advance.

A third approach is to perform the total abdominal colectomy laparoscopically, and then make a lower midline or Pfannenstiel's incision to complete the restorative proctectomy by way of the open incision. This technique has been termed the "hybrid approach" as outlined above.

Outcomes

Published literature regarding laparoscopic restorative proctocolectomy is not extensive [37–39,41–44]. Most studies are small retrospective series; some make comparisons with an open surgery control group [38,39,44]. Outcomes following laparoscopic restorative proctocolectomy have not been markedly different from outcomes following open procedures. Wexner and colleagues' comparison of open and laparoscopic procedures demonstrated longer operative time, greater transfusion requirements, and higher morbidity in the group that underwent laparoscopy, and similar tolerance to oral intake, time to bowel function, and length of stay in both groups [41,43]. These studies were published in 1994 and 1996, early in the laparoscopic colectomy experience, however. Marcello and colleagues [39] reported longer operative times in the group that underwent laparoscopy, but no difference in estimated blood loss and morbidity. They also demonstrated a shorter length of stay in the group that underwent laparoscopy. More recently, Maartense and colleagues [44] reported their results of a prospective, randomized trial that compared laparoscopic (hand-assisted) with open restorative proctocolectomy (n = 30 in each group). They found no significant differences in estimated blood loss, complication rates, narcotics requirement, return to normal diet, and length of hospital stay. Operating room time was longer with the laparoscopic technique.

Costs and quality of life

Common sense argues that the costs of laparoscopic pouch surgery are higher than those of open pouch operations, particularly in the short-term. Maartense and colleagues [44] found that the median cost in the operating room for a laparoscopic pouch operation was higher ($¤$3,387) than for the open operation ($¤$1,721, $P < .001$). Conversely, they also found that median overall costs, including costs of surgery plus costs of relaparotomies, hospital stay, and readmission (eg, for stoma closure), were similar ($¤$16,728 for laparoscopy versus $¤$13,405 for open technique; $P = .095$). Just as for laparoscopic operations for rectal cancer, an exact determination of the relative costs and benefits of the laparoscopic approach to restorative proctocolectomy is difficult.

Patent quality of life also was evaluated in Maartense and colleagues' study. They measured postoperative quality of life using the short form-36 and the gastrointestinal quality of life index questionnaires at 1 and 2 weeks and at 1 and 3 months. All patients had a significant decrease in quality of life, which was at its worst at 2 weeks postoperatively. Quality of life increased to baseline at 1 month, then to above baseline at 3 months. The patients who underwent laparoscopy had scores that were not significantly different from the patients who underwent open surgery.

The lack of proven benefit of the laparoscopic approach to restorative proctocolectomy may be related to a host of factors. Removal of the organ that is causing significant morbidity to the patient (in patients who have ulcerative colitis) may be more important to their overall quality of life than anything else, and may overshadow smaller differences that are made by the surgical approach. Construction of a loop ileostomy may make differences in time to resolution of ileus minor when comparing the open and laparoscopic approaches. This variable may be eliminated by forgoing temporary fecal diversion, as some surgeons have done in select patients who undergo open restorative proctocolectomy. Milsom and colleagues reported the results of just such an approach, and performed laparoscopic one-stage restorative proctocolectomy in 32 select patients [42]. In their series, there were two intraoperative complications: an inconsequential rectal perforation during mobilization and one staple line misfire. There were seven major postoperative complications: three obstruction/ileus, two strictures, one pelvic abscess, and one pouch leak. Three patients required reoperation (one temporary ileostomy, one lysis of adhesions, and one transpouch drainage). Thus, even in the most experienced of hands, this operation is challenging and associated with significant morbidity.

The major benefits of the laparoscopic approach to restorative proctocolectomy may prove to be long-term rather than short-term. As has been suggested by anecdotal experience and some prospective collected data, laparoscopy is associated with markedly less adhesion formation than is laparotomy. For patients who undergo restorative proctocolectomy, which has been associated with high rates of adhesive intestinal obstruction and infertility in women as a result of pelvic adhesions, the laparoscopic approach may prove to be of substantial value.

Laparoscopy for rectal prolapse

Although rectal prolapse has been recognized since biblical times, the optimal surgical procedure to correct rectal prolapse remains a subject of debate. A plethora of operations is used to treat rectal prolapse, and the surgeon should select one that produces the best possible functional result for an individual patient with a low complication and recurrence rate. The choice of operation depends on many factors, including the age and sex of the patient, associated constipation, degree of incontinence, history of repairs, comorbid conditions, and the expertise of the surgeon.

Patient selection

Although extremely high-risk patients who have easily reducible rectal prolapse can be managed with laxatives and manual reduction of the prolapse, most patients benefit from surgical repair. The primary goals of surgery are to restore normal anatomy and improve symptoms of constipation and incontinence. Treatment options include one or more of the following: narrow the anal orifice, obliterate the pouch of Douglas, restore the pelvic floor by plicating the levators, resect the prolapsing segment of rectosigmoid, and suspend or fix the prolapsing rectum to the sacrum.

Corrective procedures for rectal prolapse can be divided by approach: transabdominal or perineal. Most transabdominal procedures have low recurrence rates, and laparotomy allows the opportunity to perform colectomy for patients with severe constipation. Additionally, associated pelvic floor disorders, such as enterocele and rectocele, may be corrected simultaneously. Most procedures that are performed using a perineal approach can be completed using local or regional anesthesia, which minimizes cardiopulmonary and anesthetic risk. Although most procedures that are performed using a perineal approach have higher recurrence rates than do transabdominal procedures, they are excellent alternatives for high-risk patients and for patients who wish to avoid pelvic dissection, particularly men who will not accept a small risk for sexual dysfunction.

Technical aspects of laparoscopic abdominal procedures for rectal prolapse

Good-risk patients who have rectal prolapse and constipation should be considered for laparoscopic sigmoid resection and rectopexy. The left colon is mobilized from mid-descending colon to the sacral promontory. The presacral space is entered, and the rectum and mesorectum are mobilized posteriorly to the coccyx. The hypogastric nerves are preserved by sweeping them posteriorly. Anterior mobilization of the rectovaginal septum usually is unnecessary. Risk for recurrence may be lessened by dividing the lateral stalks; however, postoperative constipation may be worsened by this maneuver [45]. The rectum is elevated and straightened, and several nonabsorbable sutures are placed between the lateral perirectal tissue and the presacral fascia, just inferior to the sacral promontory. Resection of the redundant sigmoid is performed. An interesting question is whether to divide the inferior mesenteric or superior rectal artery, as opposed to sparing this vessel and dividing the sigmoid mesentery closer to the colon. An argument can be made for the latter, because if recurrence of prolapse does occur, the option of perineal rectosigmoidectomy is available. The rectopexy sutures are tied after the redundant sigmoid colon is resected and end-to-end anastomosis is performed. If a Pfannenstiel's or lower midline incision is used, the rectopexy can be performed directly through the incision. This allows the surgeon easy access in case of bleeding from the basivertebral veins. If a left lower quadrant or umbilical extraction incision is used, the rectopexy and anastomosis are performed laparoscopically.

The advantages of resection/rectopexy are preservation of the native compliant rectum, removal of redundant sigmoid colon, alleviation of constipation, and low recurrence rate ($<3\%$). Imperfect anal incontinence is not a contraindication to a rectopexy. Continence will improve in 35% to 60% of patients, and if it does not, a sphincteroplasty can be considered at a later time [46]. Disadvantages are related mainly to the magnitude of the procedure. Most patients who have rectal prolapse are older, debilitated, and tolerate abdominal surgery less well than do younger, healthy patients. Additionally, the complication of anastomotic leak can be devastating. Anterior resection of the rectosigmoid without rectal fixation is not used commonly to treat rectal prolapse, because recurrence rates are much higher than after resection/rectopexy.

An alternative transabdominal procedure that avoids the complication of anastomotic leak is sacral fixation of the prolapsing rectum (rectopexy). The rectum is mobilized to the pelvic floor as described above. The rectum is straightened and suspended from the presacral fascia. The rectopexy can be performed using nonabsorbable sutures, as described above, or by using a sling of prosthetic material. A variety of materials has been used to fashion the sling, although prosthetic mesh is used most commonly. If mesh is being used, this can be tacked to the upper rectum using endoscopic staples, as are used for laparoscopic hernia repair [47]. The original sling technique, as described by Ripstein [47a], created a circumferential wrap around the rectum. Because a substantial fraction of patients developed obstructive symptoms or stool impaction proximal to the wrap, many surgeons now leave the anterior surface of the rectum free, using a partial wrap. There is no difference in the type of mesh used with regard to complication rate, recurrence rate, or functional outcome. Laparoscopic rectopexy alone is an attractive choice for some patients who have rectal prolapse because an incision is unnecessary, and there is no risk for anastomotic leak. Patients who are unable to tolerate laparotomy should not be chosen for this procedure, because bleeding from the basivertebral veins or other complication may necessitate conversion to laparotomy.

Rectopexy is an effective procedure for rectal prolapse, with recurrence rates of less than 5% in most series; however, constipation is not relieved by rectopexy and can be worsened. Occasionally, a stricture can be demonstrated at the site of the wrap, but most cases of constipation probably are secondary to preexisting colonic dysmotility. Preoperative colonic transit studies may help to guide the selection of rectopexy alone versus resection/rectopexy for patients who have rectal prolapse and constipation [48]. Patients who have rectal prolapse and enterocele or large rectocele may be considered for a combined pelvic floor repair.

Outcomes of laparoscopic repair of rectal prolapse

Laparoscopic repair of rectal prolapse was described first in 1992, and since then numerous laparoscopic techniques have been reported, including sutureless rectopexy, suture rectopexy, proctosigmoidectomy, resection/rectopexy, and mesh rectopexy. The potential benefits of laparoscopic repair include early return of gastrointestinal function, less postoperative pain, better cosmesis, and shorter hospital stay. A recent meta-analysis combined data from six studies in the literature that compared laparoscopic with open rectopexy [49]. Not surprisingly, laparoscopic rectopexy required 60 minutes longer to perform than did open rectopexy. Laparoscopic rectopexy required 3.5 days fewer in the hospital on average. Overall operative morbidity was similar between the groups. Recurrence rates were similar;

however, follow-up generally was short, and ranged from 12 to 31 months. No studies with long-term follow-up are available.

Costs and quality of life

The costs of, and quality of life after, laparoscopic surgery for rectal prolapse have not been compared rigorously with those associated with open procedures. It would not be surprising, however, if the short-term costs are higher with the laparoscopic approach. As with other laparoscopic procedures, the long-term costs are difficult to assess. Issues, such as long-term recurrence rates and adhesive bowel obstruction rates, need to be taken into account.

Summary

With the increasing popularity of minimally invasive approaches to surgery, laparoscopic techniques are being applied increasingly to more complex procedures. Surgeons who are interested in gaining skill and confidence with the techniques of rectal mobilization and resection initially should consider attempting procedures for benign disease. Patients who have rectal prolapse, who often have wide, accommodating pelvic anatomy, are the logical choice with whom to begin the laparoscopic rectal experience. Laparoscopic restorative proctocolectomy is more technically challenging. Laparoscopic proctectomy for rectal cancer probably should remain in the hands of well-trained, high-volume, experienced surgeons who have built a dedicated team for treatment of these patients, and who track their outcomes prospectively.

References

[1] Read TE, Myerson RJ, Fleshman JW, et al. Surgeon specialty is associated with outcome in rectal cancer treatment. Dis Colon Rectum 2002;45:904–14.
[2] Holm T, Johansson H, Cedermark B, et al. Influence of hospital- and surgeon-related factors on outcome after treatment of rectal cancer with or without preoperative radiotherapy. Br J Surg 1997;84:657–63.
[3] Porter GA, Soskolne CL, Yakimets WW, et al. Surgeon-related factors and outcome in rectal cancer. Ann Surg 1998;227:157–67.
[4] McArdle CS, Hole D. Impact of variability among surgeons on postoperative morbidity and mortality and ultimate survival. BMJ 1991;302:1501–5.
[5] Kapiteijn E, Marijnen CA, Nagtegaal ID, et al. Preoperative radiotherapy combined with total mesorectal excision for resectable rectal cancer. N Engl J Med 2001;345:638–46.
[6] Pietrabissa A, Moretto C, Carobbi A, et al. Hand-assisted laparoscopic low anterior resection: initial experience with a new procedure. Surg Endosc 2002;16:431–5.
[7] Kockerling F, Gastinger I, Schneider B, et al. Laparoscopic abdominoperineal excision of the rectum with high ligation of the inferior mesenteric artery in the management of rectal carcinoma. Endosc Surg Allied Technol 1993;1:16–9.

[8] Kim J, Shim M, Kwun K. Laparoscopic-assisted transvaginal resection of the rectum. Dis Colon Rectum 1996;39:582–3.

[9] Vithiananthan S, Cooper Z, Betten K, et al. Hybrid laparoscopic flexure takedown and open procedure for rectal resection is associated with significantly shorter length of stay than equivalent open resection. Dis Colon Rectum 2001;44:927–35.

[10] Leung KL, Kwok SP, Lau WY, et al. Laparoscopic-assisted abdominoperineal resection for low rectal adenocarcinoma. Surg Endosc 2000;14:67–70.

[11] Yamamoto S, Watanabe M, Hasegawa H, et al. Prospective evaluation of laparoscopic surgery for rectosigmoidal and rectal carcinoma. Dis Colon Rectum 2002;45:1648–54.

[12] Monson JR, Darzi A, Carey PD, et al. Prospective evaluation of laparoscopic-assisted colectomy in an unselected group of patients. Lancet 1992;340:831–3.

[13] Lacy A, Garcia-Valdecasas J, Delgado S, et al. Postoperative complications of laparoscopic-assisted colectomy. Surg Endosc 1996;11:119–22.

[14] Kockerling F, Rose J, Schneider C, et al. Laparoscopic colorectal anastomosis: risk of postoperative leakage. Results of a multicenter study. Laparoscopic Colorectal Surgery Study Group (LCSSG). Surg Endosc 1999;13:639–44.

[15] Kockerling F, Scheidbach H, Schneider C, et al. Laparoscopic abdominoperineal resection: early postoperative results of a prospective study involving 116 patients. The Laparoscopic Colorectal Surgery Study Group. Dis Colon Rectum 2000;43:1503–11.

[16] Huscher C, Silecchia G, Croce E, et al. Laparoscopic colorectal resection. A multicenter Italian study. Surg Endosc 1996;10:875–9.

[17] Fleshman JW, Wexner SD, Anvari M, et al. Laparoscopic vs. open abdominoperineal resection for cancer. Dis Colon Rectum 1999;42:930–9.

[18] Lord SA, Larach SW, Ferrara A, et al. Laparoscopic resections for colorectal carcinoma. A three-year experience. Dis Colon Rectum 1996;39:148–54.

[19] Leung KL, Kwok SP, Lau WY, et al. Laparoscopic-assisted resection of rectosigmoid carcinoma. Immediate and medium-term results. Arch Surg 1997;132:761–4 [discussion 765].

[20] Patankar SK, Larach SW, Ferrara A, et al. Prospective comparison of laparoscopic vs. open resections for colorectal adenocarcinoma over a ten-year period. Dis Colon Rectum 2003;46:601–11.

[21] Morino M, Parini U, Giraudo G, et al. Laparoscopic total mesorectal excision: a consecutive series of 100 patients. Ann Surg 2003;237:335–42.

[22] Schiedeck TH, Schwandner O, Baca I, et al. Laparoscopic surgery for the cure of colorectal cancer: results of a German five-center study. Dis Colon Rectum 2000;43:1–8.

[23] Hartley JE, Mehigan BJ, Qureshi AE, et al. Total mesorectal excision: assessment of the laparoscopic approach. Dis Colon Rectum 2001;44:315–21.

[24] Lezoche E, Feliciotti F, Paganini AM, et al. Results of laparoscopic versus open resections for non-early rectal cancer in patients with a minimum follow-up of four years. Hepatogastroenterology 2002;49:1185–90.

[25] Poulin EC, Schlachta CM, Gregoire R, et al. Local recurrence and survival after laparoscopic mesorectal resection for rectal adenocarcinoma. Surg Endosc 2002;16:989–95.

[26] Scheidbach H, Schneider C, Konradt J, et al. Laparoscopic abdominoperineal resection and anterior resection with curative intent for carcinoma of the rectum. Surg Endosc 2002;16:7–13.

[27] Anthuber M, Fuerst A, Elser F, et al. Outcome of laparoscopic surgery for rectal cancer in 101 patients. Dis Colon Rectum 2003;46:1047–53.

[28] Guillou PJ, Quirke P, Thorpe H, et al. Short-term endpoints of conventional versus laparoscopic-assisted surgery in patients with colorectal cancer (MRC CLASICC trial): multicentre, randomised controlled trial. Lancet 2005;365:1718–26.

[29] Ritchie WP Jr, Rhodes RS, Biester TW. Work loads and practice patterns of general surgeons in the United States, 1995–1997: a report from the American Board of Surgery. Ann Surg 1999;230:533–42 [discussion 542–3].

[30] Wheeler HB. Myth and reality in general surgery. Bull Am Coll Surg 1993;78:21–7.

[31] Goldstein ET. Outcomes of anorectal disease in a health maintenance organization setting. The need for colorectal surgeons. Dis Colon Rectum 1996;39:1193–8.

[32] Schoetz DJ Jr. Colon and rectal surgery: a true subspecialty. Dis Colon Rectum 1998;41: 1–10.

[33] Delaney CP, Kiran RP, Senagore AJ, et al. Case-matched comparison of clinical and financial outcome after laparoscopic or open colorectal surgery. Ann Surg 2003;238:67–72.

[34] Chapman AE, Levitt MD, Hewett P, et al. Laparoscopic-assisted resection of colorectal malignancies: a systematic review. Ann Surg 2001;234:590–606.

[35] Patel NA, Bergamaschi R. Laparoscopy for diverticulitis. Semin Laparosc Surg 2003;10: 177–83.

[36] Koea JB, Guillem JG, Conlon KC, et al. Role of laparoscopy in the initial multimodality management of patients with near-obstructing rectal cancer. J Gastrointest Surg 2000;4: 105–8.

[37] Kienle P, Weitz J, Benner A, et al. Laparoscopically assisted colectomy and ileoanal pouch procedure with and without protective ileostomy. Surg Endosc 2003;17:716–20.

[38] Larson DW, Dozois EJ, Piotrowicz K, et al. Laparoscopic-assisted vs. open ileal pouch-anal anastomosis: functional outcome in a case-matched series. Dis Colon Rectum 2005; 48:1845–50.

[39] Marcello PW, Milsom JW, Wong SK, et al. Laparoscopic restorative proctocolectomy: case-matched comparative study with open restorative proctocolectomy. Dis Colon Rectum 2000;43:604–8.

[40] Rivadeneira DE, Marcello PW, Roberts PL, et al. Benefits of hand-assisted laparoscopic restorative proctocolectomy: a comparative study. Dis Colon Rectum 2004;47:1371–6.

[41] Reissman P, Salky BA, Pfeifer J, et al. Laparoscopic surgery in the management of inflammatory bowel disease. Am J Surg 1996;171:47–50 [discussion 50–1].

[42] Ky AJ, Sonoda T, Milsom JW. One-stage laparoscopic restorative proctocolectomy: an alternative to the conventional approach? Dis Colon Rectum 2002;45:207–10 [discussion 210–1].

[43] Schmitt SL, Cohen SM, Wexner SD, et al. Does laparoscopic-assisted ileal pouch anal anastomosis reduce the length of hospitalization? Int J Colorectal Dis 1994;9:134–7.

[44] Maartense S, Dunker MS, Slors JF, et al. Hand-assisted laparoscopic versus open restorative proctocolectomy with ileal pouch anal anastomosis: a randomized trial. Ann Surg 2004;240:984–91 [discussion 991–2].

[45] Scaglia M, Fasth S, Hallgren T, et al. Abdominal rectopexy for rectal prolapse. Influence of surgical technique on functional outcome. Dis Colon Rectum 1994;37:805–13.

[46] Farouk R, Duthie GS, Bartolo DC, et al. Restoration of continence following rectopexy for rectal prolapse and recovery of the internal anal sphincter electromyogram. Br J Surg 1992; 79:439–40.

[47] Solomon MJ, Young CJ, Eyers AA, et al. Randomized clinical trial of laparoscopic versus open abdominal rectopexy for rectal prolapse. Br J Surg 2002;89:35–9.

[47a] Ripstein CB. Procidentia: definitive corrective surgery. Dis Colon Rectum 1972;15(5): 334–6.

[48] McKee RF, Lauder JC, Poon FW, et al. A prospective randomized study of abdominal rectopexy with and without sigmoidectomy in rectal prolapse. Surg Gynecol Obstet 1992;174: 145–8.

[49] Purkayastha S, Tekkis P, Athanasiou T, et al. A comparison of open vs. laparoscopic abdominal rectopexy for full-thickness rectal prolapse: a meta-analysis. Dis Colon Rectum 2005;48:1930–40.

ELSEVIER
SAUNDERS

SURGICAL
CLINICS OF
NORTH AMERICA

Surg Clin N Am 86 (2006) 915–925

Transanal Endoscopic Microsurgery

Peter A. Cataldo, MD

*Department of Surgery, University of Vermont, College of Medicine,
Fletcher 462, MCHV Campus, Burlington, VT 05401, USA*

Transanal endoscopic microsurgery (TEM) involves the use of specialized equipment including an operating proctoscope, insufflation, and magnified, stereoscopic vision to improve the accessibility, visualization, and precision of resection of lesions throughout the rectum. Limitations on local resection based on the anal sphincter and boney confines of the pelvis are overcome by this equipment. Although lesions previously unreachable transanally have become accessible with the use of TEM, this does not change the indications for local excision of rectal masses, particularly rectal cancer. Careful preoperative evaluation and appropriate patient selection remain the most important predictors of outcome and must be steadfastly adhered to as new technology is used to treat old problems.

TEM is unique when compared with other minimally invasive techniques, particularly abdominal laparoscopic surgery. Laparoscopic surgery, though innovative and beneficial, does not allow surgeons to perform any procedures previously not possible. TEM allows surgeons to transanally excise lesions that previously were inaccessible. Before the advent of TEM, any large, colonoscopically unresectable polyp in the mid-rectum necessitated an anterior resection via a transabdominal approach. With TEM, these polyps can now be accessed and excised without a cutaneous incision, usually as an outpatient procedure.

TEM has been available for almost 20 years and is commonly used in Europe and Great Britain, but it has been slow to "catch on" in the United States. This is likely because the equipment is expensive, the procedure is difficult to master, and the indications are limited. With the expanding role of local excision of benign and selected malignant masses in the rectum, TEM is now gaining greater acceptance in the United States. Regional centers treating large volumes of rectal cancer are embracing TEM with early, encouraging results.

E-mail address: peter.cataldo@vtmednet.org

Indications

TEM provides access to the entire rectum, therefore any lesions or abnormalities within the rectum are potentially amenable to TEM. However, technical feasibility is not equivalent to appropriateness. Indications can be neatly divided into benign and malignant categories. In the case of benign disease, any lesion that can be safely excised or corrected with minimal functional consequences is appropriate. For malignancy, the technical ability to excise the lesion must be combined with the ability to cure the disease (particularly compared with conventional approaches) when selecting patients for TEM.

Benign diseases

The most common indication for TEM is the excision of large, colonoscopically unresectable rectal polyps. This was the reason TEM was developed. In this situation, TEM can spare patients from major abdominal surgery. Polyps throughout the rectum are amenable to this approach, and although large size and proximal rectal location make the procedure technically challenging, they are not contraindications. With experience, even circumferential polyps can be excised as full-thickness sleeve resections of the rectum with complete anastomosis being performed using TEM. In addition, other benign rectal and extrarectal masses can also be excised such as carcinoids, retrorectal cysts, and masses within the anovaginal septum. TEM has also been effectively used to treat anastomotic strictures, rectal prolapse, high extrasphincteric fistulae and for transrectal drainage of pelvic collections (Box 1).

Box 1. Indications for TEM

Benign
Rectal polyps
Carcinoid tumors
Retrorectal masses
Anastomotic strictures
Extrasphincteric fistulae
Pelvic abscess

Malignant
Malignant polyps
T_1–T_2 rectal cancer
Palliative excision of T_3 cancer

Malignant diseases

Local excision of rectal cancer continues to be a controversial topic, with advocates and detractors adamantly defending their respective positions in the absence of confirming scientific evidence. To this date, there are no randomized, prospective trials comparing local excision to radical resection stage by stage for rectal cancer. Extensive review of the available literature yields evidence for and against local excision. Some retrospective analyses indicate that local recurrence is unacceptably high following local excision [1], while others indicate similar local recurrence rates and overall survival when compared with more radical approaches [2].

A reasonable approach advocated by many is detailed below. The primary goal must be cure of the rectal cancer, minimizing local recurrence and maximizing patient survival. In potentially curable patients, transanal ultrasound or MRI should be performed to identify depth of invasion (T stage) and lymph node status (N stage). All patients with perirectal lymphadenopathy (stage III) should be offered radical resection, because TEM cannot evaluate and treat regional lymph nodes. T_1 lesions (confined to the mucosa and submucosa) are ideal candidates. In addition, T_2 lesions, although more controversial, can also be successfully treated with local excision if combined with postoperative chemoradiotherapy [3].

If final histologic evaluation identifies lymphovascular invasion or poor differentiation, even in T_1 lesions, the addition of adjuvant radiation and chemotherapy may decrease recurrence rates.

All malignant masses mandate full-thickness excision. Therefore, anatomic considerations may prevent local excision even if tumor staging is appropriate. In large lesions, full-thickness excision and primary closure can lead to loss of rectal volume or strictures creating poor functional results, particularly when combined with pelvic radiation. Proximal, anterior, or lateral tumors will be within the peritoneal cavity and full-thickness excision will result in intraperitoneal penetration. This is not a contraindication to TEM, but does make the procedure technically more challenging and the consequences of suture line disruption greater (intraperitoneal sepsis). Additionally, the theoretical disadvantages of intraperitoneal tumor cell dissemination may be potentially worrisome.

T_3 (full-thickness extension) lesions are not appropriate for TEM except in unusual circumstances. If medical comorbidity precludes a transabdominal approach, then TEM may be used in combination with chemoradiation. However, supportive evidence is limited, and survival rates are likely lower than radical approaches. Some patients with very distal tumors may refuse abdominal approaches based on the need for permanent colostomy. TEM may be used to excise these lesions, even if T_3, but recurrence rates will be higher.

Some centers advocate preoperative chemoradiotherapy followed by local excision. Significant downstaging has been identified, and these patients may benefit from local excision [4]. Experience with this approach is limited and widespread application should await further evidence.

Anatomic considerations

The rectum is both an intra- and extraperitoneal organ. The relationship between the peritoneal reflection and the rectum varies from patient to patient but follows general patterns. The peritoneum sweeps over and around the rectum from posterior to anterior in a cephalad-to-caudad fashion, creating a relatively consistent relationship between the rectum and the peritoneal cavity. Posteriorly, the entire rectum is extraperitoneal; laterally, the proximal one third is intraperitoneal and the distal two thirds are extraperitoneal. Anteriorly, the proximal two thirds are intraperitoneal and only the distal one third is extraperitoneal. The distal one third of the rectum is also immediately adjacent to the vagina in females and the prostate in the males. These anatomic factors are particularly important, because TEM allows access to proximal portions of the rectum inaccessible with traditional transanal techniques.

If anterior lesions are resected, both intraperitoneal entry (with possible subsequent peritonitis) and rectovaginal or rectourethral fistulae can occur. These lesions should be approached only if the surgeon is very comfortable and proficient in suture closure of the rectal defect. Resection of lateral and posterior lesions is less challenging, because these portions of the rectum are normally extraperitoneal (except for the most proximal rectum); furthermore, defects can be closed or left open after resection, because the extraperitoneal rectum heals well by secondary intention. It is best, however, to repair all defects as patients heal faster and surgeons gain experience and familiarity with TEM suture techniques, which are necessary in more complex resections.

Equipment

TEM equipment was developed by Wolf Surgical Instruments Company (Vernon Hills, Illinois). It is available through Wolf and just recently through Storz (Karl Storz GmbH & Co., Tuttlingen, Germany) as well. It is provided as a prepackaged set containing everything necessary to perform TEM. Visualization is facilitated by rectal insufflation and pneumorectum; therefore, the system must be air-tight. This is accomplished by using 40-mm diameter proctoscopes (of various lengths up to 20 cm) (Fig. 1) with a removable faceplate with four ports for instrument access. The four ports include one for the optical stereoscope (Fig. 2), one for suction, and two for the instruments necessary to perform TEM (Fig. 3). Attached to the stereoscope and faceplate are conduits for insufflation, irrigation (to clean the lens), a light cord, and a pressure transducer (which constantly measures

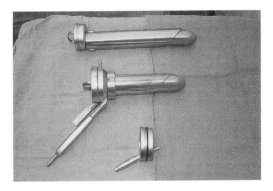

Fig. 1. Proctoscopes.

intrarectal pressure). The stereoscope is a 10-mm optical instrument with a 50-degree downward viewing angle, a 75-degree field of view, and two eyepieces for stereoscopic, three-dimensional vision (Fig. 2). A 40-degree, 5-mm scope is inserted along side the stereoscope to which a laparoscopic camera can be attached, allowing the procedure to be viewed on a standard laparoscopic monitor.

TEM is facilitated by a dedicated Wolf insufflator. This unit provides for simultaneous CO_2 insufflation and continuous measurement of intrarectal pressure. Standard laparoscopic insufflators can also be used; however, with most units, insufflation and measurement of pressure are performed through one port. This leads to intermittent changes in rectal volume each time the pressure is measured (insufflation stops to measure pressure) and is manifest by slight movements in the operating field. A dedicated roller-pump suction unit enables suction without losing pneurorectum.

All operating instruments are 5 mm in diameter, and most have tips with a downward deflection (Fig. 3). The stereoscopic lens provides 50-degree-angle viewing, thus the operating field is in the "lower half" of the rectal lumen; therefore, downward-angled instruments facilitate access to the

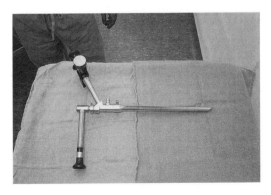

Fig. 2. Optical stereoscope.

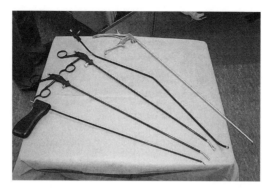

Fig. 3. Instruments necessary to perform TEM.

operative field. Instruments include graspers, cautery, needle holders, scissors, and "b.b." appliers (b.b.'s are placed at the beginning and end of each suture in place of tying knots).

The entire apparatus is held in place by the "Martin Arm," a unique "multi-elbowed" holder attached to the operating table. This allows the proctoscope to be placed precisely in the desired position and to be locked in place. This device is infinitely adjustable and facilitates excellent exposure anywhere in the rectum (and can be readjusted throughout the operation).

A trainer is also available for training residents or fellows and for maintaining or improving skills between cases.

Setup and patient positioning

Proper positioning is essential to ensure successful removal of rectal masses with TEM. The stereoscope and the majority of the instruments are manufactured with a 50-degree downward angle. This allows the instruments to pass through the "top half" of the operating proctoscope while viewing and reaching lesions in the "bottom half" of the exposed rectum. Therefore, it is important that the lesion be located in the bottom half of the viewing field or in the portion of the rectum closest to the operating room floor. This is accomplished by orienting the patient properly on the operating room table as follows: For posterior lesions, the patient is positioned in modified lithotomy; for anterior lesions, the patient is prone; for left-sided lesions, the left side is down; and so forth. This is facilitated by the use of "split leg" attachments for lateral and prone positions, and with padded stirrups for lithotomy.

Once the patient is positioned properly, the anus is gently dilated and the proctoscope inserted. The scope is manipulated until the lesion is visible in the lower half of the operating field and secured in place with the Martin Arm. The external monitor is positioned where it can be comfortably viewed. The insufflator and suction are positioned at the foot of the table where the tubing can easily reach the operating field. The scrub nurse is positioned at the opposite foot. The surgeon sits between the patient's legs with the table adjusted to a comfortable operating height.

Proper setup and positioning is essential and can be the difference between a simple, well-performed TEM and a difficult operative struggle. If the lesion is properly positioned in the operative field and is not overly large, the entire resection can often be performed without repositioning the equipment.

Operative technique

TEM can be separated into three distinct components, all equally important: patient positioning, equipment setup, and lesion removal. As previously mentioned, the orientation of the lesion should be confirmed (by way of digital examination or rigid proctoscopy) and the patient should be positioned so that the tumor is oriented toward the floor. The patient's legs should then be positioned appropriately so that the anal area is accessible and unencumbered movement of the TEM instruments is possible.

Once this is accomplished, the TEM instrumentation can be set up and inserted. The anus is gently dilated with 3 fingers and the operating proctoscope inserted. The windowed faceplate and manual bellows are attached, allowing the surgeon to operate the operating proctoscope identical to a standard rigid proctoscope. The scope is advanced until the lesion is visible in the lower half of the viewing field. The scope is then attached to the Martin Arm, which is tightened to fix the operating proctoscope in the desired position.

The standard TEM faceplate is then attached to the operating proctoscope and the stereoscope and remote viewing scopes are inserted. Following this, the TEM insufflator/pressure monitor/roller-pump suction apparatus is activated, and the TEM tubing is attached (which, incidentally, is no simple task). There are four separate pieces of tubing, each of which must be properly attached in the proper sequence—otherwise, the equipment will not function properly. One tube is responsible for continuous insufflation, a second for continuous monitoring and regulation of intrarectal pressure, a third for irrigation of the optical lens and the operative field, and a fourth for roller-pump suction (standard suction will deflate the rectal lumen instantly).

Once the equipment has been properly set up and satisfactory visualization of the lesion has been confirmed, the excision can begin. Local anesthetic containing epinephrine is infiltrated around and under the lesion to aid in hemostasis through a long needle (a laparoscopic needle for gallbladder decompression works well). Five-millimeter margins are then marked by way of electrocauterization. The excision can be performed in the submucosal plane or through the full-thickness of the rectal wall. Full-thickness excisions are technically easier and appropriate for all malignant lesions or in any lesions where malignancy is suspected. Large benign polyps can be excised in the submucosal plane.

For both submucosal and full-thickness excisions, the dissection proceeds from distal to proximal and from right to left. The mass is elevated with a grasper, and electrocauterization is applied to enter the correct operative plane; the yellow perirectal fat indicates the proper full-thickness plane, and the transversely oriented inner circular rectal muscular fibers confirm proper submucosal resection. Once the proper plane has been entered, the lesion is further elevated and the dissection continues from proximal to distal and from right to left. It is important to correctly identify the proximal extent of resection to avoid unnecessary proximal dissection and extrarectal resection. (It is easy to undermine too far proximally if care is not taken to frequently visualize the premarked proximal resection margin). After the lesion is excised, the faceplate is removed and the lesion is retrieved through the operating proctoscope.

After excising the mass, the defect is closed. Distal posterior rectal defects can be left open if necessary, because this portion of the rectum is extraperitoneal and intraperitoneal extension is highly unlikely. All other defects should be closed, because unrecognized intraperitoneal penetration will lead to peritonitis if the defect is not closed completely. It is best to close all defects if possible, because this will improve operative technique and hasten postoperative recovery.

Defects are closed with intraluminal suturing. Silver b.b.'s are attached at the beginning and end of each suture in lieu of knots, because the narrow operating space makes knot-tying difficult. All defects are closed transversely to prevent narrowing of the lumen. Large defects are bisected with a single suture to bring the proximal and distal ends into proximity and to ensure proper orientation. Once this is accomplished, the defect is closed with running suture from the lateral margins to the middle. With large resections and closures, it is possible to become disoriented and to completely occlude the lumen. Therefore, it is essential to perform rigid proctoscopy following closure to ensure an adequate postoperative lumen. With these techniques, the experienced operator can excise very large rectal masses. For large, benign, circumferential lesions, a complete sleeve resection of the rectum with full-thickness intestinal anastomosis can be performed. Following resection, the specimen is pinned to a cork board to facilitate pathologic evaluation (Fig. 4).

Results

Outcomes or results following TEM can be divided into three categories: (1) early postoperative complications and outcomes, (2) functional results, (3) and (in the treatment of malignancy) oncologic outcomes. All three are distinct and individually important. A patient with a smooth, uncomplicated, postoperative recovery receives little benefit if left with long-term

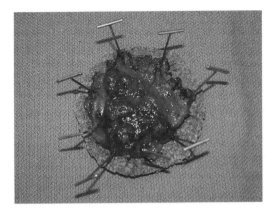

Fig. 4. Specimen pinned to corkboard to facilitate pathologic evaluation.

incontinence. Similarly, a patient with perfect postoperative functional results gains little from TEM if recurrent cancer develops.

TEM is generally performed as an outpatient procedure in the United
States and is associated with a brief inpatient stay in Europe. Average
lengths of stay vary. Cataldo and colleagues [5] reported a 0.9-day mean
length of stay in a previous series, Smith and colleagues [6] reported a range
of 0 to 3 days, and Demartines and colleagues (in Switzerland) [7] reported
a mean 5.5-day length of stay.

Complications are rare but can be significant; they include intraperitoneal
sepsis, rectovaginal fistula, suture line disruption, and hemorrhage. Demartines and colleagues [7] identified a 14% complication rate in 50 patients,
including intraperitoneal entry in 2 patients (4%), urinary tract infection
in 4 patients (8%), and myocardial infarction in 1 patient (2%). Steele noted
5 complications in 100 patients. Intraperitoneal entry in 1 patient required
conversion to a laparotomy; there were 2 cases of incontinence, 1 case of rectal stenosis, and a single postoperative cardiac death [8]. In 334 patients,
Mentges and colleagues [9] reported a 0.3% mortality rate and a 5.5% major complication rate (3 intraperitoneal sepsis; 3 rectovaginal fistulae; 7 postoperative hemorrhage requiring reoperation). In a systematic review of 55
reports, Middleton and colleagues [10] identified a complication rate of
10.3%, compared with 17% for standard local excision.

Several investigators have studied the functional consequences following
TEM. Kreis and colleagues [11] found anal dilatation and insertion of the
40-mm TEM proctoscope to be associated with a temporary decrease in
postoperative continence. Kennedy and colleagues [12] identified decreased
anal resting pressure (as identified with manometry) postoperatively, but no
diminution in clinical continence. Herman and colleagues [13] identified preoperative alterations in continence to be predictive of poor postoperative
function. In addition, resections of greater than 50% of the rectal wall

caused decreased rectal compliance and poor functional outcome. Cataldo and colleagues [5] compared the validated functional assessment and quality of life tools Fecal Incontinence Severity Index and Fecal Incontinence Quality of Life Scale preoperatively and at 6 weeks postoperatively (each patient serving as his/her own control) and found no decrease in clinical continence following TEM. In summary, most authors found TEM to be associated with some minor temporary changes in defecatory function, but permanent dysfunction was rare.

Regarding oncologic results, many studies report results with early stage rectal cancers. Some report results following excision of benign adenomas as well. With respect to local excision of rectal cancer, results are widely reported and are variable. Several authors specifically report their outcomes following TEM. Buess reported a 4% local recurrence rate following TEM for T_1 rectal cancer (2/46) and a 20% local recurrence rate (1/5) following resection of T_3 lesions. All patients were salvaged with radical surgery [10]. Steele and colleagues [9] followed 23 patients with carcinoma undergoing TEM and found 0% recurrence for T_1 lesions, 14% recurrence for T_2 lesions, and 0% recurrence for T_3 lesions. T_2 and T_3 lesions were treated with postoperative chemoradiotherapy. Floyd and Saclarides [14] identified 2 recurrences in 75 patients undergoing TEM for T_1 rectal cancer, both of which were salvaged with radical resections, for a 0% cancer specific mortality. In a systematic review of 58 reports, Middleton and colleagues [11] found local recurrence to be significantly less common (6%) following TEM when compared with traditional transanal approaches (22%).

It is clear that TEM is a safe procedure associated with a shorter hospital stay and lower perioperative morbidity and mortality when compared with transabdominal rectal resections. No studies have compared functional results between TEM and abdominal/rectal resections, but TEM appears to be associated with minimal functional consequences.

Finally, oncologic results vary, but TEM seems to be associated with lower local recurrence rates when compared with standard transanal excisions, and for early stage rectal cancer may provide identical oncologic outcomes to radical resection.

Summary

TEM has been used effectively to treat large rectal polyps and early rectal malignancy for more than 20 years in Europe. Until recently, only a few specialized centers offered TEM in the United States, where it is now gaining popularity. Many hospitals have purchased equipment and are offering TEM; however, the equipment is expensive and the learning curve is steep. Therefore, it is essential that anyone performing TEM have an adequate number of cases to develop and maintain expertise in this technique. That being said, TEM remains unique when compared with laparoscopy and other minimally invasive techniques that incorporate less invasive methods of performing old operations. TEM allows surgeons to perform operations that were impossible before the development and acceptance of this technique.

Acknowledgment

I would like to thank Tina Blais-Armell for her help in preparing the manuscript.

References

[1] Rothenberger RA, Garcia-Aguilar J. Role of local excision in the treatment of rectal cancer. Sem Surg Oncol 2000;19:367–75.

[2] Rosenthal SA, Yeung RS, Weese JL, et al. Conservative management of extensive low-lying rectal carcinomas with transanal local excision and combined preoperative and postoperative radiation therapy: a report of a phase I–II trial. Cancer 1992;69:335–41.

[3] LeVoyer TE, Hoffman JP, Cooper H, et al. Local excision and chemoradiation for low rectal T1 and T2 cancers is an effective treatment. Am Surg 1999;65:625–31.

[4] Lezoche E, Guerrieri M, Paganini AM, et al. Long-term results in patients with T2–3 N0 distal rectal cancer undergoing radiotherapy before transanal endoscopic microsurgery. Br J Surg 2005;92:1546–52.

[5] Cataldo PA, O'Brien S, Osler T. Transanal endoscopic microsurgery: a prospective evaluation of functional results. Dis Col Rectum 2005;48:1366–71.

[6] Smith LE, Ko ST, Saclarides T, et al. Transanal endoscopic microsurgery: initial registry results. Dis Col Rectum 1996;39:S79–84.

[7] Demartines N, von Flüe MO, Harder FH. Transanal endoscopic microsurgical exicision of rectal tumors: indications and results. World J Surg 2001;25:870–5.

[8] Steele RJ, Hershman MJ, Mortensen NJ, et al. Transanal endoscopic microsurgery: initial experience from three centers in the United Kingdom. Br J Surg 1996;83:207–10.

[9] Mentges B, Buess G, Schäfer D, et al. Local therapy of rectal tumors. Dis Col Rectum 1996; 39:886–92.

[10] Middleton PF, Sutherland LM, Maddern GJ. Transanal endoscopic microsurgery: a systematic review. Dis Col Rectum 2005;48:270–84.

[11] Kreis ME, Jehle EC, Haug V, et al. Functional results after transanal endoscopic microsurgery. Dis Col Rectum 1996;39:1116–21.

[12] Kennedy ML, Lubowski DZ, King W. Transanal endoscopic microsurgery excision. Dis Col Rectum 2002;45:601–4.

[13] Herman RM, Richter P, Walega P, et al. Anorectal sphincter function and rectal barostat study in patients following transanal endoscopic microsurgery. Int J Colorectal Dis 2001; 6:370–6.

[14] Floyd ND, Saclarides TJ. Transanal endoscopic microsurgical resection of pT_1 rectal tumors. Dis Col Rectum 2006;49:1–5.

ELSEVIER
SAUNDERS

Surg Clin N Am 86 (2006) 927–936

SURGICAL
CLINICS OF
NORTH AMERICA

Robotics in Colorectal Surgery: Telemonitoring and Telerobotics

Richard M. Satava, MD

Department of Surgery, University of Washington Medical Center,
1959 Pacific Street NE, Seattle, WA 98195, USA

Robotics was introduced into the surgical world in 1996 when Computer Motion, Inc. (Goleta, California) produced the first surgical robot called Aesop, a device to control the position of a laparoscopic camera, and later, Zeus, a full-function teleoperated robotic system. Shortly thereafter, Intuitive Surgical, Inc. (Menlo Park, California) introduced the DaVinci system. The result was a flurry of specialties that investigated which procedures would benefit from the advantages of robotics. Initially, cardiac surgery benefited the most, first by using the enhanced dexterity and tremor reduction to perform the arterial anastomoses of coronary artery bypass grafting (CABG); later, cardiac surgeons explored the use in many different procedures, such as mitral valve replacement and atrial septal defect. Urology also discovered the advantages in applying robotics to radical prostatectomy, while a few gynecologists began using it for hysterectomy. Surprisingly, general surgeons have been slow to pick up robotic surgery, possibly because they had had more than a decade of experience with laparoscopic surgery. This experience, along with the fact that most procedures did not require the high precision of anastomoses of CABG or radical prostatectomy, has resulted in a slow adoption within general and gastrointestinal surgery.

The opinions or assertions contained herein are the private views of the author and are not to be construed as official, or as reflecting the views of the Departments of the Army, Navy, or Air Force, the Defense Advanced Research Projects Agency, or the Department of Defense.

This is a declared work of the US Government and as such is not subject to copyright protection in the United States.

E-mail address: rsatava@u.washington.edu

0039-6109/06/$ - see front matter. Published by Elsevier Inc.
doi:10.1016/j.suc.2006.05.005
surgical.theclinics.com

Uses of robotics in surgery

Robotics in colorectal surgery is beginning to gain acceptance slowly. Most of the common procedures have been reported. There are numerous reasons why robotic procedures are not more widespread, including cost, time for set-up, applicability for all cases, and learning curve. Like general surgery, the high precision in anastomosing millimeter and submillimeter structure is required infrequently—colorectal surgery is more on a macro scale than on the micro scale that benefits greatly from robotic enhancement. Additionally, there is not a single "work space" because the colon is distributed throughout the abdomen, and, hence, requires repositioning during surgery. Several surgeons question whether the postoperative recovery is improved significantly over laparoscopic or even open procedures. Yet for those surgeons who have accepted robotic systems, there is strong advocacy.

Other applications for robotics invoke the "tele" part of telerobotics, which permits viewing, monitoring, collaborating, and even performing surgery from a distance. Teleconsultation was the first to be used, which permits a centrally located expert surgeon at a medical center to provide assistance or collaboration during a difficult procedure to a less experienced surgeon at a remote site. There are a few such programs that are thriving, especially in regions where there are underserved populations. It was envisioned that robotics would be used in telementoring, telemonitoring, and teleproctoring to help train and certify surgeons in the new robotic procedures. The reports of these applications have been rather sporadic, and the much anticipated use in teleproctoring for new procedures has not materialized. This is likely due to the amount of time that is required by the centrally located proctor, as well as to the cost of the equipment.

The use for robotics to perform surgery at a distant location (telesurgery) was developed experimentally in the 1990s by Satava and Green [1] and Bowersox and colleagues [2], and was demonstrated clinically first in September, 2001 by Jacques Marescaux of Strasbourg, France. While sitting at the surgical console in New York City, he performed a telerobotic cholecystectomy on his patient in Strasbourg, who was 4000 km away [3]. This truly was a technical tour de force that required an enormous amount of planning and execution to keep the latency (time from hand motion to actual cutting) to within acceptable limits—certainly not a procedure that was able to be reproduced for daily use. There is one remarkable success in actual telesurgery by Mehran Anvari, a general surgeon at McMasters University in Hamilton, Ontario, Canada. On a routine basis Dr. Anvari performs remote surgery in advanced minimal access procedures with a colleague in North Bay, Ontario Canada—approximately 300 miles away [4]. One factor that contributes to this success is that the Canadian health care system provides appropriate reimbursement for the procedure, whereas the system in the United States has a complex arcane reimbursement system that discourages the use of such new advanced systems.

The most common use of telerobotic surgery is during medical conferences. It has become commonplace to have a live video session of a robotic procedure, frequently with interactive audience participation through asking questions of the surgeon during the procedure. The educational value is unquestionable, and, invariably, these sessions are attended heavily.

One use that has not migrated into the colorectal surgery specialty is image-guided surgery. This is common in neurosurgery, urology (kidney and prostate), general surgery (liver and breast), endovascular surgery (carotid, aortic other vessels), and other specialties in which high precision is required for solid organ surgery or precise intravascular localization, usually combined with ablation (eg, thermal, cryo, high-intensity focused ultrasound) or interventional catheter procedures (eg, balloons, stents). The most likely potential use by colorectal surgeons would be for liver metastases, although one might speculate that image guidance could be of value in endoluminal surgery.

Concepts in robotic surgery

One of the most important, but least appreciated, aspects of robotics is its underlying fundamental principle. Most people perceive robots as a machine that is computer controlled. A robot is not a machine: it is an information system with arms (manipulators), legs (locomotion), eyes (vision systems), and so forth. This fact gives robots their enormous value, for as an information system a robot can integrate all of the aspects of operative procedures. While sitting at the surgical console, the surgeon is not looking at the patient, instead one is looking at a video image, which is an information representation of the patient. When the handles are moved, the surgeon is not cutting the patient, one is sending information (electronic signals) to the remote manipulators with the instruments that are doing the cutting. (Because the robotic surgical systems send the information from surgeon to manipulator, the computer can enhance and tremor reduce the signals, which gives the surgeon capabilities that are beyond human physical limitations.) Thus, all of a surgical procedure becomes various aspects of information. For example (Fig. 1), from the surgical console, the surgeon can perform open surgery, minimally invasive surgery, remote telesurgery, and image-guided surgery (by importing CT or MRI scans and fusing them with the video image). One can telementor, telemonitor, and teleproctor. By importing graphical images, the robotic console becomes a surgical simulator and training can be done. Likewise, the hand motions of the surgeon can be recorded (Fig. 2) for feedback to the student, for quality assurance for the practicing surgeon, or potentially as an objective assessment tool for performance assessment and certification. Patient-specific images (eg, CT, MRI) also can be used for preoperative planning or rehearsing a complicated surgical procedure (see later discussion). All of these functions are performed at the console, and integrated as a seamless whole. Additionally, other information

SATAVA

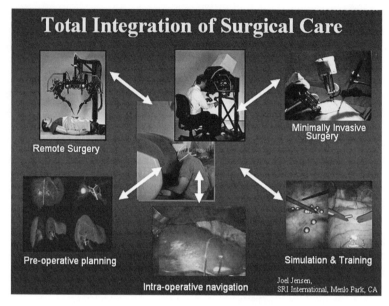

Fig. 1. The integration of surgery as an information system.

(eg, radiographs, laboratory tests, history and physical, pathology reports) can be accessed on-screen during the procedure. This is the power of robots, well beyond their mechanical and telecapabilities.

These capabilities can be augmented because more patients are receiving total body scans. These scans become the information representation of the

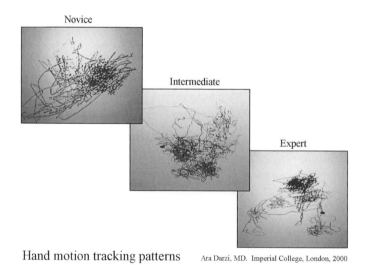

Fig. 2. The "signature" of hand motions as recorded with a tracking device. (Courtesy of Sir Ara Darzi, MD, FRCS, Imperial College, London, UK.)

patient: a holographic medical electronic representation or holomer. This holomer soon will become the electronic health record, which provides text and image as the medical record, and is viewed by the patient and surgeon as a full three-dimensional interactive image of the person. Health care has been the only major industry without a computer representation of their "product"—the patient. The billions of dollars in hardware and software that are used in other industries cannot be applied in surgery. Sophisticated computer-aided design/computer-aided manufacturing (CAD/CAM) programs permit other professionals to design, plan, and prototype their new products, then to test and evaluate the new product virtually before building the first product. Any errors are made on the image, not on the final product. They can rehearse how to use the product, and get consultation on the design or implementation before performing those expensive actions in the real world. Surgeons could learn to do the same—to do preoperative planning, test and evaluate the plan, perform a surgical rehearsal of the procedure, and make mistakes—on the virtual patient rather than upon the real patient. All the while, the robotic system is recording the performance. This cannot be done with any other nonrobotic surgical system that exists today. Surgery has been fragmented for centuries; the surgeon must look at the radiograph, plan the procedure, and operate upon the patient using different mediums and at varying times and places, and the surgeon must perform the procedure correctly the first time, or the patient suffers the consequences. With the robotic system the surgeon can plan and rehearse the procedure (on the patient's own image) until (s)he is convinced that the procedure can be performed without mistake. This has been done for decades in other industries; it is time for health care to join the Information Age.

Emerging and future surgical robotic systems

The future of robotics in colorectal surgery is mainly potential that has yet to be realized. Although there are a few brave pioneers who are pushing the boundaries of what is possible, most "pioneers" have vested heavily in laparoscopic colorectal surgery. Many surgeons want to join the minimally invasive surgery revolution through the use of the "conventional" laparoscopic approach, frequently with the idea that performing laparoscopic surgery is a preliminary step toward robotic surgery. This is a misconception in some part. True, most robotic surgery is performed through minimally invasive ports like laparoscopic surgery; however, the hand motions in robotic surgery are not "backward" as in laparoscopic surgery. The computer of the robotic system compensates for the fulcrum effect, and hand motions are the same as in performing an open procedure. Therefore, the learning curve for robotic surgery is much shorter than for laparoscopic surgery, and more importantly, expertise in laparoscopic surgery is not a prerequisite for performing robotic surgery.

Many emerging surgical systems revolve around the "operating room (OR) of the future," which is where robotic surgery will be performed. There are three variations on planning what the new ORs should be: (1) multifunctional OR—the blending of open, laparoscopic, and image-guided surgery into a single "flexible" OR; (2) perioperative OR—the incorporation of new information systems into the entire operating experience, from preoperative holding and anesthesia, to postoperative recovery; and (3) robotic OR—an OR with no people, in which robot and computer-assisted systems are integrated highly and controlled from just outside of the OR. Each system has decided advantages, and many hospitals are investigating how to incorporate one or more of these new approaches into new or renovated ORs.

Multifunctional operating rooms

Most surgeons who are advocating the multifunctional nature of ORs are focusing on the emerging image-guidance nature of interventional procedures. For solid organ surgery, neurosurgeons, urologists, and general surgeons require the use of real-time imaging (eg, CT or MRI scanning) to localize disease precisely within a solid structure, such as brain, kidney, prostate, liver, or breast. Frequently, the use of imaging is during an open surgical procedure, although interventional radiologists often use image guidance for these procedures without performing an incision. The common need is to confirm the placement of a needle, probe, or other instrument before performing the therapy, such as ablation or excision. Thus, the challenge is to develop an OR that can accommodate a huge imaging system and the needs of a surgical procedure (anesthesia, operating table, surgeon, scrub nurse, surgical instruments). There are pioneering efforts by Taylor and colleagues of Johns Hopkins to incorporate the use of a precision-guided robot with a CT scanner for prostate surgery and ablative procedures [5]. A feature in common to these procedures is the preoperative planning and surgical rehearsal before bringing the patient to the OR, and the need to update the CT or MRI image at the time of the procedure to correspond with the preoperative images and plan. Ferenc Jolesz [6] of Brigham Women's Hospital is basing the OR upon the imaging system, such as open MRI, with the approach being the capability of performing surgery in a radiology suite (rather than imaging within an OR).

Perioperative operating rooms

This emerging concept principally is about the integration of the entire surgical event, from admission to the preoperative holding area until dismissal from the postoperative recovery room, through the use of computers, robotics, and information systems. The pioneers are Sandberg of Brigham and Womens' Hospital and Ganous of University of Maryland Hospital [7]. They view the entire operating area as a single information system process, and look to industry and their current methodologies of efficiently integrating complex systems. Using business and management practices from aviation, retail, and delivery (Federal Express), the patient is viewed as a single "information object" that must be "moved" through flow of a complex process. This integration includes not only the patient and the data about the patient, but shares information among other computers, equipment (eg, OR lights, anesthesia machines), and devices (eg, surgical robots, delivery robotic systems). The technologies to support this revolution include (1) new software management systems, such as just-in-time inventory control, supply chain management, inventory tracking and (2) hardware, such as radiofrequency identification (RFID) tags, standard bar codes, robotic supply dispensers, surgical robots, and intelligent OR tables and lights. A typical scenario includes a patient arriving at the ambulatory surgery desk, registering, and receiving their plastic RFID bracelet. From this moment on, the entire operating theater (and theoretically anywhere in the hospital) could have protected access to the patient's information and location. For example, once the RFID is activated, the laboratory would be notified of the patient's registration, would check which laboratory tests still needed to be completed, detect the patient location in the preoperative holding area, and send an alert message for a technician to draw blood to complete all of the necessary tests—instantly and without a single phone call being placed. Because all patients, personnel, equipment, devices, and supplies are "tagged" with an RFID or barcode, there is instant and continuous accountability. The head nurse for the OR can track the locations of the scrub and circulatory nurses, anesthesiologists, resident, and surgeon anywhere in the hospital and have all paged simultaneously. When the patient arrives in the OR the camera above the operating table notices that the bed is green (from clean OR sheets); however, when the patient transfers to the OR table, the camera detects the change from solid green to multiple colors and shapes of the patient with standard image-recognition software, and automatically notifies everyone that the patient is on the OR table. By this time the robotic delivery system will have delivered the surgeon's "pick list" of instruments, checking to be sure they all are accounted for. Throughout the procedure the RFID tracks the instrument use, supply use, surgeon's hand motions, and so forth for quality assurance, training, and eventually maintenance of certification for surgical procedures. At any time all of this information is available through telemonitoring or telemedicine from anywhere within the hospital. At the completion of surgery, there is automatic sponge and instrument count (because everything is labeled and tracked to a location), so no sponges or instruments should be left in the patient. All of this information is collected automatically, continuously, transparently, and unobtrusively so that the operating team can concentrate upon the critical issues of performing a surgical procedure. Thus, the integration of sophisticated sensors, software analysis programs, tracking and location devices, robotics, and better business and supply management processes become a single "symphony" of surgical information exchange.

Robotic operating room

A third vision of the OR of the future is proposed by Satava [8], and focuses upon the technical challenge of replacing all of the systems inside of the OR with robotic systems. This approach is based upon currently available robotic systems in other industries. In those settings, the robots do not have people changing tools or dispensing supplies like nuts and bolts; instead there is an automatic tool changer and a parts dispenser. These robotic subsystems to the main robot perform some of the same tasks that scrub and circulating room nurses perform, especially the simple handing of instruments to the surgeon or bringing sterile supplies to the scrub nurse. Michael Treat [9] of Columbia University is performing clinical trials on Penelope (Fig. 3), a robotic scrub nurse that responds to voice commands and hands instruments to the surgeon during open surgery. Research in a military medical program, called "Trauma Pod," is developing an ambitious project to incorporate tool changers and parts dispensers with the DaVinci surgical robotic system. The result would be an OR with no people other than the patient. The surgeon and anesthesiologist would be just outside of the OR behind a glass window, controlling the robotic systems and performing surgery on the patient in the isolated sterile OR. A plausible scenario is as follows. The patient is brought to the preoperative anesthesia area, anesthetized, and placed in the proper position for surgery on an intelligent OR table. A body scan is performed and the patient is taken to the sterilization area; meanwhile, the patient image is sent to the surgeon's console to perform preoperative planning and (in the case of complicated surgical procedure) surgical rehearsal of the procedure on the patient's own

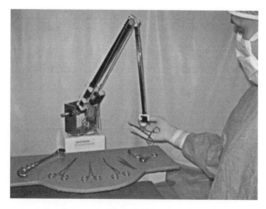

Fig. 3. Robotic surgical scrub nurse "Penelope," handing an instrument to Dr. Michael Treat, MD, PhD. (Courtesy M. Treat, New York, NY).

three-dimensional body scan, visualizing the complete anatomy and making any errors on the patient's image before operating on the patient. The patient is brought into the isolated OR, the OR table docks onto and "communicates" with the robotic surgical system to update all of the information for the surgeon. During the surgical procedure, the surgeon operates as during open surgery and requests (voice activation) surgical instruments or supplies, but from the tool changer and parts dispenser instead of nurses. Every time a supply is used, three things occur simultaneously: the patient is billed, the OR instrument pick list is updated, and a request is sent to order new supplies or instruments—all within 50 milliseconds and with 99.99% accuracy. This is standard in many industries. In the "background" on the hospital information system are all of the intelligent systems from the perioperative OR project that integrates the processes with the software, devices, personnel, and equipment to provide immediate and continuous quality assurance. Because the robotic systems are controlled from outside of the OR, this scenario could be performed as indicated, or could be used for telesurgery and telementoring to remote locations, such as the battlefield or underserved populations.

The above technologies exist and require a significant engineering effort to bring them to fruition; however, there are even greater challenges to success from nontechnical issues, such as acceptance by surgeons and other health care providers, cost-effectiveness, and legal and regulatory compliance. It is unlikely that the scenarios depicted above will occur exactly as written; however, it is highly likely that many of the components will find usefulness and acceptance in one form or another.

Summary

Surgery has just passed through the laparoscopic surgery revolution, with validation of the advantages for the patient evaluated painstakingly; however, laparoscopy is a transition phase to fully information-based surgery, which only can be accomplished when hand motions are converted to information through robotic surgery systems. The main advantage is using such systems to integrate the entire surgical process. The components that will allow such a transition exist in other industries that use robotics, so it is more a matter of applying these engineering principles to surgery, rather than inventing new technologies. Robotics cannot only improve the performance of surgery, but is providing access to surgical expertise in remote and underserved areas through telementoring, teleconsultation, and telesurgery. Colorectal surgeons should seize the opportunity to begin to use surgical robotic systems in those niche areas and procedures that have proven to be of significant benefit to the patient and are cost-effective. Over time, with the development of even more advanced systems it will become more advantageous to use robotics on a routine basis.

References

[1] Satava RM, Green PS. The next generation: telepresence surgery. Current status and impli-
    cations for endoscopy [abstract]. Gastrointest Endosc 1992;38:277.
[2] Bowersox JC, Shah A, Jensen J, et al. Vascular applications of telepresence surgery: initial fea-
    sibility studies in swine. J Vasc Surg 1996;23:281–7.
[3] Marescaux J, Clement JM, Tassetti V, et al. Virtual reality applied to hepatic surgery simula-
    tion: the next revolution. Ann Surg 1998;228:627–34.
[4] Anvari M, McKinley C. Routine use of telerobotic remote surgery. Presented at the 9th World
    Congress of Endoscopic Surgery. Cancun, February 2–7, 2004.
[5] Fichtinger G, DeWeese TL, Patriciu A, et al. System for robotically assisted prostate biopsy
    and therapy with intraoperative CT guidance. Acad Radiol 2002;9(1):60–74.
[6] Jolesz FA. Future perspectives for intraoperative MRI. Neurosurg Clin N Am 2005;16(1):
    201–13.
[7] Sandberg WS, Ganous TJ, Steiner C. Setting a research agenda for perioperative systems de-
    sign. Semin Laparosc Surg 2003;10(2):57–70.
[8] Satava RM. The operating room of the future: observations and commentary. Semin Lapa-
    rosc Surg 2003;10(3):99–105.
[9] Treat M. Intelligent robot scrubs in. Available at: http://www.cumc.columbia.edu/news/
    in-vivo/Vol3_Iss01_jan26_04/surgery.html.

ELSEVIER
SAUNDERS

SURGICAL
CLINICS OF
NORTH AMERICA

Surg Clin N Am 86 (2006) 937–967

New Techniques in the Treatment of Common Perianal Diseases: Stapled Hemorrhoidopexy, Botulinum Toxin, and Fibrin Sealant

Marc Singer, MD, Jose Cintron, MD*

*Department of Surgery (MC958), University of Illinois, Clinical Sciences Building,
#518-E, 840 S. Wood Street, Chicago, IL 60612, USA*

There have been several recent advances in the treatment of common perianal diseases. These modalities are exciting, because they represent changes in paradigm compared with more traditional treatments. Stapled hemorrhoidopexy is a procedure of hemorrhoidal fixation, combining the benefits of rubber band ligation (RBL) into an operative technique. It avoids painful surgical wounds across the highly sensitive anoderm, while restoring the normal anatomy to the anal canal.

The treatment of anal fissure has typically relied upon internal sphincterotomy. Division of the sphincter carries a risk of incontinence, as well as the pain of a surgical incision. Medical management of fissure with various smooth-muscle relaxants has been somewhat effective; however, results are variable, and less reliable than sphincterotomy. The injection of botulinum toxin represents a new form of sphincter relaxation, without division of any sphincter muscle. The morbidity is minimal and the results are quite promising.

Finally, the treatment of perianal fistulae remains a difficult challenge for surgeons. Fistulotomy remains the gold standard; however, this treatment carries significant risks of incontinence. The use of fibrin sealant to treat fistulae has been met with variable success; however, it carries no risk of incontinence and minimal postoperative pain. Traditional treatments have focused upon laying open of the tract for drainage and granulation. This new modality offers sealing of the tract, and then provides scaffolding for

---

* Corresponding author.
E-mail address: jcintron@uic.edu (J. Cintron).

doi:10.1016/j.suc.2006.06.009
surgical.theclinics.com

native tissue ingrowth. All three of these treatments offer attractive alternatives to the standard treatments for these very common perianal diseases.

Stapled hemorrhoidopexy

Introduction

Stapled hemorrhoidopexy represents the first dramatic change in the treatment of hemorrhoids in many years. Excisional hemorrhoidectomy is clearly the most definitive and reliable treatment of both internal and external hemorrhoidal disease; however, the notorious postoperative pain caused by this operation has left patients and surgeons searching for alternative treatment options. A variety of treatment options have been explored, including cyrotherapy, laser therapy, and infrared coagulation. These techniques represent alternative methods of tissue destruction, and as such, can leave patients having postoperative pain comparable to that of excisional hemorrhoidectomy. In addition, none of these techniques has been proven superior to the straightforward and cost-effective excisional hemorrhoidectomy [1–5]. RBL is a popular treatment method for internal hemorrhoids. This is a technique of fixation, as is injection sclerotherapy [6–8]. The rubber bands, placed well above the dentate line, create a local inflammatory reaction, which secures the internal hemorrhoids in place, prevents prolapse, and thus promotes resolution of symptoms. This technique has been very successful, and causes the patient little or no discomfort. RBL does not address external disease, however, and often requires multiple treatments. In addition, some internal hemorrhoids are simply too large and redundant to make RBL a feasible option. These are the types of patients typically referred for excisional hemorrhoidectomy. There have been multiple attempts to decrease postoperative pain after hemorrhoidectomy, such as altering the intraoperative anesthesia, adding sphincterotomy, or using postoperative nitroglycerine or metronidazole. Intraoperative techniques, such as using the Harmonic Scalpel (Ethicon Endo-Surgery, Cincinnati, OH) bipolar cautery, or ligasure device, have been attempted, although none is clearly superior or more cost-effective than excisional hemorrhoidectomy [9–11]. Multiple studies comparing the open (Milligan-Morgan) technique and the closed (Ferguson) technique have been conducted, revealing little or no difference in pain or outcomes. None of the supplemental maneuvers has been very popular or successful in ameliorating the postoperative pain. The underlying reason for this is that excisional hemorrhoidectomy leaves wounds across the highly sensate anoderm. This causes significant pain, which leads to muscle spasm, and thus starts the viscous cycle of postoperative pain.

In 1997, Antonio Longo introduced a novel technique. This operation made use of a modified circular stapler, traditionally used for creating a circular end-to-end intestinal anastomosis. This modified circular stapler (Ethicon Endo-Surgery) is inserted across the anus, and used to excise a circular ring of mucosal tissue from the anal canal, well above the dentate line. A stapled anastomosis is created, thus lifting the redundant, prolapsing hemorrhoids back into the anal canal. This restoration of anatomy by fixation within the anal canal made use of the same principle of fixation that made RBL so successful. The details of the stapling procedure are described below. Attention to the details of this operation are necessary, as the technical aspects lead to success and can prevent highly morbid complications unique to this operation.

The name of this procedure has undergone change throughout its relatively short history. It was initially dubbed "procedure for prolapse and hemorrhoids," or PPH. This was a proprietary name used by the manufacturer, Ethicon Endo-Surgery. The operation became popularly known as "stapled hemorrhoidectomy," because it makes use of a surgical stapler, but this operation is not truly a hemorrhoidectomy, because the hemorrhoidal tissue is not necessarily excised. The operation is a procedure of fixation; therefore the name "staple hemorrhoidopexy" was finally adopted. Some publications use "stapled anopexy," which is also appropriate. Stapled hemorrhoidopexy was accepted by an international working committee [12], and subsequently has been the name most commonly used.

Indications

Stapled hemorrhoidopexy is an alternative to excisional hemorrhoidectomy; therefore the indications should be similar. Patients being considered for a Ferguson or Milligan-Morgan hemorrhoidectomy would also be eligible for stapled hemorrhoidopexy, with some exceptions. Patients who have fourth-degree hemorrhoids—that is, irreducible internal hemorrhoids—may not be good candidates. The manufacturer of the stapling instrument does not typically recommend that fourth-degree internal hemorrhoids be treated with this procedure. The concern is that unless the hemorrhoids can be reduced, then adequate retraction back into the anal canal may not be achieved. In addition, if the internal hemorrhoids are thrombosed, they should be excised. Stapled hemorrhoidopexy returns the hemorrhoidal cushions back into the anal canal. The majority of the hemorrhoidal tissue remains in place. If there are thrombi within the hemorrhoids, then they may slough or cause gangrenous changes in the first few postoperative days. Also, patients who have thrombosed external hemorrhoids may benefit from excisional hemorrhoidectomy. As is discussed later, the restoration of normal anatomy and venous return does in fact yield improvements in external hemorrhoids; however, thrombosed external hemorrhoids would continue to cause symptoms to the patient if not excised. Patients who have undergone previous anorectal surgery may not be good candidates for stapled hemorrhoidopexy. If there is significant scarring at the anal canal, then adequate anorectal mucosa may not be drawn into the head of the stapling device. This is certainly a relative contraindication, because minor scarring should not pose a problem, and the safety and efficacy of stapled hemorrhoidopexy in patients who have undergone previous anorectal procedures has been previously demonstrated [13,14]. Otherwise, the indications should be similar. Patients eligible for RBL should continue to be treated with RBL, unless they choose otherwise or are not suitable candidates for that procedure.

Some patients who have significant Grade II (prolapsing, but spontaneously reducing) hemorrhoids may be eligible for stapled hemorrhoidopexy. The treatment of hemorrhoids is dictated by symptoms, therefore the grade by itself does not necessitate one particular treatment type. Large bulky circumferential hemorrhoids that spontaneously prolapse may be very good candidates for stapled hemorrhoidopexy. If the surgeon believes that they will not be well treated by RBL, or if the patient desires single-session treatment, then excisional hemorrhoidectomy or stapled hemorrhoidopexy may be good options.

One additional exclusion criteria is anal stenosis. The circular anoscope used has an outside diameter of 37 mm. The authors have not encountered any patients who could not accommodate this anoscope, but if a patient had anal stenosis, then potentially he could not undergo this operation. Abscess or gangrenous hemorrhoids are absolute contraindications, because these conditions will not be treated by stapled hemorrhoidopexy. Suspicion of cancer or unidentified lesions are relative contraindications, because the suspicious tissue may not be excised by stapled hemorrhoidopexy. Full-thickness rectal prolapse also should not be treated by this operation, and should undergo other surgical therapy.

Additional anorectal pathology may be treated in conjunction with stapled hemorrhoidopexy. Concomitant fistulotomies, sphincterotomies, biopsies, and excisions can safely be performed, along with stapled hemorrhoidopexy. The patient and surgeon must realize that the benefit of decreased pain compared with excisional techniques may be diminished by any additional procedures performed outside of the dentate line.

Technical aspects

Strict attention to the details of this operation are essential to maximize the desired results as well as prevent complications, some of which are common to other anal operations, and some of which are unique to stapled hemorrhoidopexy.

The instrument used for stapled hemorrhoidopexy is the Proximate HCS (hemorrhoidal circular stapler), manufactured by Ethicon Endo-surgery. The PPH03 kit includes all of the required components of the procedure, except for a suture. This stapler contains modifications from the first version of the hemorrhoid stapler. The newer stapler itself is more ergonomic for the surgeon, and also the staple height is shorter, which reduces the incidence of staple line bleeding. The kit also contains a circular anoscope (with an obturator), a suturing anoscope, which facilitates the placement of the purse string, and a suture threader, which is a hook-shaped instrument used to pull the tail of the purse string through the head of the stapling instrument.

The patient can be positioned in prone jackknife, lithotomy, or even left-lateral position, based on surgeon preference and body habitus of the patient. It is the authors' preference to place the patients in prone jackknife position, because this allows for retraction of the buttocks, and for the best visualization down the anal canal from a standing position. In addition, this is the best position to view the anterior aspect of the anal canal, which is critical to avoiding complications involving the rectovaginal septum in women.

The surgeon and patient may also choose general, regional, or even local anesthesia. All three types have been demonstrated as safe and effective. It is the authors' preference to use spinal. because this gives the patient very good relaxation of the sphincter without requiring excessive sedation, which can be problematic while the patient is in the prone position.

Once properly positioned, the anal canal should be thoroughly examined for pathology other than hemorrhoids. The sphincter should then be progressively dilated to three fingers so that the circular anoscope can be easily inserted without tearing any muscle fibers. The circular anoscope is translucent, which allows for visualization of the dentate line at all times .This is critical, because the purse string suture must be placed well above the dentate line, so that the staple line resides cephalad to the dentate line. The anoderm and perianal skin should be pulled out from under the hub of the circular anoscope so that the scope is seated deep into the anal canal. Some surgeons elect to suture the hub of the scope to the perianal skin with several nylon sutures, but this maneuver is entirely optional. Next, the purse string suture anoscope is inserted through the circular anoscope. This anoscope is a semicircular instrument that facilitates the placement of the purse string suture. This is the critical aspect of the entire operation, because the purse string drives the remainder of the operation. The purse string is placed approximately 2 cm cephalad, or proximal, to the apex of the hemorrhoids. The authors use a 2-0 polypropelene suture on a CT needle (Ethicon). The suture should be placed into the mucosa and submucosa only. Once placed circumferentially, the purse string suture anoscope is removed from the circular anoscope, and the stapler is inserted through the circular anoscope, with the head of the stapler maximally opened. The head is then passed through the purse string suture. The suture is then tightened and tied around the shaft of the stapler. This draws redundant mucosa into the head of the stapler. The suture threader is then passed through each of the side channels on the stapler head, and the tails of the purse string suture are brought out from either side of the head of the stapler. The tissue captured by the suture is the tissue that will be excised. The height of the staple line above the dentate line is dictated by the purse string suture. The staple line will lie 1 to 2 cm distal to the suture height. Once the tails of the suture are brought through the side channels of the stapler head, then several actions occur simultaneously. Gentle traction is applied to the suture, thus drawing the redundant mucosa into the head of the stapler. The stapler itself is advanced into the anal canal such that the 4 cm mark on the head of the stapler is at the level of the anal verge, and the stapler head is tightened. When fully closed, the stapler is fired. A 1 to 3 cm circular band of mucosa/submucosa is excised and the defect stapled closed. Again, this partial-thickness anastomosis is proximal to the dentate line; thus the patient experiences little somatic pain sensation. Once fired, the stapler, purse string, and circular anoscope should all be removed as a single unit so as to prevent pinching or trapping of any tissue between the stapler and the anoscope. The purse string suture anoscope or a Hill-Ferguson anoscope is then inserted back into the anus, and the circular staple line is inspected for bleeding. The new stapler has a reduced staple height, which should presumably reduce the incidence of bleeding. If bleeding is identified, then it should be addressed by oversewing that aspect of the staple line with an absorbable suture, such as a 3-0 Vicryl (Ethicon).

The purse string suture is the critical element because it drives the remainder of the procedure. If the purse string contains the full thickness of the rectum, then the entirety of the rectal wall will be drawn into the stapler head, and at least part of the staple line will be a full-thickness anastomosis. This is likely the cause of such complications as rectal perforation and rectovaginal fistula. In women, a finger should be inserted into the vagina as the purse string is being placed, when it is tightened around the shaft of the stapler, and when the stapler is closed but not yet fired. Examining the vagina for dimpling or pulling of tissue into the stapler head at these three steps should prevent inadvertent inclusion of the vagina into the staple line. If the purse string suture is placed too superficially, that is, mucosa only, then part of the staple line may dehisce. Fortunately, because this is only designed to be a partial-thickness anastomosis, serious complications such as perforation should not occur. The hemorrhoids in the area of dehiscence may continue to prolapse, but the feared complication of rectal perforation should not occur, because the outer muscular portion of the rectum remains intact. If the suture, and thus staple line, is placed too proximal, then the hemorrhoids may not be retracted far enough up into the anal canal and the result may be less than desirable. If the suture, and thus staple line, are too low, or too distal, then the patient may experience extreme pain, thus losing the main advantage of this operation compared with excisional hemorrhoidectomy.

Once the circular staple line is formed, the internal hemorrhoids are returned to their normal anatomic position, up within the anal canal. The staple line prevents prolapse of the internal hemorrhoids. With time, a fibrotic band will form and prevent the hemorrhoids from prolapsing. In addition, the restoration of the hemorrhoids to their normal anatomic position is thought to improve venous drainage from the hemorrhoids; therefore they shrink in size. It is also hypothesized that the division of the submucosal layer divides the arterial supply to the internal hemorrhoids, again helping toward regression of the enlarged cushions.

The external hemorrhoids are also drawn up into the anal canal. The interrupted arterial supply or the restored venous drainage usually cause the external hemorrhoids to resolve with time. If the external hemorrhoids have been chronically thrombosed and hard fibrotic tags are present, these will not resolve. The authors, however, recommend delaying treatment of any external pathology until a later date. The large majority of patients will not request further treatment of these pathologies after stapled hemorrhoidopexy [14]. Efforts should be made to minimize procedures performed on the anoderm, because the premise of stapled hemorrhoidopexy is reduced pain. Even if patients complain of external disease in the future, tags can easily be excised with local anesthesia in the office at a later time if necessary.

Results

There is a rapidly growing body of evidence regarding the efficacy of stapled hemorrhoidopexy. Table 1 contains a summary of prospective randomized trials comparing stapled hemorrhoidopexy to excisional hemorrhoidectomy. A detailed recounting of all 25 trials is too cumbersome for this article. First, a review of the largest trial in the United States is included. Next, the critical outcome measures are discussed as they are supported by data from the other trials. Finally, two recent meta-analyses are reviewed, which include some of the data contained within these 25 trials.

American trial

The initial experience with stapled hemorrhoidopexy in Europe led to an explosion in the popularity of the operation. The number of published trials was expanding; however, there were no large-scale, multicenter, randomized trials. The PPH Multicenter Study Group designed such a trial in the United States [14]. A prospective, randomized trial was conducted at 17 centers, including 30 colorectal surgeons. Each surgeon demonstrated competence with stapled hemorrhoidopexy before enrolling in the trial. Seventy-seven patients were randomized to stapled hemorrhoidopexy and 79 to Ferguson hemorrhoidectomy. All patients were followed for 1 year postoperatively. Patients in the Ferguson group were more likely to return to the operating room for complications (12% versus 0%, $P = .007$). Patients in the stapled group experienced significantly less pain; in fact, they had less pain than the preoperative assessment by postoperative day 14. Pain at first bowel movement and the need for postoperative analgesics were also significantly less in the stapled group. At 1-year follow-up, the patients in the two groups reported similar rates of recurrent or persistent symptoms. The trial demonstrated that stapled hemorrhoidopexy offers the benefits of less postoperative pain, less analgesic requirements, and less pain at bowel

Table 1
Table of randomized controlled trials of stapled hemorrhoidopexy

Author	Year	PPH	Excisional	Pain	Follow-up	Notes
Ho et al [15]	2000	57	62	Less	-	
Mehigan et al [16]	2000	20	20	Less	10 weeks	
Rowsell et al [27]	2000	11	11	Less	1 week	
Brown et al [18]	2001	40	40	Less	6 weeks	Included thrombosed internal hemorrhoids
Shalaby et al [19]	2001	100	100	Less	1 week	
Ganio et al [39]	2001	50	50	Less	16 months	
Racalbuto et al [42]	2001	50	50		48 months	
Boccasanta et al [17]	2001	40	40	Less	54 weeks	
Correa-Rovelo et al [25]	2002	42	42	Less	6 months	
Ortiz et al [21]	2002	27	28	Less	16 months	
Pavlidis et al [22]	2002	40	40	Less	12 months	
Krska et al [43]	2002	25	25		1 month	
Wilson et al [26]	2002	32	30	Similar	8 weeks	
Hetzer et al [20]	2002	20	20	Less	12 months	
Cheetham et al [28]	2003	15	16	Less	18 months	Some PPH patients with persistant pain
Palimento et al [23]	2003	37	37	Less	18 months	
Racalbuto et al [42]	2003	50	50	Less	48 months	
Kairaluoma et al [30]	2003	30	30	Less	12 months	
Senagore et al [14]	2003	77	79	Less	12 months	
Smyth et al [41]	2003	20	16	Less	18 months	
Gravie et al [31]	2005	63	63	Less	2.2 years	
Bikhchandani et al [29]	2005	42	42	Less	11 months	
Kraemer et al [24]	2005	25	25	Similar	6 weeks	Ligasure
Ortiz et al [33]	2005	15	16	Less	1 year	4th degree hemorrhoids
Chung et al [32]	2005	43	45	Less	15 months	Harmonic scalpel used

movement, while providing similar control of symptoms and less frequent need for additional anorectal treatments at 1-year follow-up. Because this trial was conducted at many of the major colorectal centers in the United States, and the data widely publicized, it generated significant interest in the operation in this country.

Outcomes measures from other trials

Review of Table 1 makes it clear that a great number of randomized trials have been published to date. Most trials examine similar outcomes.

The operative time for stapled hemorrhoidopexy has been demonstrated to be shorter than excisional hemorrhoidectomy in several trials [15–26]. The operative time is generally reported at 15 to 25 minutes. The length of stay in the hospital is difficult to assess because in the United States, hemorrhoid operations are frequently performed on an outpatient basis. In many other countries, patients spend several days in the hospital. This phenomenon is related to differences in the reimbursement systems of other countries, and therefore may not reflect American practices. This makes length-of-stay data variable and difficult to interpret or compare. The return to usual activities is also difficult to assess, but is crucial in the analysis of stapled hemorrhoidopexy. The main benefit of this operation is reduced pain, which also translates into quicker return to work or normal daily activities. The true benefit, in a broader sense, may not be appreciated by an assessment of the operative costs of stapled hemorrhoidopexy, because the cost of the stapler far exceeds the cost of the supplies required to perform an excisional hemorrhoidectomy. The costs are recovered, however, because patients can return to work significantly sooner. Multiple trials have documented a faster return to activity [15–20,23,26–32]. Reduction in postoperative pain is the driving force behind the search for this new hemorrhoid operation, so careful attention must be paid toward this result. Most studies assess pain using some variety of visual analog scale. Most studies demonstrated reduced pain at some time within the first 2 weeks postoperatively [14–23,25,27–30]. Ho and colleagues [15] also reported less pain at 3 months postoperatively. After longer follow-up (> 6 months), pain was also assessed by several investigators. Pain at this time is multifactorial, because postoperative wounds should have healed. Persistent pain from surgery, recurrent hemorrhoids, or additional anorectal pathology can all contribute to pain at this time. At least three trials demonstrated similar pain in the late postoperative period [23,25,33].

Reduction in the prolapse of hemorrhoidal tissue is certainly an important end point. Because stapled hemorrhoidopexy does not remove the redundant internal hemorrhoids, there has been concern that this tissue may continue to prolapse. Multiple trials have documented that stapled hemorrhoidopexy controls prolapse as least as well as excisional hemorrhoidectomy [14,19,21,25,27,28,30,31]. Ortiz and coworkers [33] enrolled patients who had fourth-degree hemorrhoids into a randomized trial. At 1-year follow-up, patients in the stapled group complained of significantly more frequent prolapse as well as tenesmus; therefore Grade IV hemorrhoids may not be a suitable indication.

Postoperative bleeding is a well-described complication of excisional hemorrhoidectomy [34], occurring with less than a 5% incidence. Stapled hemorrhoidopexy also carries a risk of bleeding both from the staple line and from the remaining internal hemorrhoids. This tissue is not excised, and therefore may continue to bleed in the early postoperative period. The number of patients who had clinically significant postoperative bleeding—that is, requiring admission, transfusion, or return to the operating room—was similar after stapled procedure compared with excisional techniques [14,15,17,18,21,22,25,26,28]. Delayed postoperative bleeding (> 30 days) is most likely caused by persistent or recurrent hemorrhoidal disease, because most surgical wounds would have healed by this time. Most trials report similar incidence of delayed bleeding between stapled and excisional groups [14,15,18,19,23,25,26,28,33].

As with any anorectal operation, preservation of continence is imperative. Sphincter injuries have been reported after transanal stapling procedures for other indications [35–37]. The circular anoscope included in the PPH kit has a 37 mm outer diameter, which could theoretically cause stretch injuries. Also, the loss of a circumferential band of anal mucosa may effect sensation or function. Boccasanta and colleagues [17] evaluated resting and squeeze pressure and found no differences between hemorrhoidopexy and hemorrhoidectomy patients. Shalaby and Desoky [19] concluded that hemorrhoidectomy patients had reduced pressures compared with the hemorrhoidopexy patients. Wilson and coworkers [26] found no differences between groups at 6 weeks postoperatively. Ho [15] found no differences in the manometric data between operative groups. By 6 weeks postoperative, the resting and squeeze pressures were decreased in the hemorrhoidectomy patients only.

Gravie and colleagues [31] conducted a randomized trial comparing hemorrhoidopexy with Milligan-Morgan hemorrhoidectomy. Results were similar to other trials; however, this group followed patients for 2 years postoperatively. At that time, there were no differences regarding control of symptoms. The two operations were equally effective in controlling prolapse, discharge, and itching, as well as skin tags and external hemorrhoids. The rates of fecal urgency, incontinence, and tenesmus were similar between groups as well. Recurrence of prolapse was 7% in the stapled group and 2% in the Milligan-Morgan group not significant (NS) [31]. This trial provides the longest follow-up data, and suggests that the two techniques provide similar longer-term results with regards to symptom control, sphincter function, and recurrent disease.

Meta-analyses

Because many of the data generated regarding stapled hemorrhoidopexy are derived from small trials, two recent meta analyses were performed. Nisar and colleagues [38] conducted a systematic review in 2004 to determine whether stapled hemorrhoidopexy had an advantage in the safety or efficacy outcomes versus excisional techniques. Fifteen trials, containing 1077 patients, were included in this review [15–20,22,23,25–28,30,33,39]. There were no differences in total complications, although immediate postoperative hemorrhage was more common in hemorrhoidopexy patients (9.6% versus 4.2%, $P = 0.02$). Hemorrhage at 2 weeks and procedures required for hemorrhage were similar between groups. There were no differences between groups with respect to transfusions, sphincter injuries, thrombosed hemorrhoids, anal stenosis, residual skin tags, fissures, or urinary retention. Recurrent prolapse after at least 6 months was reported by 9 trials, and was significantly worse in hemorrhoidopexy patients ($P = .008$). Length of hospital stay was significantly shorter in hemorrhoidopexy patients, as was return to normal activity. Pain at 24 hours was significantly improved with hemorrhoidopexy compared with conventional surgery. Nisar and colleagues conclude that the data were variable, but the meta-analysis suggested that hemorrhoidopexy is less painful than excisional hemorrhoidectomy. It may be less effective, however, as demonstrated by a high rate of recurrent prolapse. The study authors admit that the amount of long-term follow-up for this parameter is limited and warrants further investigation [38].

Lan and coworkers [40] also conducted a systematic review. This review included 10 prospective randomized trials comparing stapled hemorrhoido-pexy with Milligan-Morgan hemorrhoidectomy for Grade III and IV hem-orrhoids [16,18,19,22,23,26,39,41–43]. There were no significant differences in the safety outcomes. Postoperative bleeding within 2 weeks, at 2 to 8 weeks, or at 3 months was similar between groups. The incidence of bleeding requiring intervention, urinary retention, difficulty defecating, and anal fis-sure were similar between groups. The operative times and length of hospital stay were significantly reduced in the stapled groups. The pooled data re-garding postoperative pain revealed less pain in the stapled group (OR 0.37 95% CI, .20–.7). The analysis suggests that stapled hemorrhoidopexy is as safe as Milligan-Morgan hemorrhoidectomy. There was evidence fa-voring hemorrhoidopexy with regard to operative time, length of stay, post-operative pain, and patient satisfaction. Postoperative skin tags and prolapse did occur more frequently in the hemorrhoidopexy groups. The groups were similar in postoperative bleeding, urinary retention, anal fis-sures, and anal stenosis, sphincter injuries, resumption of daily activities, in-continence, and resting/squeeze pressures. The study authors concluded that hemorrhoidopexy is a safe and reasonable alternative to hemorrhoidectomy; however longer follow-up is required [40].

Complications

Many of the complications of stapled hemorrhoidopexy are similar to those of hemorrhoidectomy or any anorectal operation, such as urinary retention, which occurred in 10% to 15% of patients [14–17,19–21,23,25,26,30]; however, there are several serious complications, some unique to hemorrhoi-dopexy, that warrant discussion.

Rectovaginal fistula has been reported after stapled hemorrhoidopexy [25,44,45]. This complication is also known to occur after the formation of coloanal anastomoses, and even excisional hemorrhoidectomy, but is ex-ceedingly rare. This represents a potentially devastating complication of treatment for a benign disease and therefore must be avoided. It can be avoided by carefully and frequently examining the vagina at multiple times during the application of the purse string and insertion of the stapler. The rectovaginal septum can be as thin as several millimeters; therefore precise placement of the purse string is essential to avoid this complication.

Maw and colleagues [46] conducted a randomized trial comparing the rates of bacteremia in patients undergoing stapled hemorrhoidopexy and hemorrhoidectomy. Blood cultures were obtained immediately preopera-tively and then again postoperatively. There were no significant differences in the rates of bacteremia (11 versus 5%, $P = .19$) and no differences in clin-ical infectious complications.

Perforation of the rectum has been reported and was likely caused by a very low peritoneal reflection incorporated in to the anastomosis [47]. Pneumoretroperitoneum has been reported [48], as well as pelvic sepsis [49]. Despite these potentially fatal complications, they are sufficiently rare that prophylactic antibiotics are not warranted. Rectal obstruction has also been reported because the lumen was obliterated by the staples [50]. This complication is also most likely related to faulty application of the purse string. If the suture closes the anal canal, then the stapler will subsequently staple the lumen closed, further emphasizing the precision required when placing the suture.

Discussion

The postoperative pain related to excisional hemorrhoidectomy is notorious. Patients will frequently avoid definitive treatment of their disease for many years [13] so as to avoid this very problem. Stapled hemorrhoidopexy now offers a significantly less painful alternative that provides patients definitive treatment of their disease in a single setting. The Ferguson or Milligan-Morgan hemorrhoidectomies are certainly effective operations that have withstood the test of time; however, the problem of postoperative pain has never been satisfactorily addressed. Modifications, analgesics, sphincterotomies, botulinum toxin injections, and the like have never really made excisional hemorrhoidectomy an appealing option.

The method by which stapled hemorrhoidopexy addresses prolapsing internal hemorrhoids has transformed the treatment of hemorrhoids. This operation combines elements of fixative techniques with the single-setting convenience of excisional treatments. It eliminates the need for the painful wounds at the highly sensate anoderm that all excisional techniques require. It avoids tissue destruction, and simply restores the normal anatomy of the hemorrhoids. The vascular cushions that become hemorrhoids are a normal part of anorectal anatomy. Stapled hemorrhoidopexy returns these cushions to their normal location within the anal canal, and secures the position of the internal hemorrhoids with a partial-thickness staple line. At the same time, the interruption of the arterial inflow and restoration of the venous outflow cause the internal hemorrhoids to reduce their size. The prolapse is prevented, and ultimately the symptoms disappear. By avoiding excision, the patient is not burdened with extremely painful wounds across the highly sensate anoderm.

This review of the literature, as well as two meta-analyses, confirms that stapled hemorrhoidopexy is a safe and effective procedure for hemorrhoids that offers a less painful alternative to excisional hemorrhoidectomy. Because the procedure is relatively new compared with excisional techniques, the very long-term outcomes remain unknown. If the results continue as they are presently, then stapled hemorrhoidopexy may become the new standard of care for the operative treatment of internal hemorrhoid.

Fibrin glue for fistula-in-ano

Introduction

The treatment of fistula-in-ano remains a difficult problem for surgeons. Fistulotomy continues to be the gold standard to which other therapies must be compared. The goal of fistulotomy is division of all tissue, including sphincter, overlying the fistula tract. If all tissue can be completely divided, then the wound can granulate from the base and the healing rate is very high. Preservation of continence is also an important goal of any anorectal operation, however. Wide laying open of the tract puts the patient at significant risk of incontinence, as has been documented by many series [51–56]. This is particularly true for fistulae with high internal openings, because the tracts of these fistulae will encompass significant amounts of sphincter muscle. In addition, the fistulotomy leaves the patient having an open wound at the anoderm, which can be very painful, and can sometimes take weeks or months to fully heal. This has led surgeons to search for alternative methods of treating fistulae. Cutting setons, loose setons, staged division of the sphincters, endorectal advancement flaps, and dermal advancement flaps have all been used as alternatives to primary fistulotomy with variable success rates; however, each of these procedures carries risks of pain, wound healing complications, and incontinence [52–67]. For this reason, surgeons have been searching for an alternative treatment modality. The ideal treatment of a fistula would effectively close the tract without significant pain and without impairment of sphincter function, and allow the patient an early return to activities. These objectives led to the concept of obliteration of the fistula tract with fibrin sealant.

The theory behind the treatment of fistulae with fibrin sealant is twofold. First, occlusion of the fistula tract with sealant immediately halts the ongoing contamination of the tract with stool, mucus, blood, and pus. Second, the proteins contained within the sealant stimulate native tissue ingrowth, and provide a biologic scaffolding for the wound-healing process. The sealant is degraded as the fibrotic reaction progresses, and ultimately the sealant is entirely replaced by native tissues. Thus, no foreign body persists and the tract simply scars closed. Because the tract is obviously contaminated by fecal flora, it is highly desirable that no foreign bodies persist within the fistula. Because the tract is simply obliterated by the sealant, and there is no division of sphincter muscle, then there is no significant risk of incontinence. The procedure is simple and repeatable. These factors make it a highly desirable treatment option. This use of sealant has grown in popularity over the last 10 years, although its appeal may be waning because of the variable results published over time. An examination of the technical aspects of the procedure as well as the published literature is warranted. The technique may effect the results, and the patients in the published studies are variable with respect to the etiology of their disease.

Technical aspects

Fibrin sealant

Fibrin sealant has been used in a variety of forms for decades. The original products were simple mixtures of thrombin and fibrinogen. These mixtures were used during surgery for many years with poor success rates. This was in part caused by the variability of the concentration of the components. By the 1970s, highly concentrated fibrinogen became widely available, as did Factor XIII and aprotinin, which served to stabilize the clot. In 1978, however, the United States Food and Drug Administration (FDA) prohibited the use of fibrinogen concentrates derived from pooled donors because of the risk of viral transmission of hepatitis (and later HIV). After this time, surgeons were left to use single-donor fibrinogen products and bovine aprotinin. By 1998, donor screening, reliable testing methods, and viral deactivation techniques made pooled fibrinogen products safe again. The FDA approved the use of commercially produced products for patients. Since that time, the use of fibrin sealant has been described in nearly every organ system.

The combination of the two components of fibrin sealant reproduces the final stage of the native clotting cascade. The two essential components are fibrinogen and thrombin. The thrombin converts the fibrinogen into active fibrin. The commercial product most commonly available is Tisseel VH fibrin sealant (Baxter Healthcare, Deerfield, IL). The sealant is available as a two-component system. One component contains a solution of fibrinogen, Factor XIII, and bovine aprotinin. The second contains thrombin and calcium, which acts as a cofactor. The two components are maintained in separate syringes until a specially designed dual syringe applicator (Duploject, Baxter Healthcare) delivers the products to the surgical site. The two components remain separated until they are mixed at the tip of the applicator device. The clot begins to organize within seconds of the two components mixing.

The fibrin matrix contained within the clot serves as a scaffolding for tissue ingrowth into the healing wound. The human proteins within the sealant may in fact serve as chemotactic agent, attracting native fibroblasts and other cells critical to wound healing. The fibrin as well as the fibronectin and glycoproteins that migrate into the clot stimulate activate fibroblasts, collagen deposition, re-epithelialization, and neovascularization of the wound. Thus the sealant facilitates the wound healing process. With time, native plasminogen will destabilize the clot. Within 2 weeks, the entire synthetic clot is likely destabilized and replaced by host tissues [68,69]. Surgeons have attempted to treat urogenital, enteric, pancreatic, tracheoesophagel, bronchopleural, and cerebrospinal fistulae [70]. Early reports of perineal fistulae treated with sealant began to appear in the literature in the 1980s [71,72], although published treatment of fistula-in-ano did not appear until later.

Operative procedure for fistula-in-ano

The operative procedure can be performed as an outpatient procedure. Patients do not undergo preoperative mechanical bowel preparation, other than an enema on the morning of surgery to evacuate distal stool. Oral or intravenous antibiotics are not necessary for this procedure. The patient may be positioned in the prone, lithotomy, or lateral position, so long as the internal and external openings of the fistula are visible. The external opening is usually obvious, as this is the site of symptoms. Identification of the internal orifice is mandatory for this procedure, because the catheter must be passed all the way through the tract, or at least up to the internal opening. The tract should then be gently debrided using a method that will not increase the diameter of the tract. Either an unfolded gauze sponge, a silk suture with a series of knots, a small curette, or a cytology brush works well. Aggressive curettage or debridement should be avoided so as to keep the tract as narrow as possible. The tract should also be irrigated with saline or hydrogen peroxide to further cleanse the tract. Iodine irrigation should be avoided because the manufacturer of the sealant states that iodine solutions can destabilize the fibrin clot.

After the glue is prepared according to the included instructions, the dual syringe applicator is prepared. The authors prefer to use a long, flexible catheter tip, (Duploject 25). The catheter tip is then delivered from through the external orifice, through the tract, and into the anal canal. This often requires the placement of a suture through the tract, which can then be tied to the catheter. The suture is then pulled into the fistula, and drags the catheter with it (Fig. 1). The sealant is injected at the internal opening and allowed to set. (Fig. 2) Once the clot stabilizes, the catheter is slowly backed out through the tract as sealant is being injected, thus obliterating the entire tract. (Fig. 3). The clot is allowed to cure for 5 to 10 minutes. The external orifice is then dressed with a no adherent dressing. The patients are typically discharged home on the day of surgery, because there is minimal or no postoperative pain. Patients are instructed to avoid strenuous activity and to take stool softeners for at least 2 weeks. Patients are instructed not to take baths for 2 weeks, so as not to soak out the clot. Showering is permitted.

Complete obliteration of the tract with sealant is the critical feature of the procedure. If an abscess is identified during the examination, then it should be drained or a sexton placed, and the sealant deferred for a later date. Failure to fill the entire tract, or side branches, will potentially leave pockets of untrained pus. This will put the patient at high risk of failure.

Results

The literature now contains substantial evidence in favor of using fibrin sealant for anal fistulae. Unfortunately, the published studies are highly variable in design and surgical methodology. Some trials were prospective and randomized [73,74], some were prospective and nonrandomized [75–85], and

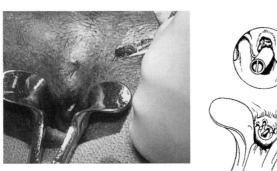
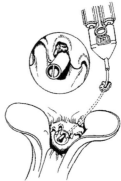

Fig. 1. Dual lumen catheter is inserted through the external opening toward the internal opening of the fistula.

some were retrospective [86,87]. The patients included in these trials were usually not standardized. They included patients who had acute and chronic fistulae, Cohn's disease, HIV-positive patients, postoperative patients, recto-vaginal fistulae, and anastigmatic fistulae. The commercial preparations of sealant are varied, and the intraoperative protocols differ in terms of preoperative preparation of the patient, management of the fistula in the operating room, and postoperative monitoring. The follow-up was relatively short in many of the trials. Nevertheless, examination of the overall data is warranted.

As previously described, it is critical to obliterate the entirety of the fistula and any attached branches. For this reason, some authors chose to exclude patients in whom additional tracts were identified [73,79,81,84], or deferred the injection until adequate drainage was achieved [74–76,86]. Other investigators chose to include these patients, and make attempts to fill all tracts and cavities with sealant [77,78,80,82,83,85].

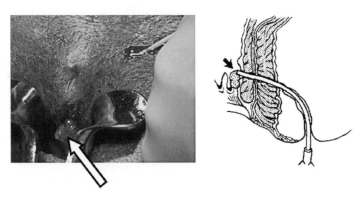

Fig. 2. Fibrin sealant is injected at the internal fistula opening. Arrow points to sealant at internal opening.

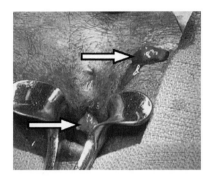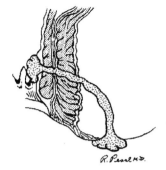

Fig. 3. Once the sealant begins to clot, the catheter is advanced out of the fistula as the sealant fills the entire tract. A second bead of sealant is left at the external opening.

Preoperative antibiotic use was also highly variable in these studies. Authors administered potential antibiotics [77,82,84,85], enterable antibiotics [80,83], or refrained from antibiotic use [73,75]. There is evidence to suggest that antibiotics mixed within the fibrin sealant will be slowly released from the matrix over 24 to 48 hours [88]. Two studies attempted to improved healing rates based on this laboratory data by including antibiotics within the sealant itself [74,81].

Table 2 contains a summary of available data and Fig. 4 represents a graphic of the healing rates of each study. Because of the variability in design, a formal systematic review or meta-analysis is not possible. The graph does give the impression that overall healing is approximately 50%. It must be emphasized that this is a crude estimate based on widely variable trials. A detailed discussion of each trial is beyond the scope of this article; however, several important conclusions brought forth by these studies are highlighted.

In 1991 Hjortrup and colleagues [79] described the first cohort of patients successfully treated with a commercial sealant. Although this group of patients was small, these were the first available data suggesting the safety and efficacy of this procedure. Abel and coworkers [77] were the next group to report success using sealant. This group included 5 patients who had rectovaginal fistulae, 4 of whom were successfully treated. Venkatesh and Ramanujam [82] examined results of 30 patients who had recurrent fistulae with various causes. Overall success was 60% in this complicated group, despite the variety of diagnoses and previous treatment failures. Patrlj and colleagues [81] enrolled 69 patients in a prospective study in which fistulae were treated with sealant that contained intra-adhesive cefotaxime. Overall healing was 74%. This was the first paper suggesting that intra-adhesive antibiotics may augment wound healing. Lindsey and coworkers [73] described 19 patients in which Beriplast (Aventis Behring, Sussex, United Kingdom; currently under clinical evaluation and not approved in the United States) was used to treat fistulae. They were offered retreatment if initial injection

Table 2
Results of treatment of fistula-in-ano with fibrin sealant

Author	Year	# Patients	Etiology	Success rate	Glue	Follow-up (months)	Notes
Hjortrup et al [79]	1991	23	Abscess, postoperative	75	Beriplast	4	First series reporting success for fistula in ano
Abel et al [77]	1993	10	Abscess, RVF, HIV, Crohn's	60	Autologous	3–12	Sealant safe and effective
Venkatesh et al [82]	1999	30	Abscess, RVF, HIV, Crohn's	60	Autologous	9–57	All patients had recurrent fistula, and success was reasonable
Aitola et al [78]	1999	10	Abscess	0	Tisseel	6	
Ramirez et al [128]	2000	9	Abscess	50	Tisseel		
Cintron et al [75]	2000	79	Abscess, HIV, RVF, Crohn's	61	Autologous, ViFuard, Tisseel	12	Autologous and commercial sealant equivalent; complex fistula heal less often
Patrlj et al [81]	2000	69	Abscess	74	Tisseel + Cefotaxime	18–36	More effective for tracts ≥ 3.5 cm
El-Shobaky et al [85]	2000	30		87			
Salim et al [80]	2001	6		100		3	
Lindsey et al [73]	2002	19	Abscess, Crohn's	63	Beriplast	3	Sealant better for complex fistulae
Chan et al [83]	2002	10		60		3	
Sentovich et al [76]	2003	48	Abscess, Crohn's, postoperative	69	Tisseel	6–46	Better healing for shorter tracts, retreated yields 89% success
Zmora et al [86]	2003	24	Abscess, Crohn's, postoperative	33	Tisseel	1–36	Sealant + flap yielded 54% healing
Buchanan et al [84]	2003	22	Abscess	14	Tisseel	14	Similar success in Crohn's patients
Loungnarath et al [87]	2004	39	Abscess, Crohn's, postoperative	31	Tisseel	26	Closure of internal opening and/or intra-adhesive cefoxitin not helpful
Vitton et al [129]	2005	14	Crohn's	14	Beriplast	23	
Singer et al [74]	2005	75	Abscess, HIV, Crohn's	35	Tisseel ± Cefoxitin	27	

Abbreviation: RVF, rectovaginal fistula.

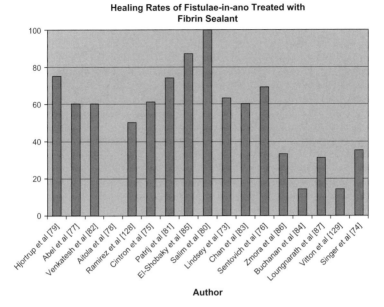

Fig. 4. Healing rates of fistulae-in-ano treated with fibrin sealant.

failed. This strategy of reinjection brought initial healing rates of 42% up to 63% overall. This confirmed that retreatment is a reasonable option in patients failing their initial injection.

Sentovich [76] reported his experience with 48 patients. All patients were initially drained with setons and subsequently injected with sealant in a delayed fashion so as to insure adequate drainage of perianal pus. The initial healing rates were 60%, and retreatment was 50% successful, thus bringing the overall healing rate to 69%. Sentovich suggests that long tracts did not heal as well as shorter tracts. Zmora and coworkers [86] performed a review of his experience with complex fistulae (high trans-sphincteric, suprasphincteric, high rectovaginal, and Crohn's fistulae). Sealant alone afforded only a 37% healing rate; however, when combined with a simultaneous endorectal advancement flap, healing was 54%.

An early trial by the authors' group [75] included 69 patients treated with autologous sealant, Vi-Guard-FS (V.I. Technologies, Watertown, MA), and Tisseel. Overall healing was 61%. There were no differences between the autologous or commercial preparations, but the commercial sealants were faster and easier to prepare [75]. The authors' most recent trial examined the use of sealant in combination with closure of the internal fistula opening or intra-adhesive cefoxitin [74]. Patients were randomized to sealant with cefoxitin, sealant with closure of internal opening, or a combined arm. There were no significant differences between groups, with healing rates of 25%, 44%, and 35% respectively.

One of the factors that may influence the rate of healing after fibrin sealant is the complexity of the fistula tract. The data regarding this parameter is mixed. The authors' group [75] reported that sealant was highly effective in intersphincteric (82%) fistulae, but less effective in complex fistulae (40%); however, Lindsay and coworkers [73] reported opposite results in a randomized study. Studies including simple fistulae [75,76,81] had higher healing rates compared with those studies including only complex fistulae [76,77,82,84,86,87], suggesting that complexity predicts failure, but this cannot be proven definitively. Sentovich [76], Zmora and colleagues [86], and Loungnarth and coworkers [87], reported that there is no difference in healing based on etiology. No study has been able to establish definitively the relationship between etiology and healing rates, likely because of the small numbers of non-cryptoglandular fistulae included in all trials.

Two trials have documented that there is no significant influence of duration of symptoms or previous operative procedures [75,87]. The length of the fistula tract has been postulated as a factor influencing healing rates. Venkatesh and Ramanujam [82] reported that short tracts predicted failure. Similarly, Patrlj and colleagues [81] reported 89% healing if the fistula was greater than 3.5 cm, but 45% if shorter. They suggested that the short tract possesses a mechanical disadvantage such that the sealant is more likely to be ejected. In contrast, Sentovich [76] concluded that long tracts were more likely to recur.

Closure of the internal opening has not been demonstrated to improve healing rates [74,87], although combining sealant with endorectal advancement flap may improve healing [86].

There are complications that can occur as a result of fibrin sealant injection. Postoperative abscesses have been reported [73,76,85]. These may be caused by incomplete obliteration of the tracts, or unidentified pus at the time of the operation. Patients have reported side effects to bovine thrombin or allergic type reactions [89–91], but not related to this specific application of fibrin sealant. It should also be noted that no cases of viral transmission have been reported after application of fibrin sealant to any surgical site after 8 million doses have been used worldwide.

Incontinence is the complication that drives the search for surgical modalities other than fistulotomy. Only three trials have specifically evaluated for incontinence [73,85,86]. None of these trials revealed any impairment of continence related to the fibrin sealant procedure. In addition, none of the other trials report procedural related incontinence.

Discussion

Fistulotomy remains the most reliable method of treating most fistulae; however, the incontinence rates make it prohibitive in many scenarios: high internal opening, anterior fistulae in women, patients who have pre-existing incontinence, and so forth. Injection of fibrin sealant carries essentially no risk of incontinence, because there is no division of sphincter muscle. This procedure causes very little postoperative pain, is easily repeatable, and does not preclude any further surgical therapy including flaps. In these respects, fibrin sealant is an ideal procedure for anal fistulae; however, the available data suggest that it yields only a 50% healing rate. This statistic is only a crude estimate. As this article has explained, the data are highly variable, and the inconsistent trial design make formal statistical analysis of the data impossible.

The operation is technically simple; however, meticulous attention to the examination remains fundamental to its success. Any significant undrained pus or unfilled side branches of the fistula will cause failure of the procedure. The surgeon should have a low threshold to place setons or drains, and should delay injection of sealant if pus is identified. If the surgeon and patient elect to undertake a course of therapy designed to avoid division of sphincter muscle, then both should be willing to return to the operating room under only the ideal circumstances.

The relationships between healing rates and fistula etiology, anatomy, length of tract, antibiotic use, and many other variables are not completely understood at this time. Many additional clinical trials may be required to properly evaluate these factors.

Given its incomparable safety profile, ease of application, and repeatability, fibrin sealant injection can be offered as first-line therapy. It is critical, however, that patients are properly counseled, and understand that this operation carries only a 50% healing rate. Fibrin sealant will likely never surpass the healing rates of fistulotomy, but as a sphincter-preserving modality, it represents a suitable alternative.

Botulinum toxin for chronic anal fissure

Introduction

Anal fissures are ulcers in the squamous epithelium of the anal canal at the mucocutaneous junction, extending cephalad toward the dentate line. They occur most commonly at the posterior midline, but may occur at any position around the anus. Anterior midline fissures occur in 10% of female patients and 1% of male patients [92]. Fissures cause severe pain during and after defecation for minutes to hours. Examination in the office setting is often impossible because of the severe pain. Bleeding from the fissure is common at the time of bowel movement. Atypical fissures will be in locations other than posterior or anterior midline, multiple, large, and irregularly shaped. They are caused by malignancies, inflammatory bowel disease, HIV, hematologic disorders, unusual infections (including tuberculosis and syphilis), trauma, or chemotherapy. The etiology of common, benign fissures is not completely understood. All fissures share the feature of internal sphincter spasm, which causes localized ischemia at the site of the fissure. This ischemia prevents healing; the open wound causes further pain, which leads to continued spasm; and thus the cycle of pain, spasm, and ischemia continues until the fissure becomes chronic [93,94]. Pain relief is an important key for patient comfort, but also to break this cycle. Pain is frequently relieved by interrupting the spasm of the internal sphincter. Traditionally, this was accomplished with surgical techniques such as anal dilation, open or closed lateral sphincterotomy, or even posterior midline sphincterotomy. These operations were successful in disrupting the sphincter and breaking the spasm; however, they carried the risk of incontinence [95]. Today, lateral internal sphincterotomy remains the gold standard as treatment for anal fissure, though concern for incontinence persists. Healing rates in excess of 95% can be expected, but alteration in continence can occur in up to 30% of patients [96]. This lead to the search for nonsurgical therapies for anal fissure.

The principle behind medical therapies for anal fissure remains the same as surgical therapy. The goal is to break the spasm of the internal sphincter, so as to reduce pain and improve blood flow to the healing ulcer. The use of nitroglycerin and calcium channel blockers have been extensively studied [97–112]. Both agents serve to relax the internal sphincter muscle, and have been met with variable success; however, these agents are well known to cause significant headaches in up to 50% of patients. This is well-described as a cause of patient noncompliance. In a recent meta-analysis of medical therapies for anal fissure, Nelson [113] questions the efficacy of nitroglycerin and calcium channel blockers because the data directly comparing these agents to placebo are limited. These agents have many side effects, with a modest rate of long-term healing of fissures.

Botulinum neurotoxins (BTX) are exotoxins produced by the bacterium *Clostridium botulinum*, and they inhibit neuromuscular transmission. The BTX inhibits acetylcholine release into the synaptic gap. The effect is temporary, and last 3 to 4 months. They have been used for the treatment of variety of conditions in which smooth muscle inhibition is desired. BTX does not block the nonadrenergic, noncholinergic responses mediated by nitric oxide, which makes it an ideal candidate for internal sphincter blockade. Because hypertonicity or spasm of the internal sphincter is one of the fundamental aspects of fissures, injection of BTX seems an ideal nonoperative therapy. The first use of BTX to treat anal fissures was in 1993 [114]. Subsequently, a large number of trials have been published.

Outcomes

The BTX injections are typically well-tolerated by most patients. Injection is contraindicated in pregnant or nursing patients. It should also be avoided in patients who have known neuromuscular transmission disorders. Side effects include a flulike syndrome, and very rarely a brachial plexopathy. These are likely caused by an immune response. There have not been any severe allergic reactions reported after anal injection, but local irritation can occur.

The injection technique is straightforward. One hundred units of Botox are mixed in 4 mL of sterile saline. The toxin is administered via an insulin syringe and 27 g needle.

Table 3 contains a summary of published series of BTX injections for anal fissure. This represents a considerably heterogeneous collection of studies; however, the data are reasonably consistent in that BTX appears to

Table 3
Summary of published series of BTX injections for anal fissure

Author	Year	# Patients	Units/site	Healing rate (%)
Gui et al [125]	1994	10	15 IAS	90
Jost et al [130]	1994	12	5 EAS	83
Jost et al [115]	1995	54	5 EAS	78
Mason et al [138]	1996	5	IAS	60
Jost et al [116]	1997	100	2.5–EAS	82
Espi et al [139]	1997	36	10 IAS/15 IAS	65/81
Maria et al [136]	1998	15	20 IAS	73
		15	Saline	13
Maria et al [120]	1998	23	15 IAS	100
		34	20 IAS	100
Minguez et al [121]	1999	23	10 IAS	83
		27	15 IAS	78
		19	21 IAS	90
Jost et al [117]	1999	25	20 EAS	76
		25	40 EAS	80
Brisinda et al [131]	1999	25	20 IAS	96
		25	Nitro	60
Fernandez et al [132]	1999	76	40 IAS	67
Gonzales et al [144]	1999	40	15 EAS	50
Madalinski et al [119]	1999	13	20 EAS	85
Khademi et al [140]	2000	11	25 IAS	82
Maria et al [137]	2000	25	20 IAS posterior	80
		25	20 IAS anterior	100
Lysy et al [133]	2001	15	20 IAS + nitrate	73
		15	20 IAS	60
Madalinski et al [118]	2001	14	25–50 EAS	54
Brisinda et al [122]	2002	75	20 IAS	100
		75	30 IAS	100
Trzcinski et al [134]	2002	13	50 IAS	85
Colak et al [142]	2002	3	30 IAS	71
		28	Lidocaine	21
Wollina et al [135]	2002	5	20–25 IAS	40
		5	50–75 IAS	100
Brisinda et al [126]	2003	6	150 IAS	100
Mentes et al [123]	2003	61	20–30 IAS	87
		50	Sphincterotomy	98
Siproudhis et al [141]	2003	22	100 IAS	32
		22	Saline	32
Giral et al [143]	2004	11	Sphincterotomy	82
		10	30 IAS	70

Abbreviations: EAS, external anal sphincter; IAS, internal anal sphincter.

afford at least an 80% healing rate. This represents simply an estimate, not a formal systematic review or formal analysis.

Most authors choose to inject into the internal sphincter, because hypertonicity of this muscle likely causes the fissure; however, several trials included injection into the external sphincter [114–119]. The authors do not recommend this type of injection; because the pathology is known to lie in the internal sphincter, we choose to direct therapy toward that muscle.

The effect of BTX on the internal sphincter is not permanent. It likely persists for 8 to 12 weeks. This is usually enough time for the fissure to heal. If healing is not completed after this time period, then a second injection of BTX can be performed. This may require a higher dose to achieve adequate sphincter relaxation.

The optimal dose of BTX has not been identified. As detailed in Table 3, most authors choose 20 to 40 units of BTX. Maria and coworkers [120] conducted a prospective trial comparing the rates of healing after injecting 15 or 20 units of BTX. There was a higher rate of healing in the 20-unit group, with a similar safety profile. Minguez and colleagues [121] compared 10, 15, and 21 units of BTX and achieved 83%, 78%, and 90% healing. In another trial, Brisinda and colleagues [122] injected either 20 or 30 units of BTX anteriorly in patients who had posterior fissures. The higher dose was associated with a higher rate of healing. The anal resting pressure was reduced in both groups. The patients receiving 30 units BTX demonstrated a lower squeeze pressure compared with this same group assessed preoperatively, suggesting that the drug diffused from the injection site at the internal sphincter into the external sphincter. It has been demonstrated that higher doses result in a greater fall in resting pressures.

Mentes and coworkers [123] conducted a randomized trial comparing BTX and internal sphincterotomy. After 2 months, the healing rate for BTX patients was approximately 75%; however, 10 of 16 failures were retreated, bringing the overall healing rate to 87%, which is not that far behind the success rate of sphincterotomy.

Complications of BTX have been reported [122,124]. Mild incontinence to gas or feces is not uncommon [116,117,120,122,123,125–127], but is transient. Perianal thrombosis may also occur [115].

Discussion

The overall results for BTX injection are encouraging, with healing rates in excess of 80%. This procedure is safe and effective. It is less expensive and better-tolerated than sphincterotomy.

References

[1] Leicester RJ, Nicholls RJ, Mann CV. Infrared coagulation: a new treatment for hemorrhoids. Dis Colon Rectum 1981;24(8):602–5.

[2] Dennison A, Whiston RJ, Rooney S, et al. A randomized comparison of infrared photoco-agulation with bipolar diathermy for the outpatient treatment of hemorrhoids. Dis Colon Rectum 1990;33(1):32–4.

[3] MacLeod JH. In defense of cryotherapy for hemorrhoids. A modified method. Dis Colon Rectum 1982;25(4):332–5.

[4] Hodgson WJ, Morgan J. Ambulatory hemorrhoidectomy with CO2 laser. Dis Colon Rectum 1995;38(12):1265–9.

[5] MacRae HM, McLeod RS. Comparison of hemorrhoidal treatment modalities. A meta-analysis. Dis Colon Rectum 1995;38(7):687–94.

[6] Murie JA, Sim AJ, Mackenzie I. Rubber band ligation versus haemorrhoidectomy for pro-lapsing haemorrhoids: a long term prospective clinical trial. Br J Surg 1982;69(9):536–8.

[7] Chew SS, Marshall L, Kalish L, et al. Short-term and long-term results of combined scle-rotherapy and rubber band ligation of hemorrhoids and mucosal prolapse. Dis Colon Rectum 2003;46(9):1232–7.

[8] Santos G, Novell JR, Khoury G, et al. Long-term results of large-dose, single-session phe-nol injection sclerotherapy for hemorrhoids. Dis Colon Rectum 1993;36(10):958–61.

[9] Armstrong DN, Frankum C, Schertzer ME, et al. Harmonic Scalpel hemorrhoidectomy: five hundred consecutive cases. Dis Colon Rectum 2002;45(3):354–9.

[10] Ramadan E, Vishne T, Dreznik Z. Harmonic Scalpel hemorrhoidectomy: preliminary re-sults of a new alternative method. Tech Coloproctol 2002;6(2):89–92.

[11] Chung CC, Ha JP, Tai YP, et al. Double-blind, randomized trial comparing Harmonic Scalpel hemorrhoidectomy, bipolar scissors hemorrhoidectomy, and scissors excision: liga-tion technique. Dis Colon Rectum 2002;45(6):789–94.

[12] Corman ML, Gravie JF, Hager T, et al. Stapled haemorrhoidopexy: a consensus position paper by an international working party—indications, contra-indications and technique. Colorectal Dis 2003;5(4):304–10.

[13] Singer MA, Cintron JR, Fleshman JW, et al. Early experience with stapled hemorrhoidec-tomy in the United States. Dis Colon Rectum 2002;45(3):360–7 [discussion: 367–9].

[14] Senagore AJ, Singer M, Abcarian H, et al. A prospective, randomized, controlled multicen-ter trial comparing stapled hemorrhoidopexy and Ferguson hemorrhoidectomy: perioper-ative and one-year results. Dis Colon Rectum 2004;47(11):1824–36.

[15] Ho YH, Cheong WK, Tsang C, et al. Stapled hemorrhoidectomy—cost and effectiveness. Randomized, controlled trial including incontinence scoring, anorectal manometry, and endoanal ultrasound assessments at up to three months. Dis Colon Rectum 2000;43(12): 1666–75.

[16] Mehigan BJ, Monson JR, Hartley JE. Stapling procedure for haemorrhoids versus Milligan-Morgan haemorrhoidectomy: randomised controlled trial. Lancet 2000;355(9206): 782–5.

[17] Boccasanta P, Capretti PG, Venturi M, et al. Randomised controlled trial between stapled circumferential mucosectomy and conventional circular hemorrhoidectomy in advanced hemorrhoids with external mucosal prolapse. Am J Surg 2001;182(1):64–8.

[18] Brown SR, Ballan K, Ho E, et al. Stapled mucosectomy for acute thrombosed circumfer-entially prolapsed piles: a prospective randomized comparison with conventional haemor-rhoidectomy. Colorectal Dis 2001;3(3):175–8.

[19] Shalaby R, Desoky A. Randomized clinical trial of stapled versus Milligan-Morgan hae-morrhoidectomy. Br J Surg 2001;88(8):1049–53.

[20] Hetzer FH, Demartines N, Handschin AE, et al. Stapled vs excision hemorrhoidectomy: long-term results of a prospective randomized trial. Arch Surg 2002;137(3):337–40.

[21] Ortiz H, Marzo J, Armendariz P. Randomized clinical trial of stapled haemorrhoidopexy versus conventional diathermy haemorrhoidectomy. Br J Surg 2002;89(11):1376–81.

[22] Pavlidis T, Papaziogas B, Souparis A, et al. Modern stapled Longo procedure vs. conven-tional Milligan-Morgan hemorrhoidectomy: a randomized controlled trial. Int J Colorectal Dis 2002;17(1):50–3.

[23] Palimento D, Picchio M, Attanasio U, et al. Stapled and open hemorrhoidectomy: randomized controlled trial of early results. World J Surg 2003;27(2):203–7.

[24] Kraemer M, Parulava T, Roblick M, et al. Prospective, randomized study: proximate PPH stapler vs. LigaSure for hemorrhoidal surgery. Dis Colon Rectum 2005;48(8):1517–22.

[25] Correa-Rovelo JM, Tellez O, Obregon L, et al. Stapled rectal mucosectomy vs. closed hemorrhoidectomy: a randomized, clinical trial. Dis Colon Rectum 2002;45(10):1367–74 [discussion: 1374–5].

[26] Wilson MS, Pope V, Doran HE, et al. Objective comparison of stapled anopexy and open hemorrhoidectomy: a randomized, controlled trial. Dis Colon Rectum 2002;45(11): 1437–44.

[27] Rowsell M, Bello M, Hemingway DM. Circumferential mucosectomy (stapled haemorrhoidectomy) versus conventional haemorrhoidectomy: randomised controlled trial. Lancet 2000;355(9206):779–81.

[28] Cheetham MJ, Cohen CR, Kamm MA, et al. A randomized, controlled trial of diathermy hemorrhoidectomy vs. stapled hemorrhoidectomy in an intended day-care setting with longer-term follow-up. Dis Colon Rectum 2003;46(4):491–7.

[29] Bikhchandani J, Agarwal PN, Kant R, et al. Randomized controlled trial to compare the early and mid-term results of stapled versus open hemorrhoidectomy. Am J Surg 2005; 189(1):56–60.

[30] Kairaluoma M, Nuorva K, Kellokumpu I. Day-case stapled (circular) vs. diathermy hemorrhoidectomy: a randomized, controlled trial evaluating surgical and functional outcome. Dis Colon Rectum 2003;46(1):93–9.

[31] Gravie JF, Lehur PA, Huten N, et al. Stapled hemorrhoidopexy versus Milligan-Morgan hemorrhoidectomy: a prospective, randomized, multicenter trial with 2-year postoperative follow up. Ann Surg 2005;242(1):29–35.

[32] Chung CC, Cheung HY, Chan ES, et al. Stapled hemorrhoidopexy vs. Harmonic Scalpel hemorrhoidectomy: a randomized trial. Dis Colon Rectum 2005;48(6):1213–9.

[33] Ortiz H, Marzo J, Armendariz P, et al. Stapled hemorrhoidopexy vs. diathermy excision for fourth-degree hemorrhoids: a randomized, clinical trial and review of the literature. Dis Colon Rectum 2005;48(4):809–15.

[34] Bleday R, Pena JP, Rothenberger DA, et al. Symptomatic hemorrhoids: current incidence and complications of operative therapy. Dis Colon Rectum 1992;35(5):477–81.

[35] Ho YH, Tsang C, Tang CL, et al. Anal sphincter injuries from stapling instruments introduced transanally: randomized, controlled study with endoanal ultrasound and anorectal manometry. Dis Colon Rectum 2000;43(2):169–73.

[36] Ho YH, Tan M, Leong A, et al. Anal pressures impaired by stapler insertion during colorectal anastomosis: a randomized, controlled trial. Dis Colon Rectum 1999;42(1):89–95.

[37] Farouk R, Duthie GS, Lee PW, et al. Endosonographic evidence of injury to the internal anal sphincter after low anterior resection: long-term follow-up. Dis Colon Rectum 1998; 41(7):888–91.

[38] Nisar PJ, Acheson AG, Neal KR, et al. Stapled hemorrhoidopexy compared with conventional hemorrhoidectomy: systematic review of randomized, controlled trials. Dis Colon Rectum 2004;47(11):1837–45.

[39] Ganio E, Altomare DF, Gabrielli F, et al. Prospective randomized multicentre trial comparing stapled with open haemorrhoidectomy. Br J Surg 2001;88(5):669–74.

[40] Lan P, Wu X, Zhou X, et al. The safety and efficacy of stapled hemorrhoidectomy in the treatment of hemorrhoids: a systematic review and meta-analysis of ten randomized control trials. Int J Colorectal Dis 2006;21(2):172–8.

[41] Smyth EF, Baker RP, Wilken BJ, et al. Stapled versus excision haemorrhoidectomy: long-term follow up of a randomised controlled trial. Lancet 2003;361(9367):1437–8.

[42] Racalbuto A, Aliotta I, Corsaro G, et al. Hemorrhoidal stapler prolapsectomy vs. Milligan-Morgan hemorrhoidectomy: a long-term randomized trial. Int J Colorectal Dis 2004;19(3): 239–44.

[43] Krska Z, Kvasnieka J, Faltyn J, et al. Surgical treatment of haemorrhoids according to Longo and Milligan Morgan: an evaluation of postoperative tissue response. Colorectal Dis 2003;5(6):573–6.
[44] Pescatori M. Prospective randomized multicentre trial comparing stapled with open haemorrhoidectomy. Br J Surg 2002;89(1):122.
[45] Roos P. Haemorrhoid surgery revised. Lancet 2000;355(9215):1648.
[46] Maw A, Eu KW, Seow-Choen F. Retroperitoneal sepsis complicating stapled hemorrhoidectomy: report of a case and review of the literature. Dis Colon Rectum 2002;45(6):826–8.
[47] Wong LY, Jiang JK, Chang SC, et al. Rectal perforation: a life-threatening complication of stapled hemorrhoidectomy: report of a case. Dis Colon Rectum 2003;46(1):116–7.
[48] Ripetti V, Caricato M, Arullani A. Rectal perforation, retropneumoperitoneum, and pneumomediastinum after stapling procedure for prolapsed hemorrhoids: report of a case and subsequent considerations. Dis Colon Rectum 2002;45(2):268–70.
[49] Molloy RG, Kingsmore D. Life threatening pelvic sepsis after stapled haemorrhoidectomy. Lancet 2000;355(9206):810.
[50] Cipriani S, Pescatori M. Acute rectal obstruction after PPH stapled haemorrhoidectomy. Colorectal Dis 2002;4(5):367–70.
[51] Mazier WP. The treatment and care of anal fistulas: a study of 1000 patients. Dis Colon Rectum 1971;14(2):134–44.
[52] Ramanujam PS, Prasad ML, Abcarian H, et al. Perianal abscesses and fistulas. A study of 1023 patients. Dis Colon Rectum 1984;27(9):593–7.
[53] van Tets WF, Kuijpers HC. Continence disorders after anal fistulotomy. Dis Colon Rectum 1994;37(12):1194–7.
[54] Lunniss PJ, Kamm MA, Phillips RK. Factors affecting continence after surgery for anal fistula. Br J Surg 1994;81(9):1382–5.
[55] Pearl RK, Andrews JR, Orsay CP, et al. Role of the seton in the management of anorectal fistulas. Dis Colon Rectum 1993;36(6):573–7 [discussion: 577–9].
[56] Garcia-Aguilar J, Belmonte C, Wong WD, et al. Anal fistula surgery. Factors associated with recurrence and incontinence. Dis Colon Rectum 1996;39(7):723–9.
[57] Nelson RL, Cintron J, Abcarian H. Dermal island-flap anoplasty for transsphincteric fistula-in-ano: assessment of treatment failures. Dis Colon Rectum 2000;43(5):681–4.
[58] Kodner IJ, Mazor A, Shemesh EI, et al. Endorectal advancement flap repair of rectovaginal and other complicated anorectal fistulas. Surgery 1993;114(4):682–9 [discussion: 689–90].
[59] Zimmerman DD, Briel JW, Gosselink MP, et al. Anocutaneous advancement flap repair of transsphincteric fistulas. Dis Colon Rectum 2001;44(10):1474–80.
[60] Jun SH, Choi GS. Anocutaneous advancement flap closure of high anal fistulas. Br J Surg 1999;86(4):490–2.
[61] Jones IT, Fazio VW, Jagelman DG. The use of transanal rectal advancement flaps in the management of fistulas involving the anorectum. Dis Colon Rectum 1987;30(12): 919–23.
[62] Garcia-Aguilar J, Belmonte C, Wong DW, et al. Cutting seton versus two-stage seton fistulotomy in the surgical management of high anal fistula. Br J Surg 1998;85(2):243–5.
[63] Hamalainen KP, Sainio AP. Cutting seton for anal fistulas: high risk of minor control defects. Dis Colon Rectum 1997;40(12):1443–6 [discussion: 1447].
[64] Schouten WR, Zimmerman DD, Briel JW. Transanal advancement flap repair of transsphincteric fistulas. Dis Colon Rectum 1999;42(11):1419–22 [discussion: 1422–3].
[65] Williams JG, MacLeod CA, Rothenberger DA, et al. Seton treatment of high anal fistulae. Br J Surg 1991;78(10):1159–61.
[66] Joo JS, Weiss EG, Nogueras JJ, et al. Endorectal advancement flap in perianal Crohn's disease. Am Surg 1998;64(2):147–50.
[67] Mizrahi N, Wexner SD, Zmora O, et al. Endorectal advancement flap: are there predictors of failure? Dis Colon Rectum 2002;45(12):1616–21.

[68] Radosevich M, Goubran HI, Burnouf T. Fibrin sealant: scientific rationale, production methods, properties, and current clinical use. Vox Sang 1997;72(3):133–43.

[69] Romanos GE, Strub JR. Effect of Tissucol on connective tissue matrix during wound healing: an immunohistochemical study in rat skin. J Biomed Mater Res 1998;39(3): 462–8.

[70] Jackson MR. Fibrin sealants in surgical practice: an overview. Am J Surg 2001;182(Suppl 2): 1S–7S.

[71] Hedelin H, Nilson AE, Teger-Nilsson AC, et al. Fibrin occlusion of fistulas postoperatively. Surg Gynecol Obstet 1982;154(3):366–8.

[72] Kirkegaard P, Madsen PV. Perineal sinus after removal of the rectum. Occlusion with fibrin adhesive. Am J Surg 1983;145(6):791–4.

[73] Lindsey I, Smilgin-Humphreys MM, Cunningham C, et al. A randomized, controlled trial of fibrin glue vs. conventional treatment for anal fistula. Dis Colon Rectum 2002;45(12): 1608–15.

[74] Singer M, Cintron J, Nelson R, et al. Treatment of fistulas-in-ano with fibrin sealant in combination with intra-adhesive antibiotics and/or surgical closure of the internal fistula opening. Dis Colon Rectum 2005;48(4):799–808.

[75] Cintron JR, Park JJ, Orsay CP, et al. Repair of fistulas-in-ano using fibrin adhesive: long-term follow-up. Dis Colon Rectum 2000;43(7):944–9 [discussion: 949–50].

[76] Sentovich SM. Fibrin glue for anal fistulas: long-term results. Dis Colon Rectum 2003; 46(4):498–502.

[77] Abel ME, Chiu YS, Russell TR, et al. Autologous fibrin glue in the treatment of rectovaginal and complex fistulas. Dis Colon Rectum 1993;36(5):447–9.

[78] Aitola P, Hiltunen KM, Matikainen M. Fibrin glue in perianal fistulas—a pilot study. Ann Chir Gynaecol 1999;88(2):136–8.

[79] Hjortrup A, Moesgaard F, Kjaergard J. Fibrin adhesive in the treatment of perineal fistulas. Dis Colon Rectum 1991;34(9):752–4.

[80] Salim AS, Ahmed TM. KTP-Laser and fibrin glue for treatment of fistulae in ano. Saudi Med J 2001;22(11):1022–4.

[81] Patrlj L, Kocman B, Martinac M, et al. Fibrin glue-antibiotic mixture in the treatment of anal fistulae: experience with 69 cases. Dig Surg 2000;17(1):77–80.

[82] Venkatesh KS, Ramanujam P. Fibrin glue application in the treatment of recurrent anorectal fistulas. Dis Colon Rectum 1999;42(9):1136–9.

[83] Chan KM, Lau CW, Lai KK, et al. Preliminary results of using a commercial fibrin sealant in the treatment of fistula-in-ano. J R Coll Surg Edinb 2002;47(1):407–10.

[84] Buchanan GN, Bartram CI, Phillips RK, et al. Efficacy of fibrin sealant in the management of complex anal fistula: a prospective trial. Dis Colon Rectum 2003;46(9): 1167–74.

[85] El-Shobaky M, Khafagy W, El-Awady W. Autologous fibrin glue in the treatment of fistula-in-ano. Colorectal Dis 2000;2(Supp):17.

[86] Zmora O, Mizrahi N, Rotholtz N, et al. Fibrin glue sealing in the treatment of perineal fistulas. Dis Colon Rectum 2003;46(5):584–9.

[87] Loungnarath R, Dietz DW, Mutch MG, et al. Fibrin glue treatment of complex anal fistulas has low success rate. Dis Colon Rectum 2004;47(4):432–6.

[88] Kram HB, Bansal M, Timberlake O, et al. Antibacterial effects of fibrin glue-antibiotic mixtures. J Surg Res 1991;50(2):175–8.

[89] Christie RJ, Carrington L, Alving B. Postoperative bleeding induced by topical bovine thrombin: report of two cases. Surgery 1997;121(6):708–10.

[90] Beierlein W, Scheule AM, Antoniadis G, et al. An immediate, allergic skin reaction to aprotinin after reexposure to fibrin sealant. Transfusion 2000;40(3):302–5.

[91] Berguer R, Staerkel RL, Moore EE, et al. Warning: fatal reaction to the use of fibrin glue in deep hepatic wounds. Case reports. J Trauma 1991;31(3):408–11.

[92] Lund JN, Scholefield JH. Aetiology and treatment of anal fissure. Br J Surg 1996;83(10): 1335–44.

[93] Schouten WR, Briel JW, Auwerda JJ. Relationship between anal pressure and anodermal blood flow. The vascular pathogenesis of anal fissures. Dis Colon Rectum 1994;37(7): 664–9.

[94] Schouten WR, Briel JW, Auwerda JJ, et al. Ischaemic nature of anal fissure. Br J Surg 1996; 83(1):63–5.

[95] Garcia-Aguilar J, Belmonte C, Wong WD, et al. Open vs. closed sphincterotomy for chronic anal fissure: long-term results. Dis Colon Rectum 1996;39(4):440–3.

[96] Nyam DC, Pemberton JH. Long-term results of lateral internal sphincterotomy for chronic anal fissure with particular reference to incidence of fecal incontinence. Dis Colon Rectum 1999;42(10):1306–10.

[97] Altomare DF, Rinaldi M, Milito G, et al. Glyceryl trinitrate for chronic anal fissure—healing or headache? Results of a multicenter, randomized, placebo-controled, double-blind trial. Dis Colon Rectum 2000;43(2):174–9 [discussion: 179–81].

[98] Antropoli C, Perrotti P, Rubino M, et al. Nifedipine for local use in conservative treatment of anal fissures: preliminary results of a multicenter study. Dis Colon Rectum 1999;42(8): 1011–5.

[99] Bacher H, Mischinger HJ, Werkgartner G, et al. Local nitroglycerin for treatment of anal fissures: an alternative to lateral sphincterotomy? Dis Colon Rectum 1997;40(7):840–5.

[100] Bailey HR, Beck DE, Billingham RP, et al. A study to determine the nitroglycerin ointment dose and dosing interval that best promote the healing of chronic anal fissures. Dis Colon Rectum 2002;45(9):1192–9.

[101] Bassotti G, Clementi M, Ceccarelli F, et al. Double-blind manometric assessment of two topical glyceryl trinitrate formulations in patients with chronic anal fissures. Dig Liver Dis 2000;32(8):699–702.

[102] Carapeti EA, Kamm MA, McDonald PJ, et al. Randomised controlled trial shows that glyceryl trinitrate heals anal fissures, higher doses are not more effective, and there is a high recurrence rate. Gut 1999;44(5):727–30.

[103] Chaudhuri S, Pal AK, Acharya A, et al. Treatment of chronic anal fissure with topical glyceryl trinitrate: a double-blind, placebo-controlled trial. Indian J Gastroenterol 2001;20(3): 101–2.

[104] Evans J, Luck A, Hewett P. Glyceryl trinitrate vs. lateral sphincterotomy for chronic anal fissure: prospective, randomized trial. Dis Colon Rectum 2001;44(1):93–7.

[105] Jonas M, Neal KR, Abercrombie JF, et al. A randomized trial of oral vs. topical diltiazem for chronic anal fissures. Dis Colon Rectum 2001;44(8):1074–8.

[106] Kennedy ML, Sowter S, Nguyen H, et al. Glyceryl trinitrate ointment for the treatment of chronic anal fissure: results of a placebo-controlled trial and long-term follow-up. Dis Colon Rectum 1999;42(8):1000–6.

[107] Kocher HM, Steward M, Leather AJ, et al. Randomized clinical trial assessing the side-effects of glyceryl trinitrate and diltiazem hydrochloride in the treatment of chronic anal fissure. Br J Surg 2002;89(4):413–7.

[108] Libertiny G, Knight JS, Farouk R. Randomised trial of topical 0.2% glyceryl trinitrate and lateral internal sphincterotomy for the treatment of patients with chronic anal fissure: long-term follow-up. Eur J Surg 2002;168(7):418–21.

[109] Lund JN, Scholefield JH. A randomised, prospective, double-blind, placebo-controlled trial of glyceryl trinitrate ointment in treatment of anal fissure. Lancet 1997;349(9044):11–4.

[110] Oettle GJ. Glyceryl trinitrate vs. sphincterotomy for treatment of chronic fissure-in-ano: a randomized, controlled trial. Dis Colon Rectum 1997;40(11):1318–20.

[111] Perrotti P, Bove A, Antropoli C, et al. Topical nifedipine with lidocaine ointment vs. active control for treatment of chronic anal fissure: results of a prospective, randomized, double-blind study. Dis Colon Rectum 2002;45(11):1468–75.

[112] Richard CS, Gregoire R, Plewes EA, et al. Internal sphincterotomy is superior to topical nitroglycerin in the treatment of chronic anal fissure: results of a randomized, controlled trial by the Canadian Colorectal Surgical Trials Group. Dis Colon Rectum 2000;43(8): 1048–57 [discussion: 1057–8].

[113] Nelson R. A systematic review of medical therapy for anal fissure. Dis Colon Rectum 2004; 47(4):422–31.

[114] Jost WH, Schimrigk K. Use of botulinum toxin in anal fissure. Dis Colon Rectum 1993; 36(10):974.

[115] Jost WH, Schimrigk K. Botulinum toxin in therapy of anal fissure. Lancet 1995;345(8943): 188–9.

[116] Jost WH. One hundred cases of anal fissure treated with botulin toxin: early and long-term results. Dis Colon Rectum 1997;40(9):1029–32.

[117] Jost WH, Schrank B. Repeat botulin toxin injections in anal fissure: in patients with relapse and after insufficient effect of first treatment. Dig Dis Sci 1999;44(8):1588–9.

[118] Madalinski MH, Slawek J, Zbytek B, et al. Topical injections and the higher doses of botulinum toxin for chronic anal fissure. Hepatogastroenterology 2001;48(40):977–9.

[119] Madalinski MH. Nonsurgical treatment modalities for chronic anal fissure using botulinum toxin. Gastroenterology 1999;117(2):516–7.

[120] Maria G, Cassetta E, Gui D, et al. A comparison of botulinum toxin and saline for the treatment of chronic anal fissure. N Engl J Med 1998;338(4):217–20.

[121] Minguez M, Melo F, Espi A, et al. Therapeutic effects of different doses of botulinum toxin in chronic anal fissure. Dis Colon Rectum 1999;42(8):1016–21.

[122] Brisinda G, Maria G, Sganga G, et al. Effectiveness of higher doses of botulinum toxin to induce healing in patients with chronic anal fissures. Surgery 2002;131(2):179–84.

[123] Mentes BB, Irkorucu O, Akin M, et al. Comparison of botulinum toxin injection and lateral internal sphincterotomy for the treatment of chronic anal fissure. Dis Colon Rectum 2003; 46(2):232–7.

[124] Tilney HS, Heriot AG, Cripps NP. Complication of botulinum toxin injections for anal fissure. Dis Colon Rectum 2001;44(11):1721–4.

[125] Gui D, Cassetta E, Anastasio G, et al. Botulinum toxin for chronic anal fissure. Lancet 1994;344(8930):1127–8.

[126] Brisinda D, Maria G, Fenici R, et al. Safety of botulinum neurotoxin treatment in patients with chronic anal fissure. Dis Colon Rectum 2003;46(3):419–20.

[127] Madalinski M, Jagiello K, Labon M, et al. Botulinum toxin injection into only one point in the external anal sphincter: a modification of the treatment for chronic anal fissure. Endoscopy 1999;31(9):S63.

[128] Ramirez RT, Hicks TC, Beck DE. Use of Tisseel fibrin sealant for complex fistulas using conscious sedation. ASCRS Annual Scientific meeting. Boston, June 2000.

[129] Vitton V, Gasmi M, Barthet M, et al. Long-term healing of Chrohn's anal fistulas with fibrin glue injection. Alimentary Pharmacology and Therapeutics 2005;21(12):1453–7.

[130] Jost WH, Schimrigk K. Therapy of anal fissure using botulin toxin. Dis Color Rectum 1994; 37(12):1321–4.

[131] Brisinda G, Maria G, Bentivoglio AR, et al. A comparison of injections of botulinum toxin and topical nitroglycerin ointment for the treatment of chronic anal fissure. New England Journal of Medicine 1999;341(2):65–9.

[132] Fernandez Lopez F, Conde Freire R, Rios Rios A, et al. Bolinum toxin for the treatment of anal fissure. Dig Surg 1999;16(6):515–8.

[133] Lysy J, Israelit-Yatzkan Y, Sestiery-Ittah M, et al. Topical nitrates potentiate the effect of botulinum toxin in the treatment of patients with refractory anal fissure. Gut 2001;48(2): 221–4.

[134] Trzcinski R, Dziki A, Tchorzewski M. Injections of botulinum A toxin for the treatment of anal fissures. European Journal of Surgery 2002;168(12):720–3.

[135] Wollina U, Konrad H. Botulinum toxin A in anal fissures: a modified technique. Journal of the European Academy of Dermatology & Venereology 2002;16:469–71.

[136] Maria G, Brisinda G, Bentivoglio AR, et al. Botulinum toxin injections in the internal anal sphincter for the treatment of chronic anal fissure: long-term results after two different dosage regimens. Ann Surg 1998;228:664–9.

[137] Maria G, Brisinda G, Bentivoglio AR, et al. Influence of botulinum toxin site of injections on healing rate in patients with chronic anal fissure. American Journal of Surgery 2000; 179(1):46–50.

[138] Mason PF, Watkins MJ, Hall HS, et al. The management of chronic fissure in ano with botulinum toxin. J R Coll Surg Edinb 1996;41:235–8.

[139] Espi A, et al. Therapeutic use of botulinum toxin in anal fissure. Int J Colorectal Dis 1997; 12:163.

[140] Khademi A, Feldman DM. A comparison of combination of botox (botulinum toxin) and nitroglycerin in the treatment of chronic anal fissure. Am J Gastroenterol 2000;95:2538.

[141] Siproudhis L, Sebille V, Pigot F, et al. Lack of efficacy of botulinum toxin in chronic anal fissure. Aliment Pharmacol Ther 2003;18:515–24.

[142] Colak T, Ipek T, Kanik A, et al. A randomized trial of botulinum toxin vs lidocain pomade for chronic anal fissure. Acta Gastroenterol Belg 2002;65:187–90.

[143] Giral A, Memisoglu K, Gultekin Y, et al. Botulinum toxin injection versus lateral internal sphincterotomy in the treatment of chronic anal fissure: a non-randomized controlled trial. BMC Gastroenterol 2004;4:7.

[144] Gonzalez Carro P, Perez Roldan F, Legaz Huidobro ML, et al. The treatment of anal fissure with botulinum toxin. Gastroenterol Hepatol 1999;22:163–6.

ELSEVIER
SAUNDERS

SURGICAL
CLINICS OF
NORTH AMERICA

Surg Clin N Am 86 (2006) 969–986

Novel Approaches in the Treatment of Fecal Incontinence

Benjamin Person, MD[a], Orit Kaidar-Person, MD[a],
Steven D. Wexner, MD, FACS, FRCS, FRCS(Ed)[a,b,c,d,*]

[a]Department of Colorectal Surgery, Cleveland Clinic Florida, 2950 Cleveland Clinic
Boulevard, Weston, Florida 33331, USA
[b]Ohio State University Health Sciences Center, Cleveland Clinic Foundation,
9500 Euclid Avenue, Cleveland, Ohio 44195, USA
[c]University of South Florida, College of Medicine, 12901 Bruce B. Downs Boulevard,
Tampa, Florida 33612, USA
[d]Department of Biomedical Science, Charles E. Schmidt College of Medicine,
Florida Atlantic University, 777 Glades Road, Boca Raton, Florida 33431, USA

Fecal incontinence (FI) usually is defined as the involuntary loss of bowel control, which normally allows the passage of gas or stool at a socially acceptable time and place. Normal continence results from an integrated activity of the anal sphincters, pelvic floor muscles, and adequate neural input. It also is influenced by stool consistency, rectal capacity and compliance, the anorectal sampling reflex, normal resting anal tone, and normal anorectal sensation. Failure of any of those factors may result in FI [1]. The tremendous physical, emotional, social, and even economic adverse effects of FI are well documented [2–5]. Owing to the social stigma that is associated with FI, this condition is usually underreported and probably underestimated. The true incidence and prevalence of FI are unknown; one community-based survey of nearly 7000 individuals reported that 2.2% of those surveyed had FI [6], although a more recent meta-analysis reported significantly higher rates ranging from 11% to 15% [7]. FI is the second leading cause of nursing home placement with up to 45% of patients in nursing homes having some form of FI [8]. The major risk factors for FI are anal sphincter and pudendal nerve injuries occurring during vaginal deliveries [9], making FI significantly more prevalent in women.

* Corresponding author. Department of Colorectal Surgery, Cleveland Clinic Florida, 2950 Cleveland Clinic Boulevard, Weston, FL 33331.
E-mail address: wexners@ccf.org (S.D. Wexner).

0039-6109/06/$ - see front matter © 2006 Elsevier Inc. All rights reserved.
doi:10.1016/j.suc.2006.06.010
surgical.theclinics.com

When planning a treatment regimen, it is extremely important to make the subjective complaints and symptoms of FI somewhat more objective. To accomplish that goal several scoring systems have been designed and validated, the Cleveland Clinic Florida FI (CCF-FI; Wexner) score being the most popular and widely cited [10]. This scale measures the frequency of incontinence to gas, liquid, and solid stool; the degree of alteration in lifestyle; and the use of protective devices (0 = total control, 20 = complete incontinence). In one of several validation studies of this scoring system it has been demonstrated that a score greater than 9 is associated with a significant alteration in quality of life and can be used as an indication for surgical therapy [11].

Because diarrhea is one of its most common aggravating factors, the mainstay of the medical management of FI is control of diarrhea through dietary modifications and a wide variety of antidiarrheal medications. Strengthening and retraining of the pelvic floor and sphincter muscles with biofeedback may be used as an adjunct to the medical treatment. The decision of which surgical modality should be undertaken is usually straightforward, depending on the condition of the anal sphincters. Patients who have obvious sphincter defects normally should undergo an overlapping sphincteroplasty; conversely, other modalities should be pursued in patients who have intact sphincters.

Injectable bulking agents

For decades, a wide variety of materials have been used successfully as bulking agents of the urinary sphincter in women who have urinary incontinence. The materials that are currently approved by the United States Food and Drug Administration (FDA) for that indication are autologous fat [12], glutaraldehyde cross-linked (GAX) collagen [13], and carbon beads [14]. These materials, when injected adjacent to the bladder neck, provide additional bulk to the malfunctioning urinary sphincter, thus improving its function. Following the success of this treatment modality, it was only a matter of time until this concept was attempted for patients who have FI. Shafik [15] provided the first report of successful short-term outcomes of treatment of FI with submucosal injection of polytetrafluoroethylene (Teflon or Polytef; DuPont, Wilmington, DE) in 1993, and similar outcomes with the use of autologous fat in 1995 [16]. Additional materials that have been used as bulking agents for the anal sphincters with varying degrees of success include GAX collagen (Contigen; Brad, Covington, GA) [17] and injectable-silicone – PTQ implants (formerly known as Bioplastique; Uroplasty BV, Geleen, The Netherlands) [18,19]. The long-term results are less encouraging than the initial results of these small pilot trials, however. The slow deterioration in fecal continence following the initial improvement was attributed to migration or flattening of the bulking material, sometimes necessitating additional injections. There are several other bulking agents that are commonly used in the fields of urology and plastic surgery, but there are limited published reports regarding their use for the treatment of FI.

Carbon-coated beads are another compound that initially has been used as a bulking agent for treating urinary incontinence and recently applied for FI also. Durasphere FI (formerly known as ACYST; Carbon Medical Technologies, Inc., St. Paul, MN, distributed by Boston Scientific Corporation, Boston, MA) is composed of pyrolytic, carbon-coated, zirconium oxide beads suspended in a water-based carrier gel containing β-glucan (Figs. 1–3). The beads have a dimension of 212–500 μm, which has been designed specifically to be nonmigratory, nonabsorbable, and biocompatible, and the gel is approximately 97% water and 3% β-glucan. Durasphere FI is manufactured in 1 mL or 3 mL sterile syringes, and may be injected either submucosally in the anal canal and distal rectum adjacently to the anal sphincter or in the intersphincteric space.

Weiss and colleagues [20] from Cleveland Clinic Florida presented their experience with Durasphere FI. A total of 10 patients (7 women) who had severe FI were enrolled in a prospective, open-label pilot trial. The patients who were included in the trial had all failed previous attempts at standard, nonsurgical treatment of FI, and all had intact external anal sphincters. In all patients the procedure was performed as an outpatient, office-based procedure under local anesthesia. Durasphere FI was injected in the submucosal space 0.5 to 1 cm distal to the dentate line, typically 45° apart. Eight of the 10 patients (80%) experienced symptomatic improvement. The CCF-FI score decreased from an average of 13 at baseline to 10 at 3 months after the injection ($P = .012$), and to 9.3 after 6 months. Davis and coworkers [21] used Durasphere FI in a slightly different manner. The authors treated 18 incontinent patients who had internal anal sphincter defects and injected the compound submucosally only adjacently to the area of the disrupted sphincter until the regularity of the anal canal was restored. The CCF-FI score decreased from a baseline of 11.89 to 8.07 at 12 months ($P = .002$), with no reduction of the effect over time. The authors demonstrated a strong correlation between the number of sites that were injected and the degree of improvement in the incontinence scores. In both trials [20,21] there was a significant improvement in FI quality-of-life scores in addition to the symptomatic improvement.

The effects of Durasphere FI were evaluated recently in a large multicenter trial in the United States in which the investigators noted that intersphincteric

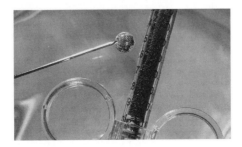

Fig. 1. Durasphere® FI. Courtesy of Carbon Medical Inc., St. Paul, Minnesota.

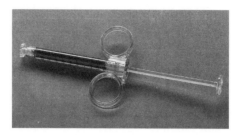

Fig. 2. Durasphere® FI. Courtesy of Carbon Medical Inc., St. Paul, Minnesota.

injection of the bulking agent may achieve significant and durable improvement with fewer mucosal complications, such as erosion or migration (EG
Weiss, personal communication, 2004), and thus may provide an attractive alternative to submucosal injection. There are several potential mechanisms in
which Durasphere FI achieves its effect: the bulk provides additional resistance to the passage of stool and allows for improved sensation and discrimination, the physical filling of sphincter defects restores the normal contour of
the anal canal, and the continuous fibrosis adds further volume to the sphincter muscles. This procedure has proven to be a safe, simple, inexpensive, and
effective technique in the treatment of moderate to severe FI.

Radiofrequency

Physicians have used thermal energy for treating a wide variety of medical conditions; electricity by far is the most prevalent energy source for generating thermal energy. For decades electrocautery has replaced cautery for
cutting tissue and controlling bleeding by coagulating blood vessels. The
radiofrequency (RF) device deploys energy by generating heat through
a high-frequency alternating current that is delivered to the tissue, causing
frictional movement of ions and heat. The immediate result is contraction

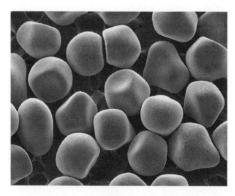

Fig. 3. Durasphere® FI: carbon-coated micro-beads. Courtesy of Carbon Medical Inc., St.
Paul, Minnesota.

of collagen fibers, with subsequent healing and remodeling processes that cause shortening of the fibers and tightening of the tissue [22]. This specific effect of RF energy has been applied for treating gastroesophageal reflux disease (GERD) [23–25], benign prostatic hypertrophy [26], joint capsule instability [27], and even obstructive sleep apnea syndrome and snoring [28–30]. Temperature-controlled RF is a modification of the technology in which a constant temperature monitoring and feedback is used to control the amount of energy delivered to the treated tissue, with a simultaneous cooling that minimizes the damage to the surface. The Stretta procedure (Curon Medical, Sunnyvale, CA) was approved by the FDA in April 2000 for treating GERD. In view of its efficacy, Curon Medical developed a similar procedure for treating FI, the Secca procedure, which was approved by the FDA in March 2002. The system consists of a central control module, a four-channel radiofrequency generator, and an anoscopic handpiece (Figs. 4 and 5). Four titanium needle electrodes that are located at the handpiece (Fig. 6) deliver the energy to the tissue. Thermocouples at the tip and base of each needle constantly monitor the temperature of the treated tissue and mucosal surface; the current is automatically interrupted if the temperature reaches the preselected target of 85°C. The procedure is typically performed in an ambulatory setting, either in the endoscopy suite or in the operating room. The patient is positioned in the prone-jackknife position, and intravenous sedation, local anesthesia, and prophylactic antibiotics are administered. The handpiece is inserted under direct visualization into the anal canal to the level of the dentate line (Fig. 7) and the four needle electrodes deliver the RF energy for 90 seconds at that level. Additional applications in all four quadrants are administered in 5-mm increments proximal to the dentate line for a total of 16 to 20 application sites depending on the height of the anal sphincter (Fig. 8).

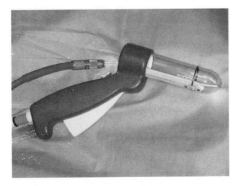

Fig. 4. The Secca® handpiece. *From* Efron JE, Corman ML, Fleshman J, et al. Safety and effectiveness of temperature-controlled radio-frequency energy delivery to the anal canal (Secca procedure) for the treatment of fecal incontinence. Dis Colon Rectum 2003;46(12):1606–18; with permission.

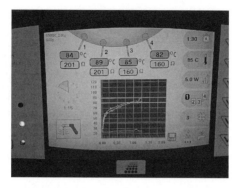

Fig. 5. The Secca® control module. *From* Efron JE, Corman ML, Fleshman J, et al. Safety and effectiveness of temperature-controlled radio-frequency energy delivery to the anal canal (Secca procedure) for the treatment of fecal incontinence. Dis Colon Rectum 2003;46(12):1606–18; with permission.

Takahashi and colleagues [31] reported the results of the first trial that assessed the efficacy of the procedure for treating FI with a subsequent report of the results at 2-year follow-up [32]. The investigators treated 10 female patients with the Secca procedure and observed a significant reduction in the CCF-FI score from 13.5 at baseline to 5 after 12 months ($P < .001$); the average CCF-FI score after 2 years was 7.3 ($P = .002$), which further emphasizes the procedure's long-term durability. Efron and coworkers [33] treated 50 patients with the Secca procedure in a multicenter trial in the United States. The average CCF-FI score decreased from 14.5 at

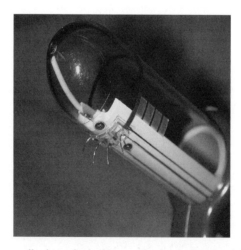

Fig. 6. Four titanium needle electrodes in the operating head of the handpiece. *From* Efron JE, Corman ML, Fleshman J, et al. Safety and effectiveness of temperature-controlled radio-frequency energy delivery to the anal canal (Secca procedure) for the treatment of fecal incontinence. Dis Colon Rectum 2003;46(12):1606–18; with permission.

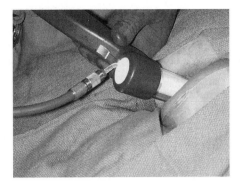

Fig. 7. Placement of the Secca® handpiece into the anal canal. *From* Efron JE, Corman ML, Fleshman J, et al. Safety and effectiveness of temperature-controlled radio-frequency energy delivery to the anal canal (Secca procedure) for the treatment of fecal incontinence. Dis Colon Rectum 2003;46(12):1606–18; with permission.

baseline to 11.1 after 6 months ($P < .0001$). Again, in both studies a significant improvement in quality of life was demonstrated. A multi-institutional single-blinded randomized prospective trial comparing the Secca procedure to a sham intervention has been completed recently and its results are pending.

Stimulated graciloplasty

The concept of substituting the anal sphincter with another muscle was attempted more than a century ago by Chetwood [34], who used the gluteus maximus muscle to replace the sphincter. A skeletal muscle that is considered as a potential candidate for this task should have a relatively negligible role in

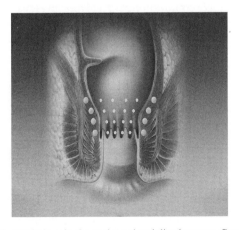

Fig. 8. Location of the RF lesions in the anal canal and distal rectum. Courtesy of Curon Medical, Inc., Fremont, California.

movement or posture, should be large enough to provide sufficient bulk, and should have a neurovascular pedicle that will allow simple handling in the process of mobilization and transposition. Since Chetwood's first experiment, several modifications to his technique of using the gluteus maximus have been made [35,36]. Although the gluteus maximus is theoretically a good option because of its strength and proximity to the anus, harvesting it for treating FI may result in significant impairment in performing simple daily activities, such as standing up or climbing stairs. The sartorius muscle has been used successfully in dogs [37], but its mobilization in humans may be complicated because of a segmental vascular supply that can be compromised easily during mobilization. The gracilis muscle is the smallest and most superficial adductor of the thigh. It has a relatively consistent proximal neurovascular pedicle and it has an insignificant role in movement. Like any other skeletal muscle, the gracilis is comprised mainly of type II fast-twitch fibers, which are prone to fatigue after prolonged contraction. Conversely, the external anal sphincter has approximately 80% type I, slow-twitch fibers, which are relatively fatigue resistant [38]. Transforming type II fibers to type I may be achieved by application of a constant low-frequency electrical current, a process that was termed muscle conditioning [39]. The technique used by most surgeons today was described initially by Pickrell and colleagues [40] in 1952, and the principle of conditioning with an electrical stimulator was independently reported in the same issue of The Lancet in 1991 by Baeten and coworkers [41] and Williams and coworkers [42]. The technique involves the transposition of the gracilis muscle from the thigh to form a muscular ring around the anus with the distal tendon anchored to the contralateral ischial tuberosity (Fig. 9). There are two phases in this procedure, with the number of required operations depending on whether the surgeon elects to create a protective stoma. The first phase usually consists of transposition of the muscle and implantation of the stimulator and electrodes (Medtronic Inc., Minneapolis, MN), and the second phase involves 8 weeks of muscle conditioning with increasing levels of neuromuscular

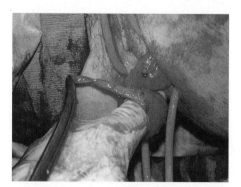

Fig. 9. The patient's left gracilis is wrapped around the surgeon's index finger. *From* Person B, Wexner SD. Advances in the surgical treatment of fecal incontinence. Surg Innov 2005;12(1): 7–21; with permission.

stimulation. The use of a diverting stoma requires additional operative inter-vention for creation and subsequent closure. On completion of the second phase, the patients can control continence with the aid of an external magnet that turns the stimulator off to allow evacuation and back on to resume mus-cular contraction and continence.

The Dynamic Graciloplasty Therapy Study Group conducted the largest prospective multi-national trial that assessed this procedure and produced both short-term and long-term data [43,44]. In the initial report [43], 60% of the patients had significant improvement in continence and quality of life; the long-term durability of the procedure was demonstrated by showing that at 2-year follow-up 62% of the patients had significant improvement in continence and quality-of-life parameters [44]. Nevertheless, stimulated gra-ciloplasty is technically demanding with considerable morbidity; a systematic review of the literature on the subject of stimulated graciloplasty [45] dem-onstrated that every patient had an average of 1.12 complications, with the most common being infection (28%), malfunctioning stimulator or elec-trodes (15%), and leg pain (13%). Efficacy ranged from 42% to 85%, and the rate of re-operation ranged from 0.14 to 1.07 per patient. Even though the complication rates of this procedure were high, most complications, with the exception of major infections, could be treated successfully without adversely affecting functional outcome.

Sadly, although this option is the best one for patients who have severe perineal tissue loss, the Medtronic Corporation decided not to pursue FDA approval and thus this beneficial procedure is no longer performed in the United States; fortunately, the stimulated graciloplasty remains a via-ble option in other parts of the world.

Artificial bowel sphincter

Another concept that was adapted from the field of urology is the use of synthetic material to replace a malfunctioning sphincter. Artificial sphinc-ters have been used to treat urinary incontinence since 1973 [46], and the first report of their use for treating FI was in 1987 [47]. The current version of the artificial bowel sphincter (ABS), the Acticon Neosphincter (American Medical Systems, Minnetonka, MN), consists of three silastic components: an inflatable cuff, a pressure-regulating balloon, and a control pump that allows activation or deactivation of the device (Fig. 10). The inflatable cuff is implanted around the anus and is connected by silastic tubing to the control pump placed in the scrotum of men or in the major labia of women, on the side of the patient's dominant hand. The control pump also is connected to the pressure-regulating balloon, which is implanted in the space of Retzius (Fig. 11). The pressure-regulating balloon constantly maintains the cuff pressure, keeping the cuff inflated and the anus closed. By manual activation of the pump, the fluid leaves the cuff into the balloon, thus deflating the cuff and allowing evacuation. The fluid subsequently

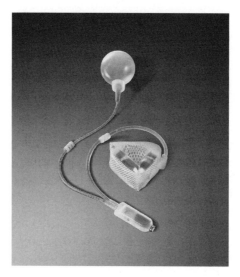

Fig. 10. The Acticon® neosphincter. Courtesy of American Medical Systems, Inc., Minnetonka, Minnesota.

returns into the cuff by the pressure that is created in the balloon. This maneuver may be repeated if evacuation is incomplete.

The Acticon Neosphincter was approved by the FDA in 1999. The largest case series to date that assessed its safety and efficacy was reported by Wong and colleagues [48] in 2002. A total of 112 patients were enrolled in a prospective multicenter nonrandomized cohort trial. At 1-year follow-up 75 of these 112 patients (67%) had a functional device; of these, 85% had significant

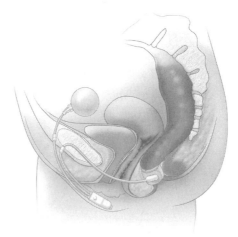

Fig. 11. The final position of the ABS in a female patient. Courtesy of American Medical Systems, Inc., Minnetonka, Minnesota.

improvement in incontinence scores and quality-of-life parameters. The overall intention to treat success rate was 53%. Ninety-nine patients (88%) had a total of 384 complications related to the ABS; 41 patients (37%) had their ABS completely explanted, and the overall infection rate that led to surgical interventions was 25%. In a recent prospective comparison of eight cases of dynamic graciloplasty and eight implantations of the ABS followed for more than 3 years, there was no difference in complications, wound healing problems, or explantation rates, all of which were considerably high in both groups, although the ABS was found to be more effective in lowering the FI scores [49]. A systematic review of the literature about ABS [50] demonstrated that approximately one third of patients have their ABS explanted by the end of the follow-up period; this number approaches 50% in series with the longest follow-up (5 years), which may be an indirect indicator of the lifespan of the device. There are no reported data on the outcomes of patients in whom the ABS was explanted. Because these patients represent a substantial percentage of all those treated by ABS, and the condition of these patients may have deteriorated following the explantation, these data may be crucial to fully appreciate the true efficacy and safety of the device. Recent modifications to the perioperative antibiotic treatment regimens resulted in a significant reduction in the rates of infectious complications to approximately 9% (unpublished data).

Despite these numerous drawbacks, ABS remains one of only a few available surgical treatment modalities for patients who have end-stage FI who otherwise would require a permanent stoma; however, it has limited or no usefulness in patients who have major perineal tissue loss. In these individuals, a nonstimulated graciloplasty before implantation of an ABS may prove beneficial as a means of bulking or replenishing the lost tissue, or a stimulated graciloplasty may be considered.

Sacral nerve stimulation

The latest and most innovative modality in the armamentarium available for treating FI is sacral nerve stimulation (SNS). Once again the concept was initially implemented for treating urinary incontinence, and subsequently the technology has been adopted by the colorectal community also. Patients who were treated by SNS for urinary incontinence and had FI also soon noted a significant improvement in both symptoms. This observation prompted investigators to attempt SNS in patients who had isolated FI. Matzel and colleagues [51] published the first report of successful outcomes in three patients who were treated with SNS in 1995; in the decade since that initial report, several hundred patients have been treated with SNS for FI in Europe; in the United States, SNS is currently under investigation in a multicenter trial.

The innervation of the pelvic floor musculature and anal sphincter apparatus is derived from both the somatic and autonomic nervous systems. Terminal nerve fibers of both nervous systems reach the target organs in the pelvis by way of the sacral plexus. The rationale behind SNS is that direct stimulation of the sacral nerves potentially will result in recruitment and arousing of additional, inactive motor units. SNS also has a beneficial effect on the sensory and autonomic components of the sacral nerves as demonstrated by improvement in rectal sensory threshold and improved balloon expulsion time [52] and an increase in the resting anal pressure and rectal blood flow [53].

The technique of SNS is unique in the sense that it includes an extremely strict patient selection process, which is an integral part of the procedure sequence itself. This selection process allows choosing patients with the best potential to benefit from the procedure. The hardware for the procedure (stimulator and electrodes) is supplied by Medtronic Inc, Minneapolis, MN. SNS is a staged procedure that consists of two stages: percutaneous nerve evaluation (PNE, the diagnostic stage), and the permanent implant (the therapeutic stage). The PNE consists of two steps: in the acute phase the feasibility of SNS is determined and the sacral nerve that elicits the best muscular response is selected; in the subchronic phase of this stage SNS is performed with an external stimulator for a period of 2 weeks, during which the therapeutic effect is assessed. The patient is placed in the prone position and local anesthesia is administered; the sacral foramina are identified using bony landmarks and the needle electrodes are inserted into the foramina with fluoroscopic guidance. Correct placement of the electrodes is determined by intermittent electrical stimulation until visual muscular contraction is obtained. Typical muscular responses include contraction of the perineal muscles and external rotation of the leg (S2), contraction of the levator ani and external sphincter with a plantar flexion of the first and second toes—the "bellows response" (S3), and contraction of the external sphincter without movement of any part of the leg (S4). When satisfactory response is achieved, the subchronic phase of the PNE is initiated. This phase involves placement of a temporary stimulator lead into the same position as the testing needle. This lead is left in place for a trial period of 2 weeks to allow evaluation of functional response. The decision to proceed from temporary to permanent stimulation is made on the basis of 50% functional improvement in either the number of episodes or incontinence-free days. Patients who experience such an improvement are offered a permanent implant. The permanent stimulator (Model 3023 InterStim implantable pulse generator; Medtronic Inc., Minneapolis, MN) (Fig. 12) is implanted in the subcutaneous tissue in the buttock; the patients may deactivate the stimulator or modulate the delivered energy with a hand-held device.

Most of the reports that assessed the efficacy of SNS for FI included small numbers of patients and had relatively short follow-up periods. A recent systematic review of SNS for the treatment of FI [54] evaluated six studies. A total of 266 patients underwent PNE, of whom 149 (56%) had a permanent stimulator implanted; follow-up periods ranged from 1 to 99 months. Complete continence was reported in approximately 55% of patients, with 90% having more than 50% improvement in incontinence; there was no deterioration of the effect of SNS over time. The reported complications were minor and

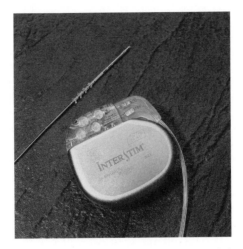

Fig. 12. The Interstim® neurostimulator. Reprinted with the permission of Medtronic, Inc., © 2003.

rare with lead migration being the most common, accounting for 8 of the 19 adverse events, and infection necessitating explantation of the stimulator occurred in 3 patients. The remaining complications were attributed mostly to pain originating either in the stimulator or leads.

The excitement surrounding SNS results from its relative simplicity, high efficacy, and safety. The procedure offers numerous advantages over almost any other surgical treatment modality for FI: it is the only modality in which the patient selection and screening process is incorporated in the procedure itself, which inevitably results in high success rates; it is a minimally invasive procedure that is usually performed in an outpatient setting and does not require mechanical bowel preparation; it does not involve physical manipulation of the rectum, anus, or the pelvic floor anatomy, and therefore has significantly fewer complications; repeat operations, explantations, and revisions following SNS are relatively simple procedures that do not necessarily obligate the patient to a stoma. It is an exciting treatment option in a population in whom conservative measures have failed and other surgical approaches may be conceptually questionable, have limited success, or are considered too risky. Again, unlike the stimulated graciloplasty, SNS has no role for patients who have significant muscle loss.

Choice of procedure

As for any other condition for which several treatment options are available, choosing the appropriate procedure for treating end-stage FI is a complicated process that depends on several factors, including patient-related comorbidities and risk factors, procedure-specific risks and contraindications, and the cause of FI. Our suggested decision-making algorithm is illustrated in Fig. 13.

Patients in poor general health who have significant comorbidities and who are poor surgical candidates, and individuals who refuse more invasive therapy, may benefit most from the least-invasive procedure, which is injection of a bulking agent. The Secca procedure and SNS are also considered minimally invasive, but they are performed in a monitored setting under some form of anesthesia, and require sophisticated instrumentation. Another patient-related aspect that needs to be addressed when planning a surgical intervention is the patient's mental capacity. ABS, SNS, and stimulated graciloplasty all are extremely high-maintenance procedures that mandate that the patients have complete appreciation of the complexity of the hardware, basic knowledge in pelvic and anorectal anatomy, and full commitment to daily operation and maintenance of the devices; they should also be educated as to the high rates of complications, be able to recognize the early signs of failure, and be mentally prepared for re-operations, including the possibility of the need for a stoma. Conversely, injectable bulking agents and RF do not require any maintenance or routine follow-up and thus may be more suitable for patients who have impaired mental capacity.

Injectable bulking agents and RF cause an increase in the physical barrier to the passage of stool through the anal canal. This feature of both procedures makes them potentially suitable for treatment of mild FI regardless of cause. SNS has been used successfully for various causes also, but it requires an intact neuromuscular architecture of the sphincter mechanism, which should be demonstrated adequately by preoperative electromyography and pudendal nerve terminal motor latency testing. Patients who

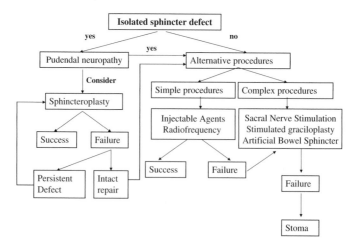

Fig. 13. Suggested algorithm for treatment of FI.

have substantial sphincter muscle loss may not benefit from SNS and should be considered as candidates for sphincter replacement techniques.

Injectable bulking agents, the Secca procedure, stimulated graciloplasty, and ABS implantation require direct manipulation of the perianal area, anal canal, or distal rectum. Consequently, any local pathology—abscesses, fistulae, fissures, perianal inflammatory bowel disease, or anorectal cancer—is a contraindication for attempting these modalities. Patients who have cardiac pacemakers or implantable defibrillators should not undergo SNS or the stimulated graciloplasty because of the obvious interference of the electrical stimulators. ABS is the most complicated and most invasive procedure currently available in the United States for treating FI. It usually is reserved for patients in whom other treatment modalities have failed. ABS requires highly motivated patients who are physically able to undergo multiple potential subsequent interventions, overcome severe infections, and be mentally prepared to live with a permanent stoma, because this is the almost inevitable consequence of failure of ABS. Implantation of an ABS may not be optimal in patients who have an artificial urinary sphincter or inflatable penile prosthesis; however, we have successfully implanted the ABS in these settings.

Summary

The availability of novel techniques to treat end-stage FI gives hope for a better quality of life in patients who were traditionally treated by a permanent stoma. The diversity of causes of FI and the different modes of action of the various treatment modalities mandate a tailored, individualized approach in each case. A meticulous preoperative evaluation process is imperative in the course of the decision-making of which procedure to perform, with full awareness that a stoma still may be the best option for some patients who have end-stage FI.

References

[1] Mavrantonis C, Wexner SD. A clinical approach to fecal incontinence. J Clin Gastroenterol 1998;27(2):108–21.
[2] Madoff RD, Parker SC, Varma MG, et al. Faecal incontinence in adults. Lancet 2004; 364(9434):621–32.
[3] Deutekom M, Terra MP, Dobben AC, et al. Impact of faecal incontinence severity on health domains. Colorectal Dis 2005;7(3):263–9.
[4] Miner PB, Jr. Economic and personal impact of fecal and urinary incontinence. Gastroenterology 2004;126(1, Suppl 1):S8–13.
[5] Mellgren A, Jensen LL, Zetterstrom JP, et al. Long-term cost of fecal incontinence secondary to obstetric injuries. Dis Colon Rectum 1999;42(7):857–65.
[6] Nelson R, Norton N, Cautley E, et al. Community-based prevalence of anal incontinence. JAMA 1995;274(7):559–61.

[7] Macmillan AK, Merrie AE, Marshall RJ, et al. The prevalence of fecal incontinence in community-dwelling adults: a systematic review of the literature. Dis Colon Rectum 2004;47(8): 1341–9.

[8] Whitehead WE, Wald A, Norton NJ. Treatment options for fecal incontinence. Dis Colon Rectum 2001;44(1):131–42.

[9] Madoff RD, Williams JG, Caushaj PF. Fecal incontinence. N Engl J Med 1992;326(15): 1002–7.

[10] Jorge JM, Wexner SD. Etiology and management of fecal incontinence. Dis Colon Rectum 1993;36(1):77–97.

[11] Rothbarth J, Bemelman WA, Meijerink WJ, et al. What is the impact of fecal incontinence on quality of life? Dis Colon Rectum 2001;44(1):67–71.

[12] Haab F, Zimmern PE, Leach GE. Urinary stress incontinence due to intrinsic sphincteric deficiency: experience with fat and collagen periurethral injections. J Urol 1997;157(4):1283–6.

[13] Monga AK, Robinson D, Stanton SL. Periurethral collagen injections for genuine stress incontinence: a 2-year follow-up. Br J Urol 1995;76(2):156–60.

[14] Lightner D, Calvosa C, Andersen R, et al. A new injectable bulking agent for treatment of stress urinary incontinence: results of a multicenter, randomized, controlled, double-blind study of Durasphere. Urology 2001;58(1):12–5.

[15] Shafik A. Polytetrafluoroethylene injection for the treatment of partial fecal incontinence. Int Surg 1993;78(2):159–61.

[16] Shafik A. Perianal injection of autologous fat for treatment of sphincteric incontinence. Dis Colon Rectum 1995;38(6):583–7.

[17] Kumar D, Benson MJ, Bland JE. Glutaraldehyde cross-linked collagen in the treatment of faecal incontinence. Br J Surg 1998;85(7):978–9.

[18] Malouf AJ, Vaizey CJ, Norton CS, et al. Internal anal sphincter augmentation for fecal incontinence using injectable silicone biomaterial. Dis Colon Rectum 2001;44(4):595–600.

[19] Kenefick NJ, Vaizey CJ, Malouf AJ, et al. Injectable silicone biomaterial for faecal incontinence due to internal anal sphincter dysfunction. Gut 2002;51:225–8.

[20] Weiss EG, Efron JE, Nogueras JJ, et al. Submucosal injection of carbon coated beads is a successful and safe office based treatment for fecal incontinence. Dis Colon Rectum 2002;45: A46–7 [abstract].

[21] Davis K, Kumar D, Poloniecki J. Preliminary evaluation of an injectable anal sphincter bulking agent (Durasphere) in the management of faecal incontinence. Aliment Pharmacol Ther 2003;18(2):237–43.

[22] Gustavson KH. On the chemistry of collagen. Fed Proc 1964;23:613–7.

[23] Richards WO, Scholz S, Khaitan L, et al. Initial experience with the stretta procedure for the treatment of gastroesophageal reflux disease. J Laparoendosc Adv Surg Tech A 2001;11(5): 267–73.

[24] Triadafilopoulos G, Dibaise JK, Nostrant TT, et al. Radiofrequency energy delivery to the gastroesophageal junction for the treatment of GERD. Gastrointest Endosc 2001;53(4): 407–15.

[25] Triadafilopoulos G, DiBaise JK, Nostrant TT, et al. The Stretta procedure for the treatment of GERD: 6 and 12 month follow-up of the US open label trial. Gastrointest Endosc 2002; 55(2):149–56.

[26] Dawkins GP, Harrison NW, Ansell W. Radiofrequency heat-treatment to the prostate for bladder outlet obstruction associated with benign prostatic hyperplasia: a 4-year outcome study. Br J Urol 1997;79(6):910–4.

[27] Hecht P, Hayashi K, Lu Y, et al. Monopolar radiofrequency energy effects on joint capsular tissue: potential treatment for joint instability. An in vivo mechanical, morphological, and biochemical study using an ovine model. Am J Sports Med 1999;27(6):761–71.

[28] Powell NB, Riley RW, Troell RJ, et al. Radiofrequency volumetric tissue reduction of the palate in subjects with sleep-disordered breathing. Chest 1998;113(5):1163–74.

[29] Steward DL. Effectiveness of multilevel (tongue and palate) radiofrequency tissue ablation for patients with obstructive sleep apnea syndrome. Laryngoscope 2004;114(12): 2073–84.

[30] Said B, Strome M. Long-term results of radiofrequency volumetric tissue reduction of the palate for snoring. Ann Otol Rhinol Laryngol 2003;112(3):276–9.

[31] Takahashi T, Garcia-Osogobio S, Valdovinos MA, et al. Radio-frequency energy delivery to the anal canal for the treatment of fecal incontinence. Dis Colon Rectum 2002;45(7):915–22.

[32] Takahashi T, Garcia-Osogobio S, Valdovinos MA, et al. Extended two-year results of radio-frequency energy delivery for the treatment of fecal incontinence (the Secca procedure). Dis Colon Rectum 2003;46(6):711–5.

[33] Efron JE, Corman ML, Fleshman J, et al. Safety and effectiveness of temperature-controlled radio-frequency energy delivery to the anal canal (Secca procedure) for the treatment of fecal incontinence. Dis Colon Rectum 2003;46(12):1606–16.

[34] Chetwood CH. Plastic operation for restoration of the sphincter ani with a report of a case. Med Rec 1902;61:529.

[35] Pearl RK, Prasad ML, Nelson RL, et al. Bilateral gluteus maximus transposition for anal incontinence. Dis Colon Rectum 1991;34(6):478–81.

[36] Devesa JM, Vicente E, Enriquez JM, et al. Total fecal incontinence - a new method of gluteus maximus transposition: preliminary results and report of previous experience with similar procedures. Dis Colon Rectum 1992;35(4):339–49.

[37] Konsten J, Baeten CG, Havenith MG, et al. Canine model for treatment of faecal incontinence using transposed and electrically stimulated sartorius muscle. Br J Surg 1994;81(3): 466–9.

[38] Konsten J, Baeten CG, Havenith MG, et al. Morphology of dynamic graciloplasty compared with the anal sphincter. Dis Colon Rectum 1993;36(6):559–63.

[39] Pette D, Vrbova G. Adaptation of mammalian skeletal muscle fibers to chronic electrical stimulation. Rev Physiol Biochem Pharmacol 1992;120:115–202.

[40] Pickrell KL, Broadbent TR, Masters FW, et al. Construction of a rectal sphincter and restoration of anal continence by transplanting the gracilis muscle; a report of four cases in children. Ann Surg 1952;135(6):853–62.

[41] Baeten CG, Konsten J, Spaans F, et al. Dynamic graciloplasty for treatment of faecal incontinence. Lancet 1991;338(8776):1163–5.

[42] Williams NS, Patel J, George BD, et al. Development of an electrically stimulated neoanal sphincter. Lancet 1991;338(8776):1166–9.

[43] Baeten CG, Bailey HR, Bakka A, et al. Safety and efficacy of dynamic graciloplasty for fecal incontinence: report of a prospective, multicenter trial. Dynamic Graciloplasty Therapy Study Group. Dis Colon Rectum 2000;43(6):743–51.

[44] Wexner SD, Baeten C, Bailey R, et al. Long-term efficacy of dynamic graciloplasty for fecal incontinence. Dis Colon Rectum 2002;45(6):809–18.

[45] Chapman AE, Geerdes B, Hewett P, et al. Systematic review of dynamic graciloplasty in the treatment of faecal incontinence. Br J Surg 2002;89(2):138–53.

[46] Scott FB, Bradley WE, Timm GW. Treatment of urinary incontinence by implantable prosthetic sphincter. Urology 1973;1(3):252–9.

[47] Christiansen J, Lorentzen M. Implantation of artificial sphincter for anal incontinence. Lancet 1987;2(8553):244–5.

[48] Wong WD, Congliosi SM, Spencer MP, et al. The safety and efficacy of the artificial bowel sphincter for fecal incontinence: results from a multicenter cohort study. Dis Colon Rectum 2002;45(9):1139–53.

[49] Ortiz H, Armendariz P, DeMiguel M, et al. Prospective study of artificial anal sphincter and dynamic graciloplasty for severe anal incontinence. Int J Colorect Dis 2003;18(4):349–54.

[50] Mundy L, Merlin TL, Maddern GJ, et al. Systematic review of safety and effectiveness of an artificial bowel sphincter for faecal incontinence. Br J Surg 2004;91(6):665–72.

[51] Matzel KE, Stadelmaier U, Hohenfellner M, et al. Electrical stimulation of sacral spinal nerves for treatment of faecal incontinence. Lancet 1995;346(8983):1124–7.

[52] Ganio E, Masin A, Ratto C, et al. Short-term sacral nerve stimulation for functional anorectal and urinary disturbances: results in 40 patients: evaluation of a new option for anorectal functional disorders. Dis Colon Rectum 2001;44(9):1261–7.

[53] Kenefick NJ, Emmanuel A, Nicholls RJ, et al. Effect of sacral nerve stimulation on autonomic nerve function. Br J Surg 2003;90(10):1256–60.

[54] Jarrett ME, Mowatt G, Glazener CM, et al. Systematic review of sacral nerve stimulation for faecal incontinence and constipation. Br J Surg 2004;91(12):1559–69.

SURGICAL
CLINICS OF
NORTH AMERICA

Surg Clin N Am 86 (2006) 987–1004

Advanced Laparoscopic Skills Acquisition: The Case of Laparoscopic Colorectal Surgery

Eric C. Poulin, MD, MSc[a,b,*], Jean Pierre Gagné, MD[c],
Robin P. Boushey, MD, PhD[a,d]

[a]Department of Surgery, University of Ottawa, 501 Smyth Road, Ottawa,
Ontario K1H 8L6, Canada
[b]Department of Surgery, The Ottawa Hospital, 501 Smyth Road, Ottawa,
Ontario K1H 8L6, Canada
[c]Centre Hospitalier Universitaire de Québec, Hôpital Saint-François d'Assise,
10 de l'Espinay, Québec G1L 3L5, Canada
[d]Department of Clinical Epidemiology, The Ottawa Hospital, 501 Smyth Road,
Ottawa, Ontario K1H 8L6, Canada

"The only constant is change"
Heraclitus, Greek philosopher
2500 years ago

Historical context

It has been almost 20 years since the introduction of laparoscopic chole-cystectomy by Eric Mühe [1] and Philippe Mouret [2] in the early 1990s, and it changed the face of surgery forever. Since then, the development and val-idation of advanced end-organ and intestinal minimally invasive procedures have occupied an ever-increasing place in the surgical literature [3–8]. More-over, multiple randomized trials have demonstrated the superiority of lapa-roscopic colon resection over the open method for short-term outcomes [9–13]. More recently, a well-publicized trial (Clinical Outcomes of Surgical Therapy; COST) showed the noninferiority of laparoscopic colon resection for colon cancer survival, whereas another even suggested better long-term

* Corresponding author. Department of Surgery, The Ottawa Hospital, 501 Smyth Road, Ottawa, Ontario K1H 8L6, Canada.
E-mail address: epoulin@ottawahospital.on.ca (E.C. Poulin).

0039-6109/06/$ - see front matter © 2006 Elsevier Inc. All rights reserved.
doi:10.1016/j.suc.2006.05.004

survival for stage III disease [14,15]. The results of more trials on various continents are expected soon, and similar trials to evaluate laparoscopic mesorectal excision in rectal cancer are being set up. This has created a sense of urgency for surgeons in training and surgeons in practice to acquire advanced laparoscopic skills. Yet, the transfer of this technology has faced many hurdles.

"The Capacity of American Surgery to Adequately Teach Advanced Minimally Invasive Surgery is Simply Overwhelmed"
    Frederick Greene, MD. World Congress of Laparoscopic Surgery, Rome, June 1998

It has taken time for the surgical community to accept that the journey of modern surgery is defined by equal or better outcomes with less surgical trauma, a vision that has been endorsed more rapidly by patients. Although solid data are difficult to obtain, it was estimated recently that the penetration of laparoscopic colon resection is limited, and varies from 5% (United States) to 15% (France) [16]. Although the routine performance of laparoscopic appendectomy is suggested by most experts as the best introduction to the performance of laparoscopic colon resection, its acceptance also is discouraging, despite the fact that multiple randomized trials and more systematic reviews than one would care to read have demonstrated its superiority. Of interest is a population study that was performed by the College of Physicians of a Canadian province (Québec, 7.8 million population) during 1 year (April 2002–March 2003). It studied 5707 appendectomies and found that a low rate of laparoscopic appendectomy (<20%) was found in 50% of teaching hospitals and 37% of nonteaching institutions (Gagné and colleagues, unpublished data). Studies also have demonstrated the poor exposure of North American surgery residents to advanced laparoscopic procedures by the end of their training (<10 advanced cases during surgical training of 4 or 5 years), a fact that correlates well with the insufficient number of teachers. The impact of hiring laparoscopic surgeons in academic health sciences centers is felt clinically by an increase in the number of advanced cases, more laparoscopic training sessions, and the number of minimally invasive surgery (MIS) research projects [17]. Furthermore, despite the recommendation by respected societies (eg, Society of American Gastrointestinal Endoscopic Surgeons; SAGES) that fellowship programs should "train teachers," some exceptional fellowship-trained laparoscopic surgeons have not been able to find work in teaching environments, which complicates the issue with political agendas even further.

    This article reviews the basic principles of technical skills acquisition, the various methods of skill transfer, and a blueprint for integration of new skills into practice. Although much is based on evidence, a significant portion also is based on the experience that has been gained in teaching advanced laparoscopic skills to residents, fellows, and surgeons over the last 15 years.

Basic principles of technical skill acquisition

Unfortunately, many teachers of surgery in the past have downplayed the technical aspect of surgery while trying to highlight the importance of sound surgical judgment, cognitive knowledge, and decision-making capability— "...you can train a monkey to operate." With the advent of advanced laparoscopic procedures, it has become evident that the difficulty of acquiring the technical skill aspect of surgery has been underestimated [18]. Although it is beyond the scope of this article to review all theories that govern skill acquisition and the development of expert performance, a brief overview of a few is relevant to understand the challenges that are faced by surgical educators in the current environment. These theories—far from being contradictory— provide complementary insights into the learning of surgical technical skills.

The Kopta Theory of Skill Acquisition

Three overlapping phases are described in the learning of any motor skill: cognitive, integrative, and autonomous. The first involves knowing what to do without necessarily being able to do it. Then the learner needs to intellectualize what one wants to do and plan the necessary steps to accomplish the task. Integration starts when the new knowledge is translated into the appropriate motor behavior. During the early integrative phase, performance is irregular with each step of the task easily identifiable. An instructor must be able to break down a task into its components and communicate those to the learner. Practice improves flow of movement to the point where routine execution no longer requires cognitive input. At this level, the autonomous phase has been attained, and performance becomes smooth and automatic. The issue with this theory is that automaticity implies satisfaction with the level of competence. Surgeons, like any other expert performers, always should be looking for ways to improve [19–21]. Practice with feedback (ie, guided practice) is essential to learning skills. A minimum exposure to error-prone alternatives also is essential for an efficient skill teaching program.

Ericsson's Model of Expert Skill Acquisition

The theory is based on research on expert performers in the fields of music, art, chess, science, and sports. It has two main parts. The first states that expert performance requires years of intensive training. The evidence supports that the highest levels of human performance (eg, world class athletes, chess players) are seen many years after physical maturation and require approximately 10 years of intensive or "deliberate practice" [21]. Boxes 1 through 3 illustrate common strategies that are used to teach skills. "Deliberate practice" requires effort. There is a world of difference between a junior resident spending 20 minutes working with a box trainer and Moe Norman (recognized as one of the world's best golf ball strikers) who from

---

Box 1. Principles of teaching surgical technical skills

Analogous to teaching competitive sport
Accuracy
Speed
Economy of effort
Adaptability

Teaching motor skills is different than teaching verbal skills
Represents a chain of responses
Requires eye-hand coordination
Requires organization of subroutines

---

age 19 to 32 routinely hit 800 balls a day, or Bobby Fisher, the famed chess player who was known to spend 5 to 10 hours a day practicing and studying games played by chess grandmasters [20].

The second part of Ericsson's model has not been studied as much. He suggests that experts do not reach a level of automaticity. Rather the appearance of automaticity is, in fact misleading. He argues that experts develop complex cognitive networks that allow them to seem to bypass normal human limits. Experts may appear to have faster reaction times. In fact, they do not have faster hands. Instead, experts have learned to find preexisting clues that allow them to predict what is likely to happen in a given situation. The change in ability is not so much physical as

---

Box 2. Instructional phases

Introductory phase
Needs assessment
Introduction of objectives
Explanation of rationale
Familiarization with equipment
Demonstration of sequential steps

Practice phase
Give specific instruction
Guide the initial attempts
Provide feedback
Allow independent practice
Certify competence

Perfecting phase
Provide for continued practice
Evaluate performance under actual conditions

Box 3. The steps to mastery by repetition

Unconsciously incompetent
Consciously incompetent
Consciously competent
Unconsciously competent

To teach a technical skill, the teacher must revert to a consciously competent state of mind.

---

cognitive. Experts can generate a complex representation and awareness of the encountered situation. This information is integrated with existing knowledge, and allows selection of action as well as evaluation, checking, and reasoning about alternative actions [20]. A good example in the world of sports is Wayne Gretzky, the best hockey player of all time. Although not a great skater, shooter, or stick handler, he seemed to have the best overall premonition of where the next play would occur and could translate that into scoring opportunities faster than anybody.

The Ericsson Theory argues against the traditional model of skill acquisition, which describes skill learning as occurring in phases that develop from cognitive to automatic (see Box 3). It also argues against the strategy of isolating technical skill as a focus separate from the cognitive aspects of surgery.

The Behaviorist School

The behaviorists unified the results of many years of research in the field of education into a conceptual framework, and classified human abilities into five categories: verbal information, intellectual skills, cognitive strategies, motor skills, and attitudes [22]. For each ability, conditions within the learner (internal conditions) and conditions within the teaching environment (external conditions) were considered essential for effective learning (Box 4). According to this theory, learning of a skill occurs through the integration of the executive routine along the previously described phases (cognitive, associative, autonomous). This involves the combination of several basic surgical skills that are performed in an orderly series of steps whereby recall of part skills is one of the most important in elaborating learning hierarchies. According to this approach, practice is another key condition of learning motor skills.

Neuropsychologic testing

Neuropsychologic tests have been conducted on surgical residents to measure pure motor skills (speed and precision of movement), imagery

---

Box 4. Conditions of learning motor skills

Internal conditions
Recall of part skills
Recall of executive routines (learning hierarchies)

External conditions
Provide verbal instructions
Provide pictures
Use demonstrations
Give opportunity to practice
Give feedback

(internal representation of an object), and visuospatial organization (ability to represent mentally a three-dimensional situation). The final score of high performance correlated significantly with complex visuospatial organization, somatosensory memory, and stress tolerance without significant correlation with tests of pure motor abilities [23,24]. The importance of visuospatial perceptual ability also has been identified by other investigators [25]. In laparoscopic surgery, the surgeon uses the two-dimensional image from the monitor to construct a three-dimensional mental representation of the anatomy before him. The quality of this representation depends on the interpretation he makes of the visual information.

Educational strategies

Advanced laparoscopic surgery is a highly intellectual activity that involves the processing of perceptual information that is received from proprioceptive, visual, tactile, olfactory, and auditory sources. DesCôteaux and colleagues [26] have suggested three strategies to help learners process, organize, and retain perceptual information: imagery, mental practice, and systematic review of performance.

Imagery

Imagery as defined as the internal representation of an object has been found best suited for learning concrete information, and, therefore, should be applicable to surgery. Ten percent to 12% of the population report being unable to create imagery. Trainees will benefit from learning to make mental images as they observe or perform surgery. These images will be made up of the visible anatomy at various stages of procedures, but perhaps more importantly, of structures yet to be exposed. This is especially important in advanced laparoscopic surgery where the tactile or visual clues are so different at first.

"Advanced laparoscopic surgery is not a science of the hands, it is a science of the eyes."

Dr. Japp Bonjër, MIS surgeon, Rotterdam, Netherlands
Halifax, Nova Scotia

Although there is constant debate as to how much time trainees should spend on observation and on actual practice, a recent study suggest that a combination of the two is complementary [27]. Observation allows concentration on the perception and processing of information to build mental images without the distraction of the many other stimuli that can reduce the concentration that is needed in building imagery.

Mental practice

Mental practice is to imagery what movies are to still photography. The procedure is rehearsed in memory several times before the actual performance. This technique improves the performance of skills that involve a large mental component (anterior resection of the rectum) rather that a single pure motor skill (inserting a trocar). This process is well understood by high-performance athletes or musicians. Without fluidity in mental practice there can be no fluidity in actual performance.

Systematic review of performance

Providing feedback as close to the actual performance as possible is an essential component of the external conditions for learning motor skills (see, external conditions, Box 4.) This should permit study, analysis, and processing of the perceptual information that is received during the procedure. This is successful only if the learner can internalize the comments by linking them to the sensory information assembled to adjust and correct the next performance. In advanced laparoscopic surgery, because of the steep learning curves that are involved, one has to admit the necessity of the "apprenticeship" model (one-on-one) of the learning environment in the operating room or the animal laboratory.

Integration of technical skills into practice

The MIS mindset

Medicine, the only profession that labors incessantly to destroy the reason for its existence.

James Bryce, British historian (1838–1922)

In the past 2 decades, the use of the least aggressive treatment that provides equivalent or better outcomes for the patient has been a clear direction of surgical therapy in all specialties. Although this vision still may seem utopian for some, it certainly depicts the philosophy of MIS surgeons, who, in every case, try to use the least aggressive approach to reduce the overall trauma of surgery. The truly MIS surgeon tries to introduce elements of surgical trauma reduction in the management of every patient, whether the surgery is urgent or elective, following the tried and true principle of "first do no harm."

In that sense, MIS not only refers to several surgical techniques, but to a surgical philosophy. The first step, in many cases, is to begin many body cavity procedures by a laparoscopic exploration. The value of diagnostic or staging laparoscopy has been well established in cases of pancreatic [28], gastric [29], and esophageal [30] cancers where 25% to 33% of patients are found to have incurable disease and more invasive surgery would be futile. In urgent situations, laparoscopy allows confirmation of diagnosis or alternatively defines another unsuspected pathology. It determines the feasibility of fully laparoscopic treatment or allows better position of incisions with a view to reduce the clinical impact for the patient. As the surgeon gains experience, more urgent abdominal conditions are dealt with entirely laparoscopically. The laparoscopic management of perforated duodenal ulcers [31], perforated diverticulitis [32,33], small bowel obstruction [34], and some cases of trauma is well accepted.

Furthermore, the integration of any advanced technical skill into practice cannot occur without creating a team approach that includes Surgery, Nursing, and Anesthesia. Although the topic is beyond the scope of this article, this approach allows standardization of processes (eg, instruments, anesthesia protocols, patient positioning, first trocar entry, fast-track postoperative care, aftercare issues) to permit provision of quality of MIS care 24 hours a day. Doing appendectomies laparoscopically during the day and the open technique at night sends the wrong message.

Lost opportunities (laparoscopic appendectomy)

> A pessimist sees the difficulty in every opportunity; an optimist sees the opportunity in every difficulty.
>
> Sir Winston Churchill (1874–1965)

Laparoscopic appendectomy certainly emerges as the ideal teaching and learning procedure to transfer advanced laparoscopic skills. With the confirmation of its value [35], one might wonder about the reason for its low use in academic health sciences centers (Gagné and colleagues, unpublished data). Given its high volume and its technical requirements, laparoscopic appendectomy is regarded by those who teach laparoscopic surgery as the ideal introduction to advanced MIS procedures. First, because the appendix is located in the area of the abdomen where the distance between the abdominal wall and the spine is shortest, it forces the surgeon to learn working in a restricted environment. Second, the procedure requires bimanual instruments handling, an essential skill to the performance of advanced MIS. The inability to use the nondominant hand represents one of the major weaknesses of novice laparoscopists. Third, for a retrocecal appendix the surgeon learns to mobilize the line of Toldt, the first step to ileocecal resection. It is a natural introduction to laparoscopic colon surgery. Finally, completion of the procedure and peritoneal cleaning require safe small bowel handling, another essential skill for most advanced laparoscopic procedures.

Colorectal surgeons or any subspecialist not taking call in General Surgery and limiting themselves to subspecialty call are forfeiting many opportunities to improve their laparoscopic skills.

Patient selection

The evolution of laparoscopic surgery over the last 15 years has seen a constant decline in the number of absolute contraindications to the performance of MIS techniques. Classic contraindications to laparoscopic cholecystectomy in the early 1990s consisted of pregnancy, obesity, previous abdominal surgery, and acute cholecystitis; however, it became evident that the contraindications were related more to the surgeon's experience than to the patient's status. Other than the inability to tolerate a general anesthetic there remains few contraindications. Laparoscopy even facilitates surgery in obese patients, once appropriate exposure is obtained.

Although patient characteristics generally are not contraindications as such, they initially serve to guide the selection of cases, because it generally is advisable to start with easier cases. Also, they will serve as a predictor of the difficulty of the procedure, the anticipated need for experienced assistance, and the risk for conversion [36].

Multiple risk factors have been reported as predicting a higher risk for conversion in various conditions. In Crohn's disease: multiple bouts, use of immunosuppressive drugs, the presence of an abscess or fistula, and the need for multiple resections [37]; in bariatric surgery: steatohepatitis, diabetes mellitus, adhesions from various causes, previous bile leaks, large waist size, and body mass index [38]; in gallbladder surgery: cholecystitis, choledocholithiasis, male sex, and obesity [39]; and in colon surgery: left colon surgery, anterior resection of the rectum, diverticulitis, and cancer [40]. Schlachta and colleagues [41] described a simple point system (0 to 4) based on surgical experience (less than or more than 50 cases), patient weight (<60 kg, 60–90 kg, >90 kg), and the diagnosis of cancer that correlates well with the likelihood of conversion to open surgery. Therefore, wise selection of appropriate cases should guide the novice in advanced laparoscopic surgery.

Learning curves

Several factors seem to impede the learning of advanced laparoscopic surgery and contribute to a steep learning curve: (1) learners usually fail to appreciate the value of sitting in the operating room to observe a few cases at first and come ill-prepared; (2) proper assistance for advanced cases is different and much more demanding than in open cases, and surgeons only experienced with open surgery often are lost at first and are almost useless as assistants during an advanced case early on; and (3) teaching advanced cases is far more challenging than is traditional surgery. The margin of error from the teacher perspective is smaller and the ability to control all aspects of the procedure is more difficult.

Most investigators consider the learning curve to be the number of cases that has to be performed to reach a plateau in outcomes, such as conversion rates, operative times, and perioperative and postoperative complications [42,43]. The number of cases that is needed to reach proficiency varies from 30 to 70 for laparoscopic colon resections [44,45]. This has been confirmed in a joint statement by the American Society of Colon and Rectal Surgeons and the Society of American Gastrointestinal Endoscopic Surgeons. Based on results from the COST trial [14], they cited that performing 20 procedures is necessary to attain the level of expertise that is required to undertake laparoscopic resection of colon cancers on a curative basis. Figures vary for other advanced procedures. Some examples are inguinal hernia repair, 50 cases [46]; Nissen fundoplications, 20 cases [47]; Roux-en-Y gastric bypass, 100 cases [43]; and Heller myotomies, 20 cases [48].

In essence, what these numbers say is that there is a peculiar challenge to MIS that is unseen in open surgery. The surgeon must be ready to invest time and patience to reach the desired level of competence. Also, at the same time, the number of cases that is attached to the learning curve of a specific procedure should not be viewed as a definite benchmark, but merely as a rough indicator of what is needed to achieve technical competence. Reality has shown the subjectivity of measures to assess technical competence. Although some surgeons will be technically facile after a few cases, others never will integrate MIS into their practice [49].

Skill sets more specific to advanced laparoscopic surgery

Several problems need to be addressed for the adequate performance of advanced laparoscopic procedures, and most advanced laparoscopists of the first generation often have learned the hard way. Laparoscopic surgery is based foremost on the prophylaxis of any errors. One cannot cut corners in laparoscopic surgery, and patience is paramount. This surgery is not for impatient surgeons.

Some skills that seem to define advanced laparoscopic surgery are reviewed. Because many laparoscopic skills are common to all advanced laparoscopic operations, experience in a specific operation enhances the acquisition of skills that are necessary to perform others.

Triangulating/sectoring

Triangulation is defined as "the location of an unknown point by the formation of a triangle having the unknown point and two known points as the vertices" [50]. There is at least three ways that the principles of triangulation (also used in global positioning systems) are used in laparoscopic surgery. First, the surgeon needs to locate the site of surgery by interpreting mental triangles that are made by drawing imaginary lines between one's eyes, the operative field, and the monitor. Second, the optimal working trocar placement follows triangulation principles. The classic arrangement for a laparoscopic procedure is to set the camera between the two working trocars of the operating surgeon, while maintaining good working angles of 45° to 75° in the process [51]. The downside of this ergonomic design is that the hand that holds the camera head necessarily has to cross over one of the surgeon's hand. This can be cumbersome and tiring for the surgeon and the assistant, unless a mechanical camera holder is used. One way to avoid this is to use the concept of sectoring; the two working trocars are side by side and the laparoscope is located to the left or to the right of the surgeon. This creates a working scheme that is different from open surgery; the surgeon is looking at his work from a lateral perspective, which is an awkward concept at first. Again, laparoscopic appendectomy is the ideal procedure with which to master sectoring because the trocars are configured this way: scope in the umbilicus and the two working trocars to the left. Mastering sectoring is essential before undertaking colon resections. Finally, triangulation principles are used less frequently to "reset" the surgeon whose working instruments are off the operating field and the view of the monitor. A quick look on the patient's abdomen to check the direction where the laparoscope is pointing facilitates "resetting" the working instruments to the operating field, again using the principles of triangulation.

Mastery of monopolar cautery

Although few will deny the monumental contribution of laparoscopic hemostatic devices, such as Harmonic Scalpel (Ethicon Endo-Surgery, Cincinnati, Ohio), Ligasure (Valleylab, Boulder, Colorado), or SonoSurg (Olympus, Orangeburg, New York) and others to the field of laparoscopic surgery, too many surgeons have succumbed to the propaganda and have forgotten the basics. It is essential for all MIS surgeons to learn all aspects of safe electrosurgery for dissection and hemostasis, and practice responsible cost containment. It is amazing that so few surgeons ignore the differences between cutting, fulguration, and desiccation currents, notions that were described initially by Cushing and Bovie almost a century ago [51a]. Many expert laparoscopists who have mastered the electrosurgery hook rarely use alternate energy sources. They can use the sides or surfaces of the instrument with all type of currents with a speed and precision that cannot be matched while reducing the cost of MIS procedures significantly. In a busy unit, it is simply too costly to "dumb down" laparoscopic procedures with expensive alternate energy sources used routinely. They should be reserved for specific indications, and surgeons should be encouraged to master cheap and safe alternatives.

Enhancing use of the nondominant hand

Training MIS surgeons in a fellowship environment has revealed that many surgeons use their nondominant hand only for secondary, noncritical roles. Although adequate open surgery can be performed in this way, the minimal use of the nondominant hand is a major obstacle in advanced MIS. In an environment in which instruments are fixed and hinged in the abdominal wall and where working angles and camera angles vary, the nondominant hand has to be trained for critical tasks (eg, dissection, cutting, tissue manipulation, suturing). Relegating the nondominant hand to retraction is not sufficient.

Intracorporeal knotting and suturing

Tying of knots and intracorporeal suturing is considered an advanced skill in laparoscopy, even though it is basic in all types of open surgery. Intracorporeal knot tying in laparoscopic surgery is time-consuming and difficult to learn, and many believe that this is one skill that tends to deteriorate if not used regularly. Experienced mentors always put in a few stitches themselves during procedures that require this skill. The environment of the skills laboratory is particularly well suited to learn laparoscopic suturing and knot tying to minimize painful intraoperative performance. Empirically, some trainers suggest that learners complete at least 50 sutures and knots before expecting decent intraoperative performance.

Intracorporeal lysis of adhesions

Managing intra-abdominal adhesions is an important skill of advanced MIS. The surgeon needs to be able to find the most avascular plane, usually in close proximity to the peritoneum, and use scissor dissection to avoid iatrogenic sparking of hidden viscera. The use of energy sources should be limited to areas of adhesions where vessels need control. Keeping the operative field blood-free, especially at the beginning of a procedure when adhesions usually are encountered, is paramount to better vision throughout the case. This is different than dissecting adhesions in open surgery where one can touch and feel the bowel.

Intraoperative mishaps and Disaster Tolerance Index

Initially, one of the most difficult skills to master in MIS surgery is the ability to gauge the gravity of intraoperative mishaps. For example, one has to get used to the magnification of the laparoscope ($10\times$–$13\times$) in the estimation of bleeding severity. All MIS surgeons have faced the question of "Can this bleeding be controlled laparoscopically or does the operation need to be converted to an open case?". If an iatrogenic enterotomy occurs while dissecting adhesions, should the case be converted or the bowel sutured laparoscopically?

With experience and training there is an increase in the ability of the MIS surgeon to deal with intraoperative adverse events laparoscopically, what the authors have termed an increase in the Disaster Tolerance Index.

It is more crucial to develop a style of careful, deliberate, and defensive surgery whereby all adverse events are prevented. Any small event that often could be taken care of easily in open surgery can be problematic in laparoscopy, and it adds significant time for a laparoscopic resolution or triggers a conversion. Most often in laparoscopic fellowship training, the first thing that has to be impressed on trainees is the need to slow themselves down and to learn "preventative" dissection in the appropriate plane.

In the authors' estimation, this aspect of surgery is most unforgiving in advanced laparoscopic surgery, and requires a degree of concentration that is greater than what is needed in traditional surgery.

Methods of skill transfer in laparoscopy

Skills laboratory and simulators

Skills and simulation laboratories have proliferated in the teaching environment of academic health sciences centers over the last few years. With regards to laparoscopic skills they offer an introduction to basic MIS skills with a spectrum of tools that ranges from box trainers to virtual reality simulators. They have been shown to improve operating room performance in basic laparoscopic procedures (eg, laparoscopic cholecystectomy), and are useful in introducing learners to laparoscopic equipment and teaching the basics of triangulation, instrument manipulation, and knot tying. Undoubtedly, this prepares learners for the operating room environment [52]. The case for the importance of practice in the acquisition of any technical skill has been made in the previous paragraphs. But presence in the skills laboratory does little to teach the seamless flow of steps and the ability to recognize anatomic planes that are required to perform a bloodless advanced MIS procedure. In the future, higher-fidelity simulators will increase the enthusiasm for practice sessions, and likely will be more helpful for the learning of advanced laparoscopic surgery.

Short courses

Short courses traditionally occur on weekends, and offer a combination of lectures, demonstrations, and hands-on experience in laboratories. Most are well organized from a pedagogical perspective. They serve as a good introduction to the topic of an advanced surgical domain; however, there is some evidence that points to the limits of short courses alone in the overall education requirements for advanced MIS [53].

Preceptorships

Preceptor is defined as a "specialist in a profession, especially medicine, who gives practical training to a student" [54]. Because of the paucity of trainers for advanced MIS procedures, arranging for significant time for preceptorship has been elusive. They tend not to occur in academic health sciences center other than in the form of observerships because of competition from other trainees (residents and fellows). Most would agree that successful preceptorships need to have one-on-one hands-on training. Although there is little literature on this topic, there are many anecdotal reports whereby expert laparoscopic surgeons have spent significant time training surgeons in the community, either by a series of single operative days or during a concentrated visit of 1 to 2 weeks (J. Mamazza, MD, personal communication, 2005). Advanced cases can be performed with the surgeons designated for the apprenticeship with good results. The trainees can leverage their experience by teaming up with other colleagues for surgery. Colleagues assisting each other until the learning curve is passed have been successful in the transfer of laparoscopic colorectal surgery skills in a community setting. A recent paper from a regional hospital illustrates the quality outcomes in a three-surgeon practice where these principles were followed for the introduction of laparoscopic colon surgery in a community environment [55]. Valuable preceptorships also are given by experienced laparoscopists in the community. So far, these initiatives have tended to exist in isolation.

There are few, if any, structured training programs for established surgeons to take on laparoscopic colorectal surgery. Several models exist. In Scotland, the Minimal Access Therapy Training Unit Scotland was set up in 1994. It involved the National Health Service releasing funds for 4-hour operating sessions for training purposes in MIS. In General Surgery, according to a 1997 report, 234 training sessions had occurred for 99 trainees who attended a median of two sessions each. During these sessions, 333 MIS operations had been performed. No colorectal resections took place in this program [56]. Another initiative between the Association of Laparoscopic Surgeons of Great Britain and Ireland and the Association of Coloproctology of Great Britain and Ireland is worthy of mention. It was scheduled to start in 2004. Candidates for this program need to have watched at least 10 live laparoscopic colorectal resections first. The entire MIS team at the trainee's hospital is required to be trained to support the development of the MIS program. Preceptors travel if requested, and it is recommended that the preceptorship involve two to four cases. Trainees are responsible for auditing their own data. Compensation and clinical liabilities are addressed.

Although it is beyond the scope of this article to evaluate the pedagogical value of these programs, it remains that for the appropriate transfer of this technology to practicing surgeons, comprehensive, funded programs need to be established and they likely will be influenced by the nature of the medical system in each country. Although such programs face many hurdles, they probably represent the best way to address the issue of transfer of technology for surgeons in practice, and the authors believe that curriculum development with input from experts in knowledge transfer needs to occur.

Mini-sabbaticals

To get the most from a mini-sabbatical, it needs to incorporate hands-on training. Profitable mini-sabbaticals usually have involved surgeons experienced in traditional open surgery spending time with an experienced laparoscopist doing enough cases to become comfortable with the performance of routine cases. Mini-sabbaticals, which usually are given in the teacher's institution, have tended to involve a commitment of a few months (2–6 months).

Fellowships

MIS fellowships in North America have proliferated from approximately 20 15 years ago to about 190 today. Whether broad-based, organ, or subspecialty focused, they have paralleled the validation of MIS surgery. Most believe that they are the best way to attain a high level of proficiency in advanced MIS. Several publications have shown that fellows have similar outcomes as do staff for spleen surgery [57]. The clinical outcomes of laparoscopic colorectal cases from an attending surgeon coming out of an MIS fellowship was equal to that of his mentor in his first year of practice [58]. Fellowships eliminate the learning curves. Although MIS fellowships have the advantage of training trainers for academic health sciences centers or surgeons who will go into the community, they have had minimal impact for the training of practicing surgeons so far.

Summary

Acquisition of advanced technical skills requires commitment, time, patience, and discipline (eg, the 10-year rule). Dabbling is not a recipe for success.

Despite the value of all other teaching methods, guided practice with feedback is essential to develop the high level of visuospatial perceptual ability (observation and performance with feedback) that is necessary for advanced MIS.

The necessary ingredients to skill acquisition for advanced MIS procedures (laparoscopic colorectal surgery) for a practicing surgeon include introduction through short courses, access to skill stations, and access to preceptorship or mini-sabbatical.

For residents in training, there is no better alternative than an MIS fellowship. In an ideal world where there are enough trainers, the residency environment should provide this training.

Comprehensive strategies of knowledge transfer for practicing surgeons should be designed with the input of experts in knowledge transfer.

References

[1] Muhe E. Laparoskopische Cholezystektomie–Spatergebnisse [Laparoscopic cholecystectomy–Late results]. Langenbecks Arch Chir Suppl Kongressbd 1991:416–23.

[2] Mouret P. La coelioscopique. Evolution ou révolution [Evolution or revolution]? Chirurgie 1990;116(10):829–32 [in French].

[3] Dallemagne B, Weerts JM, Jehaes C, et al. Laparoscopic Nissen fundoplication: preliminary report. Surg Laparosc Endosc 1991;1(3):138–43.

[4] Jacobs M, Verdeja JC, Goldstein HS. Minimally invasive colon resection. Surg Laparosc Endosc 1991;1(3):144–50.

[5] Gagner M, Lacroix A, Bolte E. Laparoscopic adrenalectomy in Cushing's syndrome and pheochromocytoma. N Engl J Med 1992;327(14):1033.

[6] Delaitre B, Maignien B. Laparoscopic splenectomy—technical aspects. Surg Endosc 1992; 6(6):305–8.

[7] Thibault C, Mamazza J, Letourneau R, et al. Laparoscopic splenectomy: operative technique and preliminary report. Surg Laparosc Endosc 1992;2(3):248–53.

[8] Carroll BJ, Phillips EH, Semel CJ, et al. Laparoscopic splenectomy. Surg Endosc 1992;6(4): 183–5.

[9] Milsom JW, Bohm B, Hammerhofer KA, et al. A prospective randomized trial comparing laparoscopic versus conventional techniques in colorectal cancer surgery: a preliminary report. J Am Coll Surg 1998;187(1):46–54 [discussion 54–5].

[10] Curet MJ, Putrakul K, Pitcher DE, et al. Laparoscopically assisted colon resection for colon carcinoma: perioperative results and long-term outcome. Surg Endosc 2000;14(11):1062–6.

[11] Veldkamp R, Gholghesaei M, Bonjer HJ, et al. Laparoscopic resection of colon cancer. Consensus of the European Association of Endoscopic Surgery (E.A.E.S.). Surg Endosc 2004;18: 1163–85.

[12] Abraham NS, Young JM, Solomon MJ. Meta-analysis of short-term outcomes after laparoscopic resection for colorectal cancer. B J Surg 2004;91:1111–24.

[13] Schwenk W, Haase O, Neudecker J, et al. Short term benefits for laparoscopic colorectal resection. Cochrane Database Syst Rev 2005;3:CD003145.

[14] Clinical Outcomes of Surgical Therapy Study Group (COST). A comparison of laparoscopically assisted and open colectomy for colon cancer. N Engl J Med 2004;350(20): 2050–9.

[15] Lacy AM, Garcia-Valdecasas JC, Delgado S, et al. Laparoscopy-assisted colectomy versus open colectomy for treatment of non-metastatic colon cancer: a randomised trial. Lancet 2002;359 (9325):2224–9.

[16] Symposium on laparoscopic colorectal surgery for cancer. European Association of Endoscopic Surgery (EAES) Annual meeting, Barcelona, Spain, June 2004.

[17] Fowler DL, Hogle N. The impact of a full-time director of minimally invasive surgery: clinical practice, education, and research. Surg Endosc 2000;14(5):444–7.

[18] Szalay D. Technical skills—lessons from occupational and sports psychology. Foc Surg Educ 1997;14(4):12–6.

[19] Kopta JA. The development of motor skills in orthopaedic education. Clin Orthop Rel Res 1971;75:80–5.

[20] Ericsson KS. The acquisition of expert performance. In: Ericksonn KA, editor. The road to excellence: the acquisition of expert performance in the arts and science, sports and games. Mahwah (NJ): Lawrence Erlbaum Associates; 1996. p. 1–50.

[21] Ericsson KA, Krampe RT, Tesch-Römer C. The role of deliberate practice in the acquisition of expert performance. Psychol Rev 1993;100(3):363–406.

[22] Gagné RM. The conditions of learning. 4th ed, Orlando (FL): Holt, Rinehart and Winston; 1985.

[23] Schueneman AL, Pickelman J, Freeark RJ. Age, gender, lateral dominance and prediction of operative skills among general surgery residents. Surgery 1985;98:506–14.

[24] Schueneman AL, Pickelman J, Heisslein R, et al. Neurophysiologic predictors of operative skills among general surgery residents. Surgery 1984;96:288–93.

[25] Risucci DA, Tortolani AJ, Leitman IM, et al. Construct validation of a visual perceptual factor in surgical technical skill. Focus Surg Educ 1993;10(3):22.

[26] DesCôteaux JG, Leclère H. Learning surgical technical skills. Can J Surg 1995;38:33–8.

[27] Shea C, Wright D, Whiteacre C. Actual and observational practice: unique perspective on learning. Res Q Exerc Sport 1993;67(March Suppl):A-79.

[28] Stefanidis D, Grove KD, Scwesinger WH, et al. The current role of staging laparoscopy for adenocarcinoma of the pancreas: a review. Ann Oncol 2005;17:189–99.

[29] Burke EC, Karpeh MS, Conlon KC, et al. Laparoscopy in the management of gastric adenocarcinoma. Ann Surg 1997;225(3):262–7.

[30] Patel AN, Buenaventura PO. Current staging of esophageal carcinoma. Surg Clin North Am 2005;85:555–67.

[31] Siu WT, Chau BKB, Tang CN, et al. Routine use of laparoscopic repair for perforated peptic ulcer. Br J Surg 2004;91:481–4.

[32] Sauerland S, Agresta F, Bergamaschi R, et al. Laparoscopy for abdominal emergencies. Evidence-based guidelines of the European association for Endoscopic Surgery. Surg Endosc 2005;20:14–29.

[33] Faranda C, Barrat C, Catheline JM, et al. Two-stage laparoscopic management of generalized peritonitis due to perforated sigmoid diverticulitis: eighteen cases. Surg Laparosc Endosc Percutan Tech 2000;10(3):135–8.

[34] Kirshtein B, Roy-Shapira A, Lantsberg L, et al. Laparoscopic management of acute small bowel obstruction. Surg Endosc 2005;19:464–7.

[35] Sauerland S, Lefering R, Neugebauer EAM. Laparoscopic versus open surgery for suspected appendicitis. Cochrane Database Syst Rev 2004;4:CD001546.

[36] Pikarsky AJ, Saida Y, Yamaguchi T, et al. Is obesity a high-risk factor for laparoscopic colorectal surgery? Surg Endosc 2002;16:855–8.

[37] Alves A, Panis Y, Bouhnik Y, et al. Factors that predict conversion in 69 consecutive patients undergoing laparoscopic ileocecal resection for Crohn's disease: a prospective study. Dis Colon Rectum 2005;48:2302–8.

[38] Schwartz ML, Drew RL, Chazin-Caldie M. Factors determining conversion from laparoscopic to open Roux-en-Y gastric bypass. Obes Surg 2004;14(9):1193–7.

[39] Livingston EH, Rege RV. A nationwide study of conversion from laparoscopic to open cholecystectomy. Am J Surg 2004;188(3):205–11.

[40] Gervaz P, Pikarsky A, Utech M, et al. Converted laparoscopic colorectal surgery. Surg Endosc 2001;15(8):827–32.

[41] Schlachta CM, Mamazza J, Seshadri PA, et al. Predicting conversion to open surgery in laparoscopic colorectal resections. A simple clinical model. Surg Endosc 2000;14(12):1114–7.

[42] Soot SJ, Eshraghi N, Farahmand M, et al. Transition from open to laparoscopic fundoplication. The learning curve. Arch Surg 1999;134:278–81.

[43] Shikora SA, Kim JJ, Tarnoff ME, et al. Laparoscopic Roux-en-Y bypass. Results and learning curve of a high-volume academic program. Arch Surg 2005;140:362–7.

[44] Schlachta CM, Mamazza J, Seshadri PA, et al. Defining a learning curve for laparoscopic colorectal resections. Dis Colon Rectum 2001;43:217–21.

[45] Dagash H, Chodhury M, Pierro A. When can I be proficient in laparoscopic surgery? A systematic review of the evidence. J Pediatr Surg 2005;38:720–4.

[46] Voitk AJ. The learning curve in laparoscopic inguinal repair for the community general surgeon. Can J Surg 1998;41(6):446–50.

[47] Voitk A, Yau P, Joffe J, et al. Effect of laparoscopic failure on outcome of laparoscopic Nissen fundoplication: independent review. J Laparoendosc Adv Surg Tech A 2002;12(1):35–9.

[48] Bloomston M, Serafini F, Boyce HW, et al. The "learning curve" in videoscopic Heller myotomy. JSLS 2002;6:41–7.

[49] McLeod RS, Stern H for the CAGS Evidence-Based Reviews in Surgery Group. Canadian Association of General Surgeons evidence-based reviews in surgery: 10. Laparoscopy-assisted colectomy versus open colectomy for treatment of nonmetastatic colon cancer: a randomized trial. Can J Surg 2003;47:209–11.

[50] The American heritage dictionary of the English language. 4th edition. Boston: Houghton Mifflin Co.; 2000.

[51] Hanna GB, Shimi S, Cuschieri A. Optimal port locations for endoscopic intracorporeal knotting. Surg Endosc 1997;11(4):397–401.

[51a] Voorhees JR, Cohen-Gadol AA, Laws ER, et al. Battling blood loss in neurosurgery: Harvey Cushing's embrace of electrosurgery. J Neurosurg 2005;102:745–52.

[52] Fried GM, Feldman LS, Vassiliou MC, et al. Proving the value of simulation in laparoscopic surgery. Ann Surg 2004;240(3):518–25 [discussion 525–8].

[53] Rogers DA, Elstein AS, Bordage G. Improving continuing medical education for surgical techniques: applying the lessons learned in the first decade of minimal access surgery. Ann Surg 2001;233(2):159–66.

[54] Soukhavov A, editor. Encarta World English dictionary. New York: St. Martin's Press; 1999.

[55] Do LV, Laplante R, Miller S, et al. Laparoscopic colon surgery performed safely by general surgeons in a community hospital: a review of 154 consecutive cases. Surg Endosc 2005;19: 1533–7.

[56] Cushieri A, Wilson RG, Sunderland G, et al. Training Initiative List Scheme (TILS) for minimal access therapy: the MATTUS experience. J R Coll Surg Edinb 1997;42:295–302.

[57] Pace DE, Chiasson PM, Schlachta CM, et al. Laparoscopic splenectomy: does the training of minimally invasive surgical fellows affect outcomes? Surg Endosc 2002;16(6):954–6.

[58] Schlachta CM, Mamazza J, Gregoire R, et al. Predicting conversion in laparoscopic colorectal surgery. Fellowship training may be an advantage. Surg Endosc 2003;17(8):1288–91.

ELSEVIER
SAUNDERS

SURGICAL
CLINICS OF
NORTH AMERICA

Surg Clin N Am 86 (2006) 1005–1022

Evolving Techniques in the Treatment of Liver Colorectal Metastases: Role of Laparoscopy, Radiofrequency Ablation, Microwave Coagulation, Hepatic Arterial Chemotherapy, Indications and Contraindications for Resection, Role of Transplantation, and Timing of Chemotherapy

Bridget N. Fahy, MD[a], William R. Jarnagin, MD[b],*

[a]Department of Surgery, Memorial Sloan-Kettering Cancer Center,
1275 York Avenue, New York, NY 10021, USA
[b]Hepatobiliary Service, Memorial Sloan-Kettering Cancer Center,
1275 York Avenue, New York, NY 10021, USA

Colorectal cancer (CRC) is a leading cause of cancer death in the United States. More than 140,000 patients were diagnosed with CRC in 2004 [1]. It has been reported that between 16% and 25% of patients have liver metastases at the time of exploration for their primary tumor [2]. Furthermore, approximately one half eventually develops liver metastases [3]. Patients who have untreated liver metastases from CRC rarely survive 5 years and have a reported median survival of 6 to 13 months [4]. The 5-year overall survival following resection of CRC liver metastases in current series is up to 58% [5,6]. Unfortunately, most patients are not candidates for resection because of the extent or distribution of disease [7]. Consequently, several alternate methods are being used to treat hepatic metastases from CRC, including microwave coagulation, radiofrequency ablation, and transplantation. Additionally, research regarding the route and timing of chemotherapy for hepatic metastases is an area of active study. This article provides

---

* Corresponding author.
E-mail address: jarnagiw@mskcc.org (W.R. Jarnagin).

0039-6109/06/$ - see front matter © 2006 Elsevier Inc. All rights reserved.
doi:10.1016/j.suc.2006.06.003
surgical.theclinics.com

a summary of the major studies that have been performed examining the modalities used in the management of hepatic metastases.

Laparoscopy

A small proportion of patients that has hepatic metastases from CRC are candidates for curative resection; therefore, accurate staging is paramount in selecting patients for resection. No currently available preoperative imaging modality is 100% sensitive and specific for the extent of hepatic disease or the presence of extrahepatic metastases. Laparoscopy has been offered as one means of evaluating the presence of extrahepatic intra-abdominal disease that would preclude curative resection. At least three studies have addressed the role of diagnostic laparoscopy in patients who have colorectal liver metastases. A report by Rahusen and colleagues [8] included 50 consecutive patients who had colorectal metastases that were deemed resectable by preoperative imaging, and subjected them to diagnostic laparoscopy and laparoscopic ultrasonography. Of the 47 patients who were able to undergo laparoscopy, 13% were found to be unresectable based upon findings at laparoscopy, and 25% were found to be unresectable based upon findings on laparoscopic ultrasound. They concluded that use of a combination of diagnostic laparoscopy and laparoscopic ultrasonography significantly improves the selection of candidates for liver resection, and, thereby, spared 38% of patients in their study an unnecessary laparotomy.

Two studies from the authors' group evaluated the role of laparoscopy before hepatic resection of colorectal metastases [9,10]. In the study by Jarnagin and colleagues [9], 103 patients who had potentially resectable colorectal metastases underwent laparoscopy before a planned laparotomy and partial hepatectomy. Laparoscopy identified 14 of 26 patients who had unresectable disease; 10 of these patients were spared an unnecessary laparotomy. Additional findings were seen at laparoscopy and changed the planned resection in 4 patients. Conversely, laparoscopy was not helpful in 68 patients, and 8 additional patients had unresectable disease that was missed at laparoscopy. Furthermore, a clinical risk score (CRS; see later discussion under "Indications and contraindications for resection") was used to stratify patients before laparoscopy [11]. In the CRS, one point is given for each of the following factors: node-positive primary disease, disease-free interval from primary disease to metastases of less than 12 months, more than one hepatic tumor, largest hepatic tumor greater than 5 cm, and carcinoembryonic antigen (CEA) level greater than 200 ng/mL. When patients were stratified into those with a CRS of up to 2 versus those with a CRS of 2, it was found that 57 laparoscopic procedures could have been avoided in low-risk patients. These findings were confirmed in a follow-up study by Grobmyer and colleagues [10], in which 63 of 264 patients (24%) had unresectable disease. Twenty-six (41%) of the patients who had unresectable disease were identified during laparoscopy, 22 (35%) were not identified during laparoscopy, and 15 (24%) had other procedures performed during a laparotomy. Once again, the CRS was able to distinguish those patients who were most likely to have unresectable disease found at laparoscopy and they were able to avoid a laparotomy. No low-risk patient (CRS ≤ 1) had unresectable disease, 11% of patients with a CRS of 2 or 3 had unresectable disease, and 24% of patients with a CRS of 4 or 5 had unresectable disease. Additionally, the percentage of patients that underwent a nontherapeutic laparotomy following laparoscopy that failed to identify unresectable disease was 4% in patients with a CRS of 1 or less, 10% in patients with a CRS of 2 or 3, and 14% in patients with a CRS of 4 or 5. A shortened interval to systemic chemotherapy in those who were found to be unresectable at laparoscopy was another benefit in those who were spared a nontherapeutic laparotomy. The authors advocate the selective use of laparoscopy before planned hepatic resection for colorectal hepatic metastases. There seems to be little role for this modality in patients with a low CRS, whereas those with a CRS of 4 or 5 have the most to gain from laparoscopy.

Radiofrequency ablation

Radiofrequency ablation (RFA) uses high-frequency alternating current to produce heat that destroys tumors by denaturing proteins. RFA has been applied for the treatment of colorectal hepatic metastases through three approaches: during laparotomy, laparoscopically, and percutaneously. Numerous reports have described the efficacy and safety of RFA in the treatment of colorectal metastases; however, no prospective randomized clinical trial has compared RFA with hepatic resection.

One of the largest series to date that described the use of RFA in CRC metastases came from the group at M.D. Anderson [12]; it reported on 172 patients who underwent resection plus RFA for primary or metastatic disease. Metastases from CRC was the most common histology treated, and it accounted for 72% of the cases overall. The median number of tumors resected per patient was two, whereas the median number of tumors treated by RFA per patient was one. The median tumor size for all patients in the study was 1.8 cm in largest dimension. The postoperative complication rate was 20%, with an operative mortality of 2.3%. No correlation was found between the extent of liver resection or number of tumors treated with RFA and the development of postoperative complications. Recurrence was seen in 57% of patients at a median of 21 months of follow-up. The site of first recurrence was the RFA site in 8%, non-RFA hepatic site in 39%, non-RFA hepatic site plus distant in 32%, and distant only in 21%. The investigators pointed out that although the RFA site recurrence rate was 8%, this translated into a recurrence rate of only 2% when considering that 350 tumors were ablated. The median time to recurrence was identical for each pattern of recurrence. Of the 8 patients who developed recurrence at the RFA site, 7 of 8 had CRC metastases. In this group of 7 patients, all but

1 patient had a single tumor treated. On univariate and multivariate analysis, the total number of tumors treated was the only factor that affected the time to recurrence significantly. The median actuarial survival in the subset of patients that had colorectal metastases was 37 months compared with the median survival of 59 months in patients who had noncolorectal metastases. The investigators concluded that RFA is a safe and effective adjunct to resection, but it cannot be viewed as a replacement for resection. At M.D. Anderson, RFA is used in conjunction with hepatic resection to increase the number of patients that is eligible for complete removal or destruction of their tumors. The four deaths in this series illustrate the risk for liver failure and death in patients who undergo RFA and resection. Careful patient and tumor selection is paramount to a favorable outcome in this combined approach to hepatic malignancies.

A follow-up study by the group at M.D. Anderson compared the recurrence and outcomes following hepatic resection alone, RFA alone, and resection plus RFA for colorectal liver metastases [6]. They reported on a cohort of 358 consecutive patients that had CRC metastases and underwent treatment with curative intent and 70 patients who had hepatic disease only who were not candidates for curative treatment. For the combined group of 428 patients, 45% underwent resection alone, 24% underwent RFA plus resection, 14% underwent RFA only, and 17% had a laparotomy with biopsy only or placement of a hepatic arterial infusion pump. Overall recurrence was significantly more common after RFA (84%) compared with resection alone (52%). Intrahepatic recurrence was significantly more common after RFA alone (44%) than after RFA plus resection (28%) or resection alone (11%). True local recurrence, recurrence at the site of resection or RFA, was significantly more common following RFA alone (9%) compared with resection alone (2%). Overall survival rate was highest after resection (58% at 5 years), but it did not differ significantly at 3 and 4 years in patients who were treated with RFA plus resection versus RFA alone. Patients who underwent RFA as a component of their treatment were compared with the 70 patients who were not candidates for curative therapy. Survival was improved significantly in patients who underwent RFA (in conjunction with resection or alone) compared with those who did not receive RFA. Tumor number was predictive of poor survival on multivariate analysis and survival was impacted significantly by mode of therapy; treatment of solitary or multiple tumors by resection alone was superior to RFA or RFA plus resection. The investigators concluded that hepatic resection is the treatment of choice for colorectal liver metastases. Additionally, RFA alone or in combination with resection for patients who do not have resectable disease does not provide survival that is comparable to resection, and provides survival that is only slightly superior to nonsurgical treatment.

Bleicher and colleagues [13] reported their results of RFA in 153 patients with 447 unresectable primary and metastatic liver lesions. Fifty-nine patients had metastases from CRC. Local recurrence at the RFA site occurred in 21% of patients and in 11.6% of individual tumors ablated. Recurrence was seen in 18% of colorectal metastases ablated. Tumor size and ablation of one versus two or more tumors were the two factors that were related most significantly to local recurrence. On univariate analysis, local recurrence also was noted to be higher following ablation of colorectal metastases and hepatocellular carcinoma compared with breast and carcinoid metastases. The overall morbidity of the procedure was 12%; the most common complications were abscess formation and biliary injury. Despite the risk for local recurrence and procedure-related complications, the investigators continue to endorse RFA as a palliative modality in selected patients.

In summary, RFA is associated with acceptable morbidity and mortality compared with surgical resection. Local recurrence in the ablation bed occurs in 8% to 18% of patients and 2% to 12% of tumors. The number and size of tumors ablated are the factors that are associated most consistently with local recurrence following RFA of colorectal metastases. It also should be emphasized that tumors that are unresectable because of their extent or location rarely are amenable to effective ablation. Conversely, tumors that are amenable to ablation usually are amenable to resection.

Microwave coagulation

Microwave coagulation for hepatic metastases was introduced by Tabuse in 1979. The microwave coagulator was designed to cut the liver and coagulate the cut end simultaneously. Similar to RFA, this technique can be applied during laparotomy or percutaneously under ultrasound guidance, it is less invasive than is surgical resection, and it can be applied to multiple tumors of the liver while sparing normal hepatic tissues.

The feasibility, safety, and efficacy of percutaneous microwave coagulation therapy for solitary metachronous hepatic metastases were studied by Seki and colleagues in 15 patients who had CRC [14]. Microwave coagulation successfully induced necrosis within the tumor as well as a margin of normal hepatic parenchyma in 13 of 15 patients. Complications during and following the procedure were minimal; 1 patient developed a right pleural effusion that was managed conservatively. No cancer cell seeding of the tract site was noted. Almost half of the patients survived for at least 2 years without recurrence. An additional 3 patients remained free of recurrence for at least 17 months. The median survival for all patients was 24 months. Four patients eventually died of disease, although none died as a result of recurrence at the previously treated microwave coagulation site. Successful application of this technique, like that of other local ablative techniques, is limited by anatomic constraints, such as proximity to the gallbladder or large vessels.

A randomized controlled trial that compared microwave coagulation with hepatic resection in patients who had multiple hepatic metastases from CRC was performed by Shibata and colleagues [15]. A total of 30 patients was included in the trial: 14 in the microwave group and 16 in the hepatectomy group. No recurrence was seen in the microwave group for at least 3 months in patients whose tumors were considered completely coagulated. The efficacy of microwave treatment was confirmed by a decrease in CEA. No intra- or postoperative deaths occurred in either group. The frequency of postoperative complications was not different between the two groups. No statistically significant difference in cumulative survival was seen; the mean survival in the microwave group was 27 months compared with 25 months in the hepatectomy group. The mean disease-free interval was 11 months in the microwave group and 13 months in the hepatectomy group. For both groups, the main cause of death during follow-up was hepatic failure; it was responsible for 6 of 9 deaths in the microwave group and 7 of 12 deaths in the hepatectomy group. The frequency of death due to hepatic failure was not correlated with the number or size of metastatic tumors. The investigators endorse microwave coagulation in patients who have multiple hepatic metastases from CRC, citing its reduced surgical invasiveness and comparable efficacy. Unfortunately, the investigators did not provide information regarding local recurrence following microwave coagulation, which is a major shortcoming in local ablative therapies when compared with surgical resection. Additionally, longer follow-up is needed to assess accurately the therapeutic equivalency of microwave coagulation to resection.

Currently, experience with this technique is limited and its potential advantage over hepatic resection or RFA awaits the results of larger studies.

Hepatic arterial infusion therapy

Hepatic arterial infusion (HAI) therapy is a form of liver-directed therapy that takes advantage of the fact that most of the vascular supply to colorectal hepatic metastases is derived from the hepatic artery. Additionally, HAI regional therapy, particularly with floxuridine, allows higher doses of chemotherapy to be delivered locally than could be tolerated systemically. There are two potential scenarios in which HAI can be applied to colorectal hepatic metastases: "neoadjuvant," before hepatic resection or in patients who have unresectable liver metastases and no evidence of extrahepatic disease, and adjuvant, following complete hepatic resection.

Neoadjuvant

The initial trials that used HAI chemotherapy exclusive of systemic therapy showed increased response rates and progression-free survival compared with systemic chemotherapy (reviewed in [16]), and this served as the impetus for exploring the potential role for HAI as neoadjuvant therapy. A summary of the clinical trials that evaluated neoadjuvant HAI chemotherapy in patients who had unresectable colorectal hepatic metastases is found in Table 1. Response rates in these trials ranged from 16% to 82%,

Table 1

Trials of neoadjuvant hepatic arterial infusional (HAI) chemotherapy in patients with unresectable hepatic metastases

Investigators	Treatment groups	N	Response rate	Complete resection (n [%])
Elias et al, 1995 [42]	5FU ± mitomycin ± piraubicin ± cisplatin	239	NR	14 (5.8)
Link et al, 1999 [43]	FUDR	168	42%	9 (5)
	FUDR HAI + IV		46%	
	5FU/LV		45%	
	MMF		66%	
Meric et al, 2000 [44]	FUDR, 5FU/LV + mitomycin	383	NR	13 (3.4)
Clavien et al, 2002 [45]	FUDR	23	39%	6 (26)
Milandri et al, 2003 [46]	5FU/LV ± mitomycin & IV 5FU	31	16%	4 (14)
Ducreux et al, 2005 [47]	Oxaliplatin + IV 5FU/LV	28	64%	4 (14)
Noda et al, 2004 [48]	5FU + IV uracil & tegafur	51	78%	24 (47)
Leonard et al, 2004 [49]	FUDR + FOLFOX or IROX	44	82%	9 (20)
Kemeny et al, 2005 [50]	FUDR/Dex + IV IROX	21	90%	7 (33)
	FUDR/Dex + FOLFOX	15	87%	NR

Abbreviations: 5FU, 5 fluorouracil; Dex, dexamethasone; FOLFOX, oxaliplatin & infusional 5FU/LV; FUDR, floxuridine; IROX, oxaliplatin & irinotecan; IV, intravenous; LV, leucovorin; MMF, mitoxantrone, mitomycin, 5FU/LV; NR, not recorded.

and demonstrated a conversion to resectability in 3% to 47%. The large variability in these results is a reflection of the small sample sizes in many of these trials and the variety of HAI and systemic chemotherapy regimens used. Sufficiently large randomized trials that compare neoadjuvant HAI with systemic chemotherapy in patients who have unresectable hepatic metastases from CRC are required to determine the optimal treatment regimen in this patient group. In particular, the advantage of adding liver-directed chemotherapy to the best combination of systemic agents needs clarification.

Adjuvant

Despite the favorable long-term outcome following liver resection for colorectal metastases, the most common site of failure after resection is within the remnant liver. Consequently, additional therapy after liver resection, either systemic or regional, may be an important adjunct to resection. There have been eight trials that were designed to evaluate the role of adjuvant HAI therapy following surgical resection of hepatic metastases (Table 2). Most of these studies included a small number of patients and used a variety

Table 2
Trials of adjuvant hepatic arterial infusional chemotherapy following surgical resection of hepatic metastases

Investigators	Treatment groups	N	Duration follow-up	DFS	OS
Lygidakis et al, 1995 [51]	Surgery + chemoimmunotherapy vs surgery alone	20 20	3 y	NR	20 mo 11 mo $P < .05$
Asahara et al, 1998 [52]	Surgery + HAI chemo vs surgery alone	10 28	NR	NR	3-y: 100% 4-y: 100% 3-y: 60%; 4-y: 47% $P < .05$
Lorenz et al, 1998 [53]	Surgery + HAI chemo vs surgery alone	113 113	NR	14.2 mo 13.7 mo NS	34.5 mo 40.8 mo NS
Rudroff et al, 1999 [54]	Surgery + HAI chemo vs surgery alone	14 16	5 y	5-y: 15% 5-y: 23% NS	5-y: 25% 5-y: 31% NS
Kemeny et al, 1999 [55]	Surgery + HAI chemo + IV chemo vs surgery + IV chemo	74 82	2 y	2-y: 57% 2-y: 42% NS	2-y: 86% 2-y: 72% $P = .03$
Tono et al, 2000 [56]	Surg + HAI chemo + oral chemo vs surgery + oral chemo	9 10	62 mo	1-, 2-, 3-y: 78%, 78%, 67%, respectively 1-, 2-, 3-y: 50%, 30%, 20%, respectively $P = .05$	1-, 2-, 3-y: 89%, 78%, 78%, respectively 1-, 2-, 3-y: 100%, 50%, 50%, respectively NS
Kemeny et al, 2002 [57]	Surgery + HAI chemo + IV chemo vs surgery alone	53 56	NR	4-y: 46% 4-y: 25% $P = 0.04$	64 mo 49 mo NS
Kemeny et al, 2003 [18]	Surgery + HAI chemo + IV chemo	96	26 mo	1-, 1.5-y: 69%, 47%, respectively	1-, 2-y: 97%, 89%, respectively

Abbreviations: chemo, chemotherapy; IV, intravenous; OS, overall survival; NR, not recorded; NS, not significant.

of regional agents with or without systemic chemotherapy regimens. Because of the heterogeneity in therapy regimens among the trials, variability in the percentage of patients who received the HAI treatment as prescribed, and the number of patients who crossed over from the control to the treatment arm, it is not possible to draw definite conclusions about the efficacy of adjuvant HAI therapy following hepatic resection. The data do suggest a general trend in support of adjuvant HAI therapy for disease-free survival (DFS), however. This improvement in DFS has not translated into a significant improvement in overall survival, however. Kemeny and Gonen [17] recently reported an update of their original study, now with a median follow-up of 10.3 years. They found that overall progression-free survival was significantly higher in the group that received HAI therapy (31.3 months) compared with those who did not receive adjuvant HAI therapy (17.2 months, $P = .02$). Median hepatic DFS was not reached yet in the group that received HAI therapy, and it was 32.5 months in patients who did not receive adjuvant HAI treatment ($P < .01$). Ten-year survival was 41% in the group that received HAI therapy compared with 27% in patients who did not receive adjuvant HAI therapy.

A significant limitation of the currently available trials of adjuvant HAI therapy after hepatic resection is the use of what is now considered to be suboptimal systemic chemotherapy. The potential benefit of combining adjuvant HAI therapy with the newer and more effective systemic chemotherapeutic agents, such as oxaliplatin and irinotecan, is beginning to be explored. A phase I/II study of HAI in combination with systemic irinotecan following hepatic resection was reported by Kemeny and colleagues [18]; these findings are summarized in Table 3. Randomized phase III trials are needed to address the usefulness of adjuvant HAI therapy after hepatic resection in this era of more effective systemic chemotherapy.

Indications and contraindications for resection

Despite the improved response rates that are associated with systemic chemotherapy regimens that contain oxaliplatin or irinotecan, surgical resection continues to be the most effective modality for treating CRC hepatic

Table 3
Adjuvant hepatic arterial infusional floxuridine/dexamethasone + systemic irinotecan versus hepatic arterial infusional floxuridine/dexamethasone + systemic 5-fluorouracil/leucovorin following hepatic resection

Variable	HAI + irinotecan (N [%])	HAI + 5FU/LV (N[%])
Primary tumor		
Colon	76 (79)	55 (74)
Rectum	20 (21)	19 (26)
Synchronous metastases	38 (40)	26 (35)
# hepatic lesions		
<4	84 (87)	60 (81)
≥4	12 (13)	14 (19)
Disease-free interval <12 mo	71 (74)	57 (77)
Previous chemotherapy	72 (75)	39 (53)
Preoperative CEA (median)	17.5 ng/mL	11.5 ng/mL
1-year disease-free survival	69%	82%[a]
1-year hepatic disease–free survival	92%	98%[a]
1-year overall survival	97%	98%[a]

[a] Determined from survival curves provided in [58].

Data from Kemeny N, Jarnagin W, Yonen M, et al. Phase I/II study of hepatic arterial therapy with floxuridine and dexamethasone in combination with intravenous irinotecan as adjuvant treatment after resection of hepatic metastases from colorectal cancer. J Clin Oncol 2003;21:3303–9.

metastases. The 5-year survival following resection of colorectal hepatic metastases is 20% to 37%, with a median survival of 24 to 40 months [19]. Cure following hepatic resection has been reported in a significant proportion of cases, and 10-year survival following resection has been reported by several investigators [5,11,20,21].

The morbidity and mortality that are associated with hepatic resections for metastatic CRC have been shown to be within acceptable limits; at major centers, mortality following major resections is uniformly less than 5% [11,19,22,23]. The major causes of perioperative death are liver failure or hemorrhage; these complications occur in 1% to 5% of patients. Hepatic resection continues to be associated with a high complication rate, however (20%–50%). The most common complication following hepatic resection is a perihepatic collection that results from a biliary leak; this complication is seen in 3% to 5% of patients.

The favorable outcome following liver resection for colorectal metastases is predicated, in part, on careful preoperative evaluation and patient selection. Based upon a review of 1001 liver resections for metastatic CRC, the authors' group was able to identify seven factors that were significant and independent predictors of poor long-term outcome on multivariate analysis [11]. They are positive hepatic margin, extrahepatic disease, node-positive primary disease, disease-free interval from primary disease to metastases of less than 12 months, more than one hepatic tumor, largest hepatic tumor greater than 5 cm, and CEA level greater than 200 ng/mL. The last five criteria were incorporated into a preoperative scoring system, a CRS, in which one point was given to each criterion. The total score was found to be highly predictive of outcome. An analysis of outcome based upon the CRS revealed that no patient with a score of 5 was a long-term survivor, and patients with up to two criteria can have a favorable outcome. The investigators recommended that patients with a CRS of 3 to 5 should not necessarily be denied resection, but may benefit from aggressive neoadjuvant or postresection chemotherapy.

A study of 226 patients who had colorectal hepatic metastases was reported recently by the group from Johns Hopkins that evaluated long-term survival following hepatic resection [5]. They reported a median overall survival of 46 months and a DFS of 63% at 1 year and 28% at 5 years. Predictors of overall survival were CEA of less than 100 ng/mL and negative microscopic hepatic margins. Predictors of recurrence included more than three metastases, positive microscopic hepatic margin, and a preoperative CEA of greater than 100 ng/mL. They noted an increase in survival in patients who underwent hepatic resection for colorectal metastases from 1993 to 1999 compared with those who underwent resection between 1984 and 1992. The investigators hypothesized that improved patient selection through better pre- and intraoperative imaging, improvements in surgical technique, increased pre- and postoperative use of systemic chemotherapy, and increased use of salvage surgical resections following hepatic recurrence may have contributed to this increase in overall survival and DFS.

The timing of hepatic resection for patients who have synchronous colorectal metastases is an area of controversy. Synchronous liver metastases are defined as tumors that occur within 12 months of diagnosis of the colorectal primary. Synchronous metastases are found in 13% to 25% of patients who have metastatic CRC [24,25]. Martin and colleagues [26] studied the safety of synchronous resection in CRC with liver metastases. The investigators found that simultaneous resection could be performed safely, and that the overall complication rate was higher in the group that underwent staged resection. Additionally, on multivariate analysis, staged resection was an independent predictor of overall complications. The increase in complications that was seen in the group that underwent staged resection was attributable to the need for two laparotomies and the complications that were associated with laparotomy itself. Procedure-specific complications that were associated with the resection of the colon or liver did not differ in either group. Overall survival, DFS, and hepatic recurrence-free survival following synchronous or staged resection of colorectal hepatic metastases are equivalent [27,28].

Close follow-up is warranted in patients who undergo resection of colorectal metastases, because recurrence occurs in up to two thirds of patients and effective therapies can be given to treat these recurrences. A study by Topal and colleagues [29] examined the pattern of recurrence following curative resection of colorectal hepatic metastases. In their study, 74 (70%) patients developed recurrent disease during the mean follow-up period of 32 months. Forty-five patients developed a hepatic recurrence, 63 patients developed an extrahepatic recurrence, and 34 patients recurred in the liver and an extrahepatic site. Early recurrence (within 18 months of hepatic resection) occurred in 48 patients; the liver was the only site of recurrence in 44% and it occurred in combination with extrahepatic metastases in 23%. The investigators found that hepatic recurrence after 2 years was uncommon, whereas extrahepatic metastases continued to develop throughout the course of follow-up. No factor independently predicted the risk for liver recurrence, whereas elevated CEA, satellitosis, bilateral liver metastases, lymph node involvement of the primary colorectal tumor, intraoperative complications, high American Society of Anaesthesiology score, and female gender were associated significantly with poor extrahepatic DFS. The high rate of early hepatic and extrahepatic metastases following curative hepatic resection reflects the imprecision of our current preoperative staging modalities, and highlights the need for improved methods to detect occult metastases, both intra and extrahepatic, before planned hepatic resection.

The role of repeat hepatic resection for recurrent hepatic metastases from CRC has been the focus of several reports as liver resection has become safer. The operative morbidity and mortality of repeat hepatic resection is comparable to that of initial resection (19%–32% and 0%–2%, respectively), and is associated with a median survival of 32 to 46 months (reviewed in [30]). A bi-institutional review of second liver resections for recurrent hepatic metastases was performed by the authors' group in conjunction with the University of Frankfurt [31]. In this study of 126 patients, the operative mortality was 1.6% and the operative morbidity was 28%. The actuarial survival rates following the second hepatic resection were 86%, 51%, and 34% for 1, 3, and 5 years, respectively. Survival was significantly better in patients with solitary lesions or when the largest lesion was smaller than 5 cm. Eighty-four patients developed recurrent metastatic disease following second hepatic resection. Liver-only recurrence occurred in 36%, liver plus other recurrence occurred in 31%, and extrahepatic recurrence only occurred in 33%. Independent factors that were associated significantly with a poorer outcome included the presence of multiple hepatic lesions and at least one lesion that was larger than 5 cm at the second resection. The most important factors in selecting patients for second liver resection seem to be medical fitness, small solitary tumors, ability to clear all disease, and, possibly, disease-free interval between the first and second hepatic resections.

Role of transplantation

Little has been written about the feasibility or efficacy of orthotopic liver transplantation for colorectal hepatic metastases. In general, liver metastases are considered an absolute contraindication to cadaveric liver transplantation [32]. A small retrospective study by Muhlbacher and colleagues [33] explored the feasibility of orthotopic liver transplantation for secondary liver malignancies. Their study cohort included 17 patients who had CRC metastases and 2 patients who had resected neuroendocrine tumors of the pancreas. The median survival for the transplanted group was 13.1 months, compared with 7.2 months in patients who received no specific therapy and 18 months in those who were treated with locoregional intra-arterial chemotherapy. The longest documented disease-free survivors were in the transplant group, with three patients surviving for 7,4, and 2 years. No patient in the group that received intra-arterial chemotherapy lived beyond 3 years. Optimal selection of patients for transplantation is paramount; unfortunately, the investigators did not specify how their patients were chosen for transplant, except to note that the primary lesion was resected successfully and extrahepatic tumors had been excluded.

Recently, Honore and colleagues [34] reported a patient who underwent liver transplantation as salvage therapy for acute liver failure after liver resection for isolated hepatic metastases from colon cancer. The patient developed isolated 5-cm liver metastases 3 years after a sigmoid colon resection for adenocarcinoma. The patient did not receive any posttransplant chemotherapy, and reportedly was cancer-free 10 years following his transplantation. Although this is a single case and definitive conclusions cannot be drawn based upon this one case, it does raise the question of whether liver transplantation might be an option for highly selected patients who have colon metastases that are limited to the liver. There is no role for transplantation in this setting outside a well-conceived clinical trial.

Timing of chemotherapy

The past 10 years have seen a dramatic change in systemic chemotherapy for metastatic CRC. The switch from bolus to infusional 5-fluorouracil (5FU) was the first major shift, and it has been associated with higher response rates and significantly longer progression-free survival [35]. In the 1990s, irinotecan and oxaliplatin emerged as effective agents against metastatic CRC. Compared with the 33% response rates that were seen with infusional 5FU/leucovorin alone, the addition of irinotecan or oxaliplatin is associated with response rates of up to 50% (reviewed in [36]). Systemic chemotherapy for hepatic metastases from CRC can be given in two settings: adjuvant therapy following hepatic resection and in the neoadjuvant setting, in patients who have unresectable liver disease.

Neoadjuvant

The concept of rendering unresectable hepatic metastases from CRC resectable through the use of neoadjuvant chemotherapy was described first by Bismuth and colleagues [37]. Of 330 patients who disease initially was considered to be unresectable, 53 patients (16%) responded to chemotherapy to the point that curative resection was considered possible. Patients received chronomodulated chemotherapy with 5FU, folinic acid, and oxaliplatin. In addition, patients underwent a variety of pre- and intraoperative techniques that was aimed at achieving a curative resection, including preoperative portal vein embolization and intraoperative cryotherapy and alcohol ablation. Twenty-three patients (43%) died with hepatic recurrence, and 36% were without evidence of disease at the time of last follow-up. The 1-, 3-, and 4-year overall survival rates were 91%, 54%, and 40%, respectively. This study showed that down-staging of unresectable hepatic metastases is possible, and it is associated with overall survival rates that are comparable to patients whose liver metastases initially were considered to be resectable. These findings were confirmed in a larger trial by the same investigators in which 95 of 701 patients, whose disease was considered initially to be unresectable, were rendered candidates for curative resection following neoadjuvant chemotherapy with a combination of 5FU, folinic acid, and oxaliplatin [38]. Results from more recent trials showed that the conversion from unresectable disease to resectable disease may approach 35% (reviewed in [36]). The most important lesson learned from this early experience with neoadjuvant chemotherapy in patients who had initially unresectable hepatic metastases is that chemotherapy can render a measurable proportion of cases resectable. Therefore, these patients should be monitored closely for this possibility, because resection continues to offer the best opportunity for long-term survival and possible cure.

The role of neoadjuvant chemotherapy in patients who have resectable liver metastases was the focus of a recent study by the authors' group [39].

One hundred and sixty-seven patients who had clinically resectable synchronous hepatic metastases from CRC were evaluated; 61 patients had a combined colon/liver resection, whereas 106 patients had a staged resection. Of these 106 patients, 54 received no preoperative chemotherapy and 52 received neoadjuvant chemotherapy that consisted of 5FU-based chemotherapy that was given in conjunction with leucovorin, irinotecan, or oxaliplatin. The two groups were well-matched with regard to their primary tumors and extent of liver metastases. Two factors were associated significantly with improved disease-specific survival: the ability to undergo complete hepatic resection and lack of disease progression while on neoadjuvant chemotherapy. Although no survival advantage was seen in patients who received neoadjuvant chemotherapy compared with those who did not, a survival advantage was evident among patients who received neoadjuvant therapy and showed stabilization or regression of disease. Additionally, no patient who received neoadjuvant chemotherapy became unresectable while on therapy. In patients who have synchronous CRC with hepatic metastases, the authors advocate considering these patients for neoadjuvant chemotherapy because response to treatment may provide important prognostic information and can help to guide future therapeutic interventions.

Adjuvant

Numerous investigators have shown that hepatic and extrahepatic recurrence is common following curative resection of hepatic metastases from CRC [29,31,40]. Therefore, adjuvant therapies that are designed to reduce the risk for local and distant recurrence are needed. The use of HAI therapy to reduce hepatic recurrences following curative resection was reviewed above. The role of adjuvant systemic chemotherapy following hepatic resection is unclear; there is little data to guide practitioners who care for patients in this setting. The primary data that are used to support adjuvant chemotherapy in this group of patients comes from extrapolation of data that support the use of chemotherapy after resection of node-positive CRCs. A handful of retrospective studies have explored the potential benefit of chemotherapy (Table 4). The largest study, by Figueras and colleagues [41], compared 81 patients who did not receive adjuvant chemotherapy after hepatic resection with 99 patients who received various systemic chemotherapy regimens following resection. The groups were well-matched with respect to number of liver metastases, presence of extrahepatic disease, preoperative CEA level, type of resection, and presence of positive margins. Patients who received adjuvant chemotherapy were significantly younger, were less likely to have received previous chemotherapy, and had more synchronous metastases compared with patients who did not receive adjuvant chemotherapy. Adjuvant chemotherapy had a protective effect and improved the prognosis of patients who received the therapy, independent of the presence of more synchronous metastases and previous treatment with chemotherapy.

Table 4
Summary of studies of adjuvant systemic chemotherapy following resection of colorectal hepatic metastases

Investigators	Treatment groups	N	Duration follow-up	Outcome	Benefit
Donato et al, 1994 [59]	Observation 5FU based	40 62	Median 28 mo	3-y DFS, OS: 29, 43.5 mo, respectively 3-y DFS, OS: 22, 47 mo, respectively	Yes
O'Connell et al, 1985 [60]	Observation vs 5FU + semustine	26 26	NR	5-y survival: 25% vs 15%	No
Butler et al, 1986 [61]	Observation 5FU based	51 11	NR	NR	No
Iwatsuki et al, 1986 [62]	Observation 5FU	38 22	Median 3 y	[a]3-y OS: 45% 3-y OS: 62%	Yes
Kokudo et al, 1998 [63]	Observation vs regional chemo vs systemic chemo	40 38 37	NR	5-y DFS, OS: 37%, 19%, respectively 5-y DFS, OS: 49%, 26%, respectively 5-y DFS, OS: 51%, 33%, respectively	Yes
Figueras et al, 2001 [41]	Observation vs 5FU/LV	81 99	Median 20 mo	5-y OS: 25% 5-y OS: 53%	Yes

Abbreviation: NR, not recorded.
[a] Variables extrapolated from published figures.

The precise role for adjuvant chemotherapy following hepatic resection continues to await the results from randomized clinical trials using current chemotherapy regimens.

Summary

The management of patients who have hepatic metastases from CRC has become increasingly complex as the number of modalities that is available to treat these tumors has increased. Surgical resection remains the mainstay of treatment, when possible, and may become an option in an increasing proportion of patients that has advanced disease and previously were considered unresectable when treated with a combination of neoadjuvant systemic or hepatic arterial chemotherapy. The role of microwave coagulation and RFA can be considered only complementary to surgical resection at this point, but they may represent the best option in highly selected patients, such as those who are at high risk for extrahepatic recurrence or who are poor surgical candidates.

References

[1] Jemal A, Murray T, Ward E, et al. Cancer statistics, 2005. CA Cancer J Clin 2005;55(1): 10–30.

[2] Bengtsson G, Carlsson G, Hafstrom L, et al. Natural history of patients with untreated liver metastases from colorectal cancer. Am J Surg 1981;141(5):586–9.

[3] Taylor I, Mullee M, Campbell M. Prognostic index for the development of liver metastases in patients with colorectal cancer. Br J Surg 1990;77(5):499–501.

[4] McCarter M, Fong Y. Metastatic liver tumors. Semin Surg Oncol 2000;19:177–88.

[5] Choti MA, Sitzmann JV, Tiburi MF, et al. Trends in long-term survival following liver resection for hepatic colorectal metastases. Ann Surg 2002;235(6):759–66.

[6] Abdalla E, Vauthey J, Ellis L, et al. Recurrence and outcomes following hepatic resection, radiofrequency ablation, and combined resection/ablation for colorectal liver metastases. Ann Surg 2004;239(6):818–27.

[7] Steele G, Ravikumar T. Resection of hepatic metastases from colorectal cancer. Biologic perspective. Ann Surg 1989;210:127–38.

[8] Rahusen F, Cuesta M, Borgstein P, et al. Selection of patients for resection of colorectal metastases to the liver using diagnostic laparoscopy and laparoscopic ultrasonography. Ann Surg 1999;230(1):31–7.

[9] Jarnagin W, Conlon K, Bodniewicz J, et al. A clinical scoring system predicts the yield of diagnostic laparoscopy in patients with potentially resectable hepatic colorectal metastases. Cancer 2001;91(6):1121–8.

[10] Grobmyer S, Fong Y, D'Angelica M, et al. Diagnostic laparoscopy prior to planned hepatic resection for colorectal metastases. Arch Surg 2004;139:1326–30.

[11] Fong Y, Fortner J, Sun R, et al. Clinical score for predicting recurrence after hepatic resection for metastatic colorectal cancer: analysis of 1001 consecutive cases. Ann Surg 1999; 230(3):309–18.

[12] Pawlik T, Izzo F, Cohen D, et al. Combined resection and radiofrequency ablation for advanced hepatic malignancies: results in 172 patients. Ann Surg Oncol 2003;10(9): 1059–69.

[13] Bleicher RJ, Allegra DP, Nora DT, et al. Radiofrequency ablation in 447 complex unresectable liver tumors: lessons learned. Ann Surg Oncol 2003;10(1):52–8.

[14] Seki T, Wakabayashi M, Nakagawa T, et al. Percutaneous microwave coagulation therapy for solitary metastatic liver tumors from colorectal cancer: a pilot clinical study. Am J Gastroenterol 1999;94:322–7.

[15] Shibata T, Niinobu T, Ogata N, et al. Microwave coagulation therapy for multiple hepatic metastases from colorectal carcinoma. Cancer 2000;89:276–84.

[16] Kemeny N, Ron I. Hepatic arterial chemotherapy in metastatic colorectal patients. Semin Oncol 1999;26(5):524–35.

[17] Kemeny NE, Gonen M. Hepatic arterial infusion after liver resection. N Engl J Med 2005; 352(7):734–5.

[18] Kemeny N, Jarnagin W, Gonen M, et al. Phase I/II study of hepatic arterial therapy with floxuridine and dexamethasone in combination with intravenous irinotecan as adjuvant treatment after resection of hepatic metastases from colorectal cancer. J Clin Oncol 2003; 21:3303–9.

[19] Fong Y, Salo J. Surgical therapy of hepatic colorectal metastases. Semin Oncol 1999;26(5): 514–23.

[20] Scheele J, Stang R, Altendorf-Hofmann A, et al. Resection of colorectal liver metastases. World J Surg 1995;19(1):59–71.

[21] Jamison R, Donohue J, Nagorney D, et al. Hepatic resection for metastatic colorectal cancer results in cure for some patients. Arch Surg 1997;132(5):505–10.

[22] Jarnagin WR, Gonen M, Fong Y, et al. Improvement in perioperative outcome after hepatic resection: analysis of 1,803 consecutive cases over the past decade. Ann Surg 2002;236(4): 397–406.

[23] Belghiti J, Hiramatsu K, Benoist S, et al. Seven hundred forty-seven hepatectomies in the 1990s: an update to evaluate the actual risk of liver resection. J Am Coll Surg 2000;191(1): 38–46.

[24] Blumgart L, Allison D. Resection and embolization in the management of secondary hepatic tumors. World J Surg 1982;6(1):32–45.

[25] Cady B, Monson D, Swinton N. Survival of patients after colonic resection for carcinoma with simultaneous liver metastases. Surg Gynecol Obstet 1970;131(4):697–700.

[26] Martin R, Paty P, Fong Y, et al. Simultaneous liver and colorectal resections are safe for synchronous colorectal liver metastasis. J Am Coll Surg 2003;197(2):233–41 [discussion 241–2].

[27] Weber J, Bachellier P, Oussoultzoglou E, et al. Simultaneous resection of colorectal primary tumour and synchronous liver metastases. Br J Surg 2003;90(8):956–62.

[28] Chua H, Sondenaa K, Tsiotos G, et al. Concurrent vs. staged colectomy and hepatectomy for primary colorectal cancer with synchronous hepatic metastases. Dis Colon Rectum 2004;47(8):1310–6.

[29] Topal B, Kaufman L, Aerts R, et al. Patterns of failure following curative resection of colorectal liver metastases. Eur J Surg Oncol 2003;29(3):248–53.

[30] Bentrem DJ, Dematteo RP, Blumgart LH. Surgical therapy for metastatic disease to the liver. Annu Rev Med 2005;56:139–56.

[31] Petrowsky H, Gonen M, Jarnagin W, et al. Second liver resections are safe and effective treatment for recurrent hepatic metastases from colorectal cancer: a bi-institutional analysis. Ann Surg 2002;235(6):863–71.

[32] Detry O, DeRoover A, Delwaide J, et al. Absolute and relative contraindications to liver transplantation. A perpetually moving frontier. Acta Gastroenterol Belg 2002;65:133.

[33] Muhlbacher F, Huk I, Steininger R, et al. Is orthotopic liver transplantation a feasible treatment for secondary cancer of the liver? Transplant Proc 1991;23(1):1567–8.

[34] Honore C, Detry O, DeRoover A, et al. Liver transplantation for metastatic colon adenocarcinoma: report of a case with 10 years of follow-up without recurrence. Transpl Int 2003;16: 692–3.

[35] de Gramont A, Bosset J, Milan C, et al. Randomized trial comparing monthly low-dose leucovorin and fluorouracil bolus with bimonthly high-dose leucovorin and fluorouracil bolus plus infusion for advanced colorectal cancer: a French intergroup study. J Clin Oncol 1997; 15(2):808–15.

[36] Leonard G, Brenner B, Kemeny N. Neoadjuvant chemotherapy before liver resection for patients with unresectable liver metastases from colorectal carcinoma. J Clin Oncol 2005;23: 2038–48.

[37] Bismuth H, Adam R, Levi F, et al. Resection of nonresectable liver metastases from colorectal cancer after neoadjuvant chemotherapy. Ann Surg 1996;224(4):509–20 [discussion 520–2].

[38] Adam R, Avisar E, Ariche A, et al. Five-year survival following hepatic resection after neoadjuvant therapy for nonresectable colorectal. Ann Surg Oncol 2001;8(4):347–53.

[39] Allen PJ, Kemeny N, Jarnagin W, et al. Importance of response to neoadjuvant chemotherapy in patients undergoing resection of synchronous colorectal liver metastases. J Gastrointest Surg 2003;7(1):109–15 [discussion 116–7].

[40] Fong Y, Cohen A, Fortner J. Liver resection for colorectal metastases. J Clin Oncol 1997;15: 938–46.

[41] Figueras J, Vallas C, Rafecas A, et al. Resection rate and effect of postoperative chemotherapy on survival after surgery for colorectal liver metastases. Br J Surg 2001;88(7):980–5.

[42] Elias D, Lasser P, Rougier P, et al. Frequency, technical aspects, results, and indications of major hepatectomy after prolonged intra-arterial hepatic chemotherapy for initially unresectable hepatic tumors. J Am Coll Surg 1995;180(2):213–9.

[43] Link K, Pillasch J, Formentini E, et al. Down staging by regional chemotherapy of nonresectable isolated colorectal liver metastases. Eur J Surg Oncol 1999;25:381–8.

[44] Meric F, Patt Y, Curley S, et al. Surgery after downstaging of unresectable hepatic tumors with intra-arterial chemotherapy. Ann Surg Oncol 2000;7(7):490–5.

[45] Clavien P, Selzner N, Morse M, et al. Downstaging of hepatocellular carcinoma and liver metastases from colorectal cancer by selective intra-arterial chemotherapy. Surgery 2002; 131(4):433–42.

[46] Milandri C, Calazolari F, Giampalma E. Combined treatment of inoperable liver metastases from colorectal cancer. Tumori 2003;89(Suppl):112–4.

[47] Ducreux M, Ychou M, Laplanche A, et al. Intra-arterial hepatic chemotherapy (IAHC) with oxaliplatin (O) combined with intravenous treatment with 5FU + folinic acid (FA) in hepatic metastases of colorectal cancer. Presented at the 2003 American Society of Clinical Oncology Annual Meeting. Chicago, May 31–June 3, 2003.

[48] Noda M, Yanagi H, Yoshikawa R, et al. Second-look hepatectomy after pharmacokinetic modulating chemotherapy (PMC) combination with hepatic arterial 5FU infusion and oral UFT in patients with unresectable hepatic colorectal metastases. Presented at the 2004 American Society of Clinical Oncology Annual Meeting. New Orleans, June 5–8, 2004.

[49] Leonard G, Fong Y, Jarnagin W, et al. Liver resection after hepatic arterial infusion (HAI) plus systemic oxaliplatin (Oxal) combinations in pretreated patients with extensive unresectable colorectal liver metastases. Presented at the 2004 American Society of Clinical Oncology Annual Meeting. New Orleans, June 5–8, 2004.

[50] Kemeny N, Eid A, Stockman J, et al. Hepatic arterial infusion of floxuridine and dexamethasone plus high-dose mitomycin C for patients with unresectable hepatic metastases from colorectal carcinoma. J Surg Oncol 2005;91(2):97–101.

[51] Lygidakis N, Ziras N, Parissis J. Resection versus resection combined with adjuvant pre- and post-operative chemotherapy—immunotherapy for metastatic colorectal liver cancer. A new look at an old problem. Hepatogastroenterology 1995;42(2):155–61.

[52] Asahara T, Kikkawa M, Okajima M, et al. Studies of postoperative transarterial infusion chemotherapy for liver metastasis of colorectal carcinoma after hepatectomy. Hepatogastroenterology 1998;45(21):805–11.

[53] Lorenz M, Muller H, Schramm H, et al. Randomized trial of surgery versus surgery followed by adjuvant hepatic arterial infusion with 5-fluorouracil and folinic acid for liver metastases of colorectal cancer. German Cooperative on Liver Metastases. Ann Surg 1998;228(6): 756–62.

[54] Rudroff C, Altendorf-Hoffmann A, Stangl R, et al. Prospective randomised trial on adjuvant hepatic artery infusion chemotherapy after R0 resection of colorectal liver metastases. Langenbecks Arch Surg 1999;384(3):243–9.

[55] Kemeny N, Huang Y, Cohen AM, et al. Hepatic arterial infusion of chemotherapy after resection of hepatic metastases from colorectal cancer. N Engl J Med 1999;341(27):2039–48.

[56] Tono T, Hasuike Y, Ohzato H, et al. Limited by definite efficacy of prophylactic hepatic arterial infusion chemotherapy after curative resection of colorectal liver metastases: a randomized study. Cancer 2000;88(7):1549–56.

[57] Kemeny MM, Adak S, Gray B, et al. Combined-modality treatment for resectable metastatic colorectal carcinoma to the liver: surgical resection of hepatic metastases in combination with continuous infusion of chemotherapy—an intergroup study. J Clin Oncol 2002;20(6): 1499–505.

[58] Kemeny N, Huang Y, Cohen A, et al. Hepatic arterial infusion of chemotherapy after resection of hepatic metastases from colorectal cancer. N Engl J Med 1999;341:2039–48.

[59] Donato N, Dario C, Giovanni S, et al. Retrospective study on adjuvant chemotherapy after surgical resection of colorectal cancer metastatic to the liver. Eur J Surg Oncol 1994;20(4): 454–60.

[60] O'Connell M, Adson M, Schutt A, et al. Clinical trial of adjuvant chemotherapy after surgical resection of colorectal cancer metastatic to the liver. Mayo Clin Proc 1985;60(8):517–20.

[61] Butler J, Attiyeh F, Daly J. Hepatic resection for metastases of the colon and rectum. Surg Gynecol Obstet 1986;162(2):109–13.

[62] Iwatsuki S, Esquivel C, Gordon R, et al. Liver resection for metastatic colorectal cancer. Surgery 1986;100(4):804–10.

[63] Kokudo N, Seki M, Ohta H, et al. Effects of systemic and regional chemotherapy after hepatic resection for colorectal metastases. Ann Surg Oncol 1998;5(8):706–12.

ELSEVIER
SAUNDERS

SURGICAL
CLINICS OF
NORTH AMERICA

Surg Clin N Am 86 (2006) 1023–1043

New Agents, Combinations, and Opportunities in the Treatment of Advanced and Early-Stage Colon Cancer

Neela Natarajan, MD, Todd D. Shuster, MD*

Department of Medical Oncology, Lahey Clinic Medical Center,
41 Mall Road, Burlington, MA 01805, USA

Colorectal cancer is the fourth most common malignancy in the United States (after prostate, breast, and lung cancer), with an anticipated 145,290 new cases, and is the second leading cause of cancer mortality (after lung cancer), with 56,290 expected deaths in 2005 [1]. Approximately 15% to 20% of newly diagnosed patients have metastatic disease at initial presentation, whereas the remaining 80% to 85% have earlier stage disease. Increasingly, patients who present with oligometastatic disease may be considered for potentially curative surgery as well. The estimated 5-year survival rates range from 90% for patients who have very early–stage disease to less than 10% for patients who have unresectable metastatic disease [2].

Until approximately 10 years ago, 5-fluorouracil (5-FU), mostly in combination with leucovorin (LV), was the only effective chemotherapeutic regimen for metastatic colorectal cancer, and achieved a median survival of less than 12 months [3]. Since then, the introduction of new combination chemotherapy regimens, as well as incorporation of new biologic agents, has led to significant improvements in median survival for these patients, which is now in excess of 20 months [4]. This article discusses these newer combinations and their efficacies and side effects, and reviews the use and investigation of these regimens in the adjuvant setting.

Treatment of metastatic disease

The old and gold standard: 5-fluorouracil

5-FU acts primarily by inhibiting thymidylate synthase, the rate-limiting enzyme in pyrimidine nucleotide synthesis [5]. Although 5-FU has

---

* Corresponding author.
E-mail address: todd.d.shuster@lahey.org (T.D. Shuster).

0039-6109/06/$ - see front matter © 2006 Elsevier Inc. All rights reserved.
doi:10.1016/j.suc.2006.06.002   *surgical.theclinics.com*

single-agent activity in colorectal cancer, combination with LV, which stabilizes the binding of 5-FU to thymidylate synthase, can double response rates and results in a statistically significant survival benefit compared with no treatment (12 months versus 6 months). The mode of administration of 5-FU and LV predominantly determines the side effect profile. A loading schedule that uses a monthly 5-day course of 5-FU plus low-dose LV (Mayo Clinic regimen) causes more stomatitis and neutropenia, whereas weekly boluses of 5-FU plus high-dose LV, given for 6 consecutive weeks with a 2-week break (Roswell Park regimen), causes diarrhea more frequently [6,7]. Hand-foot syndrome (palmar–plantar dysesthesia) occurs more frequently with infusional 5-FU regimens. The Mayo Clinic and the Roswell Park regimens have been compared and demonstrate similar response rates and survival. In comparison with the bolus regimens, infusional 5-FU shows an improved response rate (33% versus 14%) and median progression-free survival (28 weeks versus 22 weeks) [8]. Lower dose weekly LV regimens have been examined as well; they provide reduced toxicity without a significant compromise in efficacy [9].

Newer agents

Because first-generation 5-FU/LV regimens result in only a modest response rate and improvement in survival, attempts to improve these outcomes has led to incorporation of novel chemotherapeutic agents as well as biologic agents in combination with 5-FU. These agents include the chemotherapy drugs irinotecan, capecitabine, and oxaliplatin. The biologic targeted therapies include bevacizumab, a humanized vascular endothelial growth factor (VEGF) antibody, and cetuximab, a monoclonal antibody that binds to the epidermal growth factor receptor (EGFR).

Irinotecan (Camptosar) is a camptothecin that gets hydrolyzed to its active metabolite SN-38, and exerts its cytotoxic effects through interaction with topoisomerase-1 [10]. Its primary toxic effects include diarrhea, bone marrow suppression, nausea, vomiting, and alopecia. Randomized single-agent irinotecan studies in patients who were refractory to 5-FU showed a 2- to 3-month improvement in median overall survival (OS) as compared with best supportive care or infusional 5-FU [11,12]. Subsequently, irinotecan in combination with 5-FU/LV was evaluated in two randomized phase III trials as first-line treatment for metastatic colorectal cancer. The first study, led by Saltz, used a weekly bolus schedule of the combination (IFL), which resulted in a statistically significant improvement in response rate (39% versus 21%; $P < .001$), progression-free survival (7 months versus 4.3 months; $P = 0.004$) and OS (14.8 months versus 12.6 months; $P = 0.04$) [13]. The European infusional regimen, folinic acid, fluorouracil and irinotecan (FOLFIRI), using infusional 5-FU and bolus irinotecan every other week, also demonstrated a statistically significant improvement in response rate (35% versus 22%; $P < .005$), progression-free survival (6.7 months versus

4.4 months; $P < .001$), and OS (17.4 months versus 14.1 months; $P = .031$) [14]. The addition of irinotecan to 5-FU increases the likelihood of diarrhea and myelosuppression, and patients need to be selected carefully. Oral capecitabine may replace intravenous 5-FU safely with comparable response rates and OS [15], with potential ease of administration (as described below).

Capecitabine (Xeloda) is a prodrug that undergoes a three-step enzymatic conversion to fluorouracil, with the final step occurring at the level of the tumor. The side effect profile predominantly includes hand-foot syndrome but also bone marrow suppression and gastrointestinal toxicity. Two randomized clinical trials [16,17] that compared oral capecitabine with intravenous 5-FU/LV demonstrated that capecitabine was associated with significantly higher response rates and a better toxicity profile. The incidence of grade 3 or 4 diarrhea, stomatitis, nausea, and neutropenic sepsis was significantly less with capecitabine. Based on these results, oral capecitabine has been approved for first-line treatment of metastatic colorectal cancer. Combination regimens of oral capecitabine with irinotecan or oxaliplatin are more efficacious; single-agent capecitabine typically is reserved for patients with a poor performance status or patients whose disease does not warrant combination chemotherapy.

Oxaliplatin (Eloxatin) is a third-generation platinum derivative that forms bulky DNA adducts. The major toxicity of oxaliplatin is neuropathy, which can be in the form of an acute sensory toxicity that is precipitated by exposure to cold temperature and causes dysesthesias of the extremities and oropharynx, or a chronic cumulative peripheral sensory neuropathy that often is reversible after stopping therapy. Hypersensitivity reactions and cytopenias also can be associated with oxaliplatin therapy.

Single-agent oxaliplatin has only limited efficacy when administered in metastatic colorectal cancer; however, by down-regulating thymidylate synthase, it works synergistically with 5-FU [18]. Addition of oxaliplatin to infusional 5-FU/LV (FOLFOX) significantly increases response rates and time to disease progression in the first-line and in the second-line settings [19–22]. The first trial, by de Gramont and colleagues, compared infusional 5-FU/LV with the same regimen in combination with oxaliplatin. This trial showed a significantly higher objective response rate (22% versus 51%) and longer progression-free survival (6.2 months versus 9 months), but the median OS did not reach statistical significance. More recently, the North Central Cancer Treatment Group 9741 three-arm study compared FOLFOX, IFL, and a combination of irinotecan and oxaliplatin. This important trial demonstrated an improved median time to progression, response rate, and median survival with the FOLFOX regimen. FOLFOX also had a tolerable toxicity profile [23]. As a result of these studies, FOLFOX has been adopted as a standard first-line therapy by many oncologists in the United States.

Bevacizumab (Avastin) is a humanized monoclonal antibody against the VEGF that reduces the availability of the VEGF ligand and impairs receptor activation. The main toxicities include hypertension, proteinuria, thrombosis, and hemorrhage. In a pivotal phase II study that compared 5-FU/LV with or without bevacizumab, the combination improved response rate, time to progression, and OS [24]. Following this study—because IFL was emerging as a standard first-line treatment for metastatic colorectal cancer—a phase III randomized trial was conducted that compared IFL/bevacizumab, IFL/placebo, and 5-FU/LV/bevacizumab [25]. The third arm of the trial was stopped once safety with IFL/bevacizumab was established. In the final efficacy analysis, the IFL/bevacizumab arm showed a superior outcome compared with IFL/placebo in every trial end point, including response rate (45% versus 35%; $P < .003$), progression-free survival (10.6 months versus 6.2 months; $P < .00001$), and overall survival (20.3 months versus 15.6 months; $P < .00003$).

The two randomized phase II Three Regimens of Eloxatin Evaluation trials investigated the efficacy of three different regimens that contained oxaliplatin in the first-line setting. FOLFOX, bolus 5-FU/LV plus oxaliplatin, and capecitabine plus oxaliplatin were compared in the first cohort of patients; in the second cohort, the same regimens, with the addition of bevacizumab, were compared. Although oxaliplatin plus infusional, bolus, or oral fluoropyrimidine regimens were active, FOLFOX seemed to have a better response rate and better toxicity profile than did bolus therapy [26]. The addition of bevacizumab also improved response rates by 10% to 15% across all three arms.

More recently, the use of bevacizumab also was established in the second-line setting in a randomized phase III study, E3200 [27]. In this study, patients who had progressed on first-line irinotecan and 5-FU were randomized to FOLFOX, FOLFOX with bevacizumab, or bevacizumab alone. The bevacizumab monotherapy arm was closed early because of inferiority. There was superiority to the combined FOLFOX/bevacizumab arm with improved response rates (21.8% versus 9.2%; $P < .001$), progression-free survival (7.2 versus 4.8 months; $P < .0001$), and a statistically significant improvement in median OS (12.9 months versus 10.8 months; $P = 0.0018$). Reporting of the safety and efficacy of the combination of FOLFOX/bevacizumab in the second-line setting supported the already widely adopted use of this regimen in the first-line setting.

Finally, cetuximab (Erbitux), a chimeric monoclonal antibody that is directed against the EGFR, has demonstrated clinical activity in pretreated metastatic colorectal cancer. By binding to this receptor, it promotes apoptosis and prevents initiation of several intracellular events that are related to angiogenesis, proliferation, and invasion. Preclinical models have demonstrated single-agent activity of cetuximab, but its efficacy is enhanced significantly when used in combination with chemotherapy. Common side effects of this EGFR inhibitor include acnelike rash, diarrhea, and hypersensitivity infusion reactions.

A multicenter phase II trial that was conducted in patients who were treated previously with irinotecan showed that retreatment with irinotecan in combination with cetuximab offered a 22.5% major objective response rate [28]. Encouraged by these results, Cunningham and colleagues [29] randomly assigned 329 patients to irinotecan with cetuximab or cetuximab alone in a 2:1 schema. A nearly identical 22.9% response rate was observed in the irinotecan/cetuximab arm, with a time to progression of 4.1 months. This trial led to the approval of this drug in combination with irinotecan in the salvage setting after progression on irinotecan. Cetuximab also is approved for use as a single agent in patients who are intolerant of irinotecan.

No randomized first-line phase III trials of cetuximab have been reported, although phase II studies using cetuximab in combination with effective chemotherapy regimens, such as FOLFOX or FOLFIRI, have resulted in response rates of up to 81% [30,31]. Phase III studies are ongoing to confirm these results, but until those studies are completed, use of this drug in the first-line setting should be considered investigational.

Choice of first-line therapy in metastatic colorectal cancer

Compared with weekly bolus 5-FU/LV, combination regimens that incorporate the newer agents irinotecan or oxaliplatin have improved response rates, time to progression, and OS. Modification of the administration of 5-FU to an infusional schedule also may contribute to better outcomes with less toxicity. The choice between an oxaliplatin- and an irinotecan-based regimen is not clear-cut. FOLFOX, in comparison with IFL (a bolus regimen) in the N9741 trial, led to an improvement in response rate and progression-free survival; however, there were confounding imbalances in second-line therapies that were available to these patients. A fairer comparison between optimized oxaliplatin- and irinotecan-based combination regimens can be seen in the trial by Tournigand and colleagues [32], in which patients were randomized to FOLFOX or FOLFIRI for first-line therapy, and received the alternate regimen upon progression. There was no appreciable difference in outcome between these two arms. Thus, either of these regimens could be chosen as first-line chemotherapy based upon the anticipated side effects and patient comorbidity.

Compared with chemotherapy alone, the addition of bevacizumab has resulted in an improvement in response rates, progression-free survival, and OS in the first-line setting as well as in the second-line setting. Bevacizumab may be combined with any 5-FU–based regimen to enhance response rates and time to progression [33].

Based on the data outlined, the combination of an oxaliplatin-based regimen (FOLFOX) with bevacizumab can be considered the preferred first-line therapy for most patients who have metastatic colon cancer. An irinotecan-based regimen (FOLFIRI) is used in certain clinical situations: significant underlying sensory neuropathy, renal insufficiency, or hypersensitivity to oxaliplatin. Enrollment in clinical trials, such as Intergroup study C80405, which incorporates newer biologic agents or combinations of biologic agents, is encouraged strongly (Fig. 1).

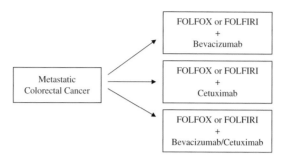

Fig. 1. CALGB 80405.

Second-line regimens in metastatic colorectal cancer

In a patient who has progressed on FOLFOX and bevacizumab, there are no data to support continuing bevacizumab with a second-line chemotherapy regimen. Switching to an irinotecan-based regimen, initially with cetuximab or followed by the combination, is recommended routinely. Although most patients without specific contraindications are receiving bevacizumab with their first-line therapies, a patient who has not received bevacizumab previously should be considered for this drug in combination with chemotherapy as a second-line regimen. The specific order in which the available agents are used does not seem to be as critical as ensuring that all of the active agents are used at some point in the patient's course [4]. In this way, prolonged survival with metastatic colon cancer can be achieved frequently. With continued advances and new drug development, metastatic colon cancer may be considered a chronic disease that is managed with a variety of active agents that are administered on an intermittent basis.

Adjuvant therapy for colon cancer

Staging and prognosis

The remarkable improvement in treatment outcomes in advanced colon cancer, with enhanced time to progression and survival, has led to trials with new agents and combinations in earlier stages of disease, where long-term survival and cure are the objectives. Although these newer regimens are associated with enhanced efficacy and a greater chance of cure, there also is a greater risk for acute and long-term toxicity. An accurate assessment of prognosis based on surgical stage is critical to determine the potential risks and benefits of any adjuvant regimen.

The most recent American Joint Committee on Cancer staging system reflects the most frequently used tool for predicting long-term survival [34]. A revised TNM classification, which divides the four stages of colorectal cancer into seven distinct subgroups based on refined definitions of T and N stage, allows a more precise estimation of prognosis. Specifically, patients who have stage II disease have been subdivided into IIa (T3N0) and IIb (T4N0), and patients who have stage III have been subdivided into stage IIIa (T1/2N1), IIIb (T3/4N1), and IIIc (TxN2) [35]. Using surveillance, epidemiology and end results data from 1991 to 2000, with approximately 120,000 patients who had colon cancer, 5-year colon cancer–specific survival by stage was determined (Table 1) [2]. Of particular interest is the finding that patients who have stage IIIa disease have a statistically significant improvement in survival compared with patients who have stage IIb disease, possibly because of the use of adjuvant therapy in patients who have stage III disease, but not in patients who have stage II disease, as recommended in the National Institutes of Health's 1990 Consensus Conference guidelines [36]. Surgical technique, without en bloc resection in patients who have stage II disease, inadequate or inaccurate staging, or real differences in biology also may explain these differences in survival.

Web-based prognostic and predictive tools are available that allow informed and shared decision making when considering adjuvant therapies for patients who have resected colon cancer. The Mayo Clinic site [37] uses patient age, T and N stage, and grade to estimate disease-free survival (DFS) and OS with surgery alone and with adjuvant therapy. Another useful tool incorporates patient age, comorbidity, T and N stage, grade, and the number of lymph nodes examined to determine prognosis with surgery alone or with the addition of a fluorouracil- or FOLFOX-based adjuvant regimen [38]. The example shown in Fig. 2 illustrates the data regarding prognosis and predictive value of treatment for a 72-year-old gentleman in good general health with a resected T3N1 moderately differentiated tumor with adequate lymph node sampling. These graphs can be printed and provided to patients during an office visit following surgical staging to facilitate discussions regarding prognosis and the absolute benefit expected with adjuvant therapy.

Table 1
Five-year colon cancer–specific survival by stage

AJCC stage	T stage	N stage	M stage	Survival
I	T1 or T2	N0	M0	93%
IIa	T3	N0	M0	85%
IIb	T4	N0	M0	72%
IIIa	T1 or T2	N1	M0	83%
IIIb	T3 or T4	N1	M0	64%
IIIc	Any T	N2	M0	44%
IV	Any T	Any N	M1	8%

Abbreviations: AJCC, American Joint Committee on Cancer. T1, tumor invades submucosa; T2, tumor invades muscularis propria; T3, tumor invades through the muscularis propria into the subserosa or nonperitonealized pericolic tissues; T4, tumor directly invades other organs/ structures or perforates visceral peritoneum; N0, no regional lymph node involvement; N1, one to three positive nodes; N2, four or more positive nodes; M0, no distant metastasis; M1, distant metastasis present.

Shared Decision Making

Name: _____ (Colon Cancer)

Age: 72   General Health: Good
Derived Tumor Stage: 3
Depth of Invasion: T3   Histologic Grade: 2
Nodes Examined: > 10   Nodes Involved: 1 - 3
Chemotherapy Regimen: FOLFOX4 Based

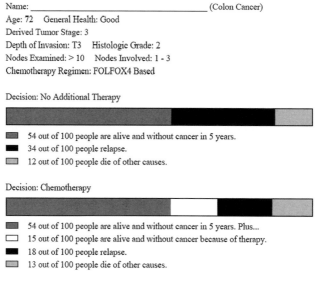

Decision: No Additional Therapy

■ 54 out of 100 people are alive and without cancer in 5 years.
■ 34 out of 100 people relapse.
□ 12 out of 100 people die of other causes.

Decision: Chemotherapy

■ 54 out of 100 people are alive and without cancer in 5 years. Plus...
□ 15 out of 100 people are alive and without cancer because of therapy.
■ 18 out of 100 people relapse.
□ 13 out of 100 people die of other causes.

Fig. 2. Example of adjuvant treatment analysis.

Historical perspective

Benefit with adjuvant therapy for stage III colon cancer was reported initially in the 1980s based on trials using a combination of 5-FU and the purported immunostimulatory agent levamisole [39,40]. Randomization in Intergroup trial 0035 was to observation, levamisole, or 1 year of 5-FU and levamisole. The combined regimen reduced the risk for cancer recurrence by 40% ($P < .0001$) and the overall death rate by 33% ($P < .0007$), and this regimen became the standard of care for adjuvant treatment of stage III colon cancer from 1989 until 1996. In 1996, the results of Intergroup trial 0089 were released in abstract, which again changed the standard of care for adjuvant treatment [41]. In 3700 patients who had stage II or III disease, 5-FU and levamisole was compared with a 6-month regimen of 5-FU with low-dose (Mayo Clinic) or high-dose (Roswell Park) LV. There was a fourth arm that used all three drugs (5 FU, LV, and levamisole). The regimens that contained LV (5-year OS 66%) proved to be as effective as the levamisole regimen (5-year OS 63%) and could be administered over 6 months instead of 12 months; there was no advantage to a three-drug regimen. A new standard of care for stage III adjuvant therapy was established, and the choice of 5-FU with low-dose or high-dose LV was based primarily on anticipated toxicities (myelosuppression and mucositis versus diarrhea). These regimens remained the standard of care for nearly a decade, and they continue to remain a therapeutic choice for many patients in the adjuvant setting.

New combination regimens

Since 2003, the results of five phase III trials that compared 5-FU/LCV with or without a new cytotoxic agent have been released. Two of these trials included oxaliplatin and three used irinotecan (Table 2).

Oxaliplatin plus fluorouracil/leucovorin

The Multicenter International Study of Oxaliplatin/5-Fluorouracil/Leucovorin in the Adjuvant Treatment of Colon Cancer (MOSAIC) trial randomized 2246 patients who had stage II (40%) or stage III (60%) resected colon cancer to a de Gramont regimen of bolus 5-FU/LCV followed by continuous infusion of 5-FU for two consecutive days every 2 weeks, without (LV5FU2) or with oxaliplatin (FOLFOX) over a period of 6 months (12 cycles). DFS at 3 years, a primary end point, was reported first at the 2003 American Society of Clinical Oncology (ASCO) meeting [42] and was published in 2004 [43]. Three-year DFS was improved significantly in the FOLFOX arm compared with the control arm (78.2% versus 72.9%; $P = .002$). Updated results of this trial at the 2005 ASCO meeting showed that the differences in DFS were maintained with a median follow-up of approximately 4.5 years (76.4% versus 69.8%; $P = .0008$) [44]. For patients who had stage III disease, 4-year DFS was 69.7% versus 61%—favoring FOLFOX, and for patients who had stage II disease, 4-year DFS was 85.1% versus 81.3%, again favoring FOLFOX.

Thus far, the differences in OS in the MOSAIC trial do not meet statistical significance (4-year OS 84.9% versus 82.8%). Three-year DFS was demonstrated previously to be an appropriate end point for assessment of adjuvant therapy trials in colon cancer, with a significant correlation with 5-year OS (correlation coefficient 0.94) [45]. This led to US Food and Drug Administration (FDA) approval of the FOLFOX regimen for adjuvant therapy in colon cancer, despite the lack of an OS benefit thus far. The FDA approved this regimen only for patients who have stage III disease, despite the inclusion of significant numbers of patients who had stage II disease in the MOSAIC trial. Toxicity with the FOLFOX regimen included a higher rate of neutropenia and neuropathy, with 12% of patients suffering grade 3 neuropathy. Significant peripheral sensory neuropathy, however, resolved in almost all of the patients; 3% had persistent grade 2 neuropathy and less than 1% had persistent grade 3 neuropathy at 18 months of follow-up.

A second randomized adjuvant study that compared an oxaliplatin/5-FU/LV regimen with 5-FU/LV was reported in abstract form by the National Surgical Adjuvant Breast and Bowel Project (NSABP) at the 2005 ASCO meeting [46]. Twenty-four hundred patients who had stage II (29%) or III (71%) resected colon cancer were randomized to standard Roswell Park bolus 5-FU/LV or the same regimen with the addition of oxaliplatin on weeks 1, 3, and 5 of the 8-week cycle (FLOX regimen). The

Table 2
Selected adjuvant chemotherapy trials

Trial (patients-stage)	Arms	3-y DFS	3-y OS	4-y DFS	4-y OS	5-y DFS	5-y OS
INT-0035 (929-III)	Observation					43%	47%
	Lev					44%	49%
	5-FU/Lev (1-y)					61%	60%
						P = .0001	P = .0007
INT-0089 (3759-II/III)	5-FU/Lev (1-y)					56%	63%
	5-FU/LV (high)					60%	66%
	5-FU/LV (low)					60%	66%
	5-FU/LV/Lev					60%	67%
MOSAIC (2246-II/III)	LV5FU2	72.9%	86.6%	69.8%	82.8%		
	FOLFOX	78.2%	88.2%	76.4%	84.9%		
		P = .002	NS	P < .001	NS		
St II only	LV5FU2	84.3%		81.3%			
	FOLFOX	87.0%		85.1%			
St III only	LV5FU2	65.3%		61.0%			
	FOLFOX	72.2%		69.7%			
NSABP C-07 (2407-II/III)	5-FU/LV	71.6%					
	FLOX	76.5%					
		P = .004					
X-ACT (1987-III)	5-FU/LCV	60.6%	77.6%				
	Capecitabine	64.2%	81.3%				
		P = .053	P = .071				
CALGB 89803 (1264-III)	5-FU/LV	NS					
	IFL						
PETACC-3 (2333-III)	LV5FU2	60.3%					
	FOLFIRI	63.3%					
		P = .09					
FNCLCC (400-III)	LV5FU2	60%					
	FOLFIRI	51%					
		NS					

Abbreviations: C, CCALGB, cancer and leukemia group B; FLOX, bolus 5-FU+LV+Oxaliplatin; FNCLCC, Fédération Nationale des Centres de Lutte Contre le Cancer; FOLFIRI, bolus/infusional 5-FU+LV+Irinotecan; FOLFOX, bolus/infusional 5-FU+LV+Oxaliplatin; INT, Intergroup; Lev, levamisole; LV5FU2, infusional 5-FU+LV; MO-SAIC, Multicenter International Study of Oxaliplatin/5-Fluorouracil/Leucovorin in the Adjuvant Treatment of Colon Cancer; NS, not significant; NSABP, National Surgical Adjuvant Breast and Bowel Project; PETACC-3, Pan European Trial of Adjuvant Colon Cancer; St, Stage; X-ACT, Xeloda in Adjuvant Colon Cancer Therapy.

results of C-07 were similar to those seen in the MOSAIC trial, which confirmed the benefit of a combination regimen. Three-year DFS was increased from 71.6% to 76.5% with FLOX, which corresponded to a 21% relative risk reduction in recurrence or death; this was comparable to the 23% risk reduction that was seen in the MOSAIC trial with FOLFOX.

Complete toxicity data have not been presented from C-07, although there seems to be a higher rate of diarrhea but a lower rate of neutropenia and neuropathy with the FLOX regimen compared with FOLFOX. Aside from differences in toxicity, the convenience of bolus therapy instead of infusional treatment by way of a portable pump makes FLOX an attractive option. A switch from an infusional FOLFOX regimen to bolus FLOX as adjuvant treatment for colon cancer remains premature until the complete data set has been presented.

Irinotecan plus fluorouracil/leucovorin

In contrast to the positive results that were seen with the addition of oxaliplatin to 5-FU/LV, phase III trials of irinotecan-based combination regimens have failed to demonstrate a significant advantage over standard therapy. CALGB 89803 used IFL [47], a regimen that had been demonstrated to provide incremental benefit in the metastatic setting. Unexpectedly, IFL proved to be no more effective than bolus 5-FU/LV, and it was associated with increased toxicity, specifically a significantly greater risk for neutropenia and death during treatment.

Two other studies were presented recently that compared infusional 5-FU/LV (LV5FU2) without or with irinotecan (FOLFIRI). The Pan European Trial of Adjuvant Colon Cancer enrolled more than 3000 patients who had stage II or III colon cancer [48]. The primary study end point of 3-year DFS for patients who had stage III disease was not met (63.3% versus 60.3%, $P = .091$); however, a post hoc analysis that adjusted for imbalances in the T and N staging revealed a trend toward improvement with irinotecan. Some investigators have interpreted the results of this trial as justification to use an irinotecan-based regimen with infusional 5-FU/LV in situations in which there is a compelling clinical reason to avoid an oxaliplatin-based regimen (hypersensitivity or preexisting neuropathy). Finally, no benefit from adding irinotecan to infusional 5-FU could be demonstrated in the Fédération Nationale des Centres de Lutte Contre le Cancer (FNCLCC) trial, which had a similar design [49]. This smaller trial enrolled 400 high-risk patients who had stage III disease (N2 or N1 with perforation/obstruction). Three-year DFS was 60% versus 51%, and favored the arm that did not contain irinotecan, although there were some imbalances in prognostic factors.

Capecitabine

Recently, the results of the Xeloda in Adjuvant Colon Cancer Therapy trial, which was conducted in Europe and Canada, were published [50]. Approximately 2000 patients who had stage III disease were randomized to receive Mayo Clinic intravenous 5-FU/LV or oral capecitabine for 6 months of adjuvant treatment. The trial was designed to demonstrate equivalence between the two regimens. Three-year DFS favored the capecitabine arm (64.2% versus 60.6%; $P = .05$) as did 3-year OS (81.3% versus 77.6%; $P = .07$). The investigators concluded that capecitabine is at least equivalent to 5-FU/LV as an adjuvant regimen for patients who have stage III disease, and the side effect profile favored the oral capecitabine arm, with less diarrhea, stomatitis, neutropenia, nausea, and alopecia. As expected, there was more hand-foot syndrome with capecitabine, which resulted in dose reductions in a significant number of patients.

Recommendations for stage III adjuvant therapy

First-generation 5-FU regimens with LV modulation have resulted in a 35% to 40% proportional risk reduction in colon cancer–specific mortality for patients who have stage III disease. With the addition of oxaliplatin, there is an additional 20% reduction in the risk of relapse beyond that seen with first-generation regimens. This results is an almost 50% reduction in recurrence with a second-generation regimen compared with no adjuvant treatment in stage III disease.

Based on the significant improvement in DFS that was seen with two different oxaliplatin/5-FU/LCV regimens (MOSAIC and C-07 trials), a FOL-FOX infusional regimen is the best option for adjuvant treatment in most patients who have stage III colon cancer. If port placement or ambulatory pump therapy is not feasible or is refused by the patient, a FLOX regimen of oxaliplatin and bolus 5-FU is a reasonable alternative, although the incidence of diarrhea may be increased. For patients who have a contraindication to the use of oxaliplatin (hypersensitivity, preexisting peripheral neuropathy, renal insufficiency), 5-FU/LCV alone as a bolus regimen (Roswell Park, Mayo Clinic), or an infusional regimen (de Gramont) is appropriate. If oxaliplatin is not going to be part of the regimen, then capecitabine is a good option for patients who prefer oral therapy, and there seems to be a favorable toxicity profile when compared with intravenous therapy.

Adjuvant therapy for patients who have stage II disease

Adjuvant treatment for patients who have stage II disease remains a controversial area. Studies that used first-generation chemotherapy regimens (5-FU/LV) failed to demonstrate a survival advantage for these patients. The 1999 International Multicenter Pooled Analysis of Colon Cancer Trials analysis of more than 1000 patients in five different trials showed a nonsignificant difference in 5-year OS (82% versus 80%) [51]. This led the investigators to conclude that chemotherapy is not standard treatment for patients who have B2 (IIA) colon cancer.

In the same issue of the *Journal of Clinical Oncology*, the NSABP presented a controversial analysis of combined data from four trials (C-01, 02, 03, and

04), and pooled and compared outcomes for patients on the "superior" arm with those on the "inferior" arm of each trial [52]. When data from all four trials were examined in a combined analysis, the mortality reduction was 30% for patients who had Dukes' B colon cancer and 18% for patients who had Dukes' C colon cancer. The investigators concluded, "patients with Dukes' B colon cancer benefit from adjuvant chemotherapy and should be presented with this treatment option," regardless of clinical prognostic factors.

The Quick and Simple and Reliable (QUASAR) trial randomized more than 3200 patients with "uncertain indications" for adjuvant treatment (92% had stage II disease) to chemotherapy or observation. With a median follow-up of 4.5 years, there was a statistically significant improvement in freedom from recurrence (77.8% versus 73.8%; $P = .001$) and in 5-year survival (80.3% versus 77.4%; $P = .02$) [53].

In the MOSAIC study, a subgroup analysis of patients who had stage II disease did not demonstrate a significant DFS advantage; however, the study was not powered to detect such differences. In 2004, ASCO published guidelines recommending against routine treatment with adjuvant therapy for average risk patients who have stage II disease. It was suggested, however, that chemotherapy be considered for patients who have high-risk features (T4 disease, perforation, high-grade tumors, or fewer than 12 lymph nodes examined) [54].

Regarding adjuvant therapy for patients who have stage II disease, the National Comprehensive Cancer Network, an alliance of 19 of the leading cancer centers in the United States, offers some guiding principles [55]. Several elements need to be considered when determining whether adjuvant therapy should be administered: number of lymph nodes examined, poor prognostic features (high-grade tumor, lymphatic or vascular invasion, bowel obstruction), and assessment of comorbidities. For patients who have low-risk T3N0 disease, observation or a clinical trial is recommended. Adjuvant therapy is an option, however, for high-risk patients who have T3 or T4 disease using 5-FU/LV or a FOLFOX regimen. Patients should be informed of the potential risks and benefits of therapy, and it should be recognized that the absolute survival benefit does not exceed 2% to 5%. Although the improvement seems to be small, this is similar to the magnitude of benefit that is seen with the use of adjuvant chemotherapy in patients who have node-negative breast cancer—an accepted practice in academic and community oncology.

A randomized phase III trial in stage II colon cancer is being conducted by the Intergroup, led by the Eastern Cooperative Oncology Group. In E5202, risk stratification is performed prospectively by tumor analysis for microsatellite instability status (MSI) and loss of heterozygosity (LOH) at chromosome 18q. Patients who have high-risk tumors, defined as having microsatellite stability [56] and 18q LOH [57], are randomized to FOLFOX with or without bevacizumab. The low-risk patients will be assigned to an observation arm and followed (Fig. 3).

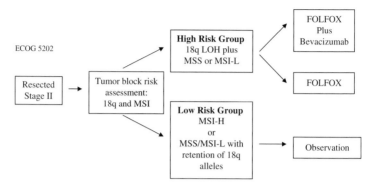

Fig. 3. Adjuvant study for stage II colon cancer. MSI-H, microsatellite instability high; MSI-L, microsatellite instability low; MSS, microsatellite stability.

Adjuvant and neoadjuvant therapy for resectable metastatic disease

Given the potential to eradicate microscopic metastatic disease in some patients who have stage II and III disease with adjuvant therapy, there has been significant interest in extrapolating the use of adjuvant therapies to patients who have resected stage IV disease. Surgical resection of hepatic metastases has resulted in long-term relapse-free survival of approximately 35%. More recently, a retrospective review from Johns Hopkins showed that in 226 consecutive patients who underwent potentially curative liver resection, 5-year OS was 31% for 93 patients who were operated on between 1984 and 1992 compared with 58% for 133 patients who were operated on between 1993 and 1999 [58]. Of the multiple factors that were analyzed to explain these differences in survival rates between the two time periods, only resection type, use of intraoperative ultrasonography, and administration of perioperative chemotherapy differed between the early and late cohorts.

Small series have reported upon use of 5-FU/LV after resection of metastases, without demonstrating a significant survival benefit [59]. National Comprehensive Cancer Network guidelines recommend 6 months of adjuvant therapy after resection of metastatic disease [60]. Because hepatic artery infusion plus systemic chemotherapy was superior to systemic chemotherapy alone after hepatic resection in a single institution trial [61], hepatic artery infusion with or without systemic 5-FU-based therapy also is an option; however, there is no consensus on this recommendation. The NSABP is conducting a trial (C-09) to examine the usefulness of regional chemotherapy when added to a systemic regimen of capecitabine and oxaliplatin following resection or radiofrequency catheter ablation of hepatic metastases.

As a result of the significant activity of multiagent regimens in the metastatic setting, neoadjuvant therapy has been an increasingly attractive approach, not only for patients who have initially unresectable disease, but also as a means to improve survival in those who have resectable metastases. Although randomized trials that compare preoperative treatment with postoperative treatment are lacking, patients frequently tolerate chemotherapy better before surgery, and earlier treatment of micrometastatic disease provides a theoretic advantage toward eradication of residual disease. Systemic therapy before surgery also permits an assessment of efficacy, which may guide the choice of additional postoperative chemotherapy. Although the best type of neoadjuvant chemotherapy is undefined, a retrospective review of patients who underwent resection of metastases after treatment in Intergroup N9741 revealed that 22 of the 24 patients (92%) had been treated with an oxaliplatin-based regimen [62]. Bevacizumab, a monoclonal antibody that inhibits VEGF, increases response rates and survival when added to chemotherapy in the metastatic setting. The use of this angiogenesis inhibitor along with chemotherapy in the preoperative setting may present some unusual hepatotoxicities for the hepatic surgeon.

Vascular alterations with "blue liver syndrome," which is characterized by discoloration from veno-occlusive disease, edema, and a spongiform consistency similar to that seen in early cirrhosis, have been described in association with the preoperative use of an oxaliplatin-based regimen [63]. Steatohepatitis also has been reported with the use of oxaliplatin- or irinotecan-based regimens [64], which may contribute to postoperative complications, including hepatic insufficiency. Individualized care with consideration of potential hepatotoxicities suggests that initial surgery should be considered for those with a good prognosis pattern of resectable disease. Preoperative therapy is recommended for patients who have borderline resectable or unresectable disease, and the duration of preoperative therapy should be limited to the time that is required to render the disease resectable. When bevacizumab is used along with chemotherapy, elective surgery should be delayed until at least 6 weeks after the last dosage because of concerns regarding delayed wound healing and impaired hepatic regeneration.

Current trials

Based on the results that were observed in the metastatic setting, future directions in adjuvant therapy focus on the integration of new biologic agents (cetuximab and bevacizumab). The Intergroup N0147 study will enroll patients who have stage III colon cancer with randomization to FOLFOX or FOLFOX plus cetuximab. NSABP C-08 is comparing FOLFOX with FOLFOX plus bevacizumab in patients who have stage II or III colon cancer (Fig. 4).

Assessment of molecular markers and gene expression is another active area of research to facilitate selection of patients for adjuvant therapies. Genetic polymorphisms in dihydropyrimidine dehydrogenase and the UGT1A1 gene predict increased toxicity with 5-FU and irinotecan, respectively, because of diminished clearance of the chemotherapeutic agent or its

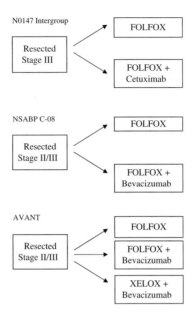

Fig. 4. Current adjuvant trials in colon cancer. AVANT, Avastin adjuvant study.

active metabolite (SN38). In addition to 18q LOH and MSI being used to assess prognosis in stage II disease, MSI also may be a predictor of benefit with adjuvant therapy [65]. Ultimately, as is being done in breast cancer, gene microarray technology will be used to determine prognosis and to predict response to individual chemotherapy agents.

Surveillance for patients who have stage II/III colon cancer

Based on recent meta-analyses of randomized trials that compared "low intensity" and "high intensity" follow-up strategies, which reported a 20% to 33% reduction in all-cause mortality with intensive follow-up, ASCO recently updated its guidelines for surveillance [66]. Surveillance strategies, including periodic history and physical examination, carcino embryonic antigen and endoscopy, had only minor changes. Recommendations for imaging procedures, however, represent a major modification in the current guidelines. For patients who are believed to be at "higher risk of recurrence, and who would be candidates for curative-intent surgery," annual CT imaging of the chest and abdomen for 3 years after primary therapy is now recommended. Chest radiographs, complete blood cell counts, and liver function tests are not recommended.

Summary

There has been a dramatic improvement in outcomes for patients who have colon cancer over recent years. These improvements have come about largely because of the availability of new chemotherapy agents (irinotecan, oxaliplatin and capecitabine) and new biologic agents (bevacizumab and cetuximab). Large, well-designed clinical trials have resulted in the routine use of all of these agents in the treatment of patients who have metastatic disease, and this has led to improved survival for these patients. In earlier stage disease, oxaliplatin/5-FU–based chemotherapy has become a new standard of adjuvant therapy for many patients. Clinical research efforts are investigating the use of biologic agents along with chemotherapy for adjuvant treatment; it is hoped that this will translate into a greater cure rate for these patients.

References

[1] Jemal A, Murray T, Ward E, et al. Cancer statistics, 2005. CA Cancer J Clin 2005;55(1): 10–30.

[2] O'Connell JB, Maggard MA, Ko CY. Colon cancer survival rates with the new American Joint Committee on Cancer sixth edition staging. J Natl Cancer Inst 2004;96(19): 1420–5.

[3] Thirion P, Michiels S, Pignon JP, et al. Modulation of fluorouracil by leucovorin in patients with advanced colorectal cancer: an updated meta-analysis. J Clin Oncol 2004;22(18): 3766–75.

[4] Grothey A, Sargent D, Goldberg R, et al. Survival of patients with advanced colorectal cancer improves with the availability of fluorouracil-leucovorin, irinotecan, and oxaliplatin in the course of treatment. J Clin Oncol 2004;22(7):1209–14.

[5] Sobrero A, Guglielmi A, Grossi F, et al. Mechanism of action of fluoropyrimidines: relevance to the new developments in colorectal cancer chemotherapy. Semin Oncol 2000;27 (5)(Suppl 10):72–7.

[6] Buroker TR, O'Connell MJ, Wieand HS, et al. Randomized comparison of two schedules of fluorouracil and leucovorin in the treatment of advanced colorectal cancer. J Clin Oncol 1994;12(1):14–20.

[7] Wang WS, Lin JK, Chiou TJ, et al. Randomized trial comparing weekly bolus 5-fluorouracil plus leucovorin versus monthly 5-day 5-fluorouracil plus leucovorin in metastatic colorectal cancer. Hepatogastroenterology 2000;47(36):1599–603.

[8] de Gramont A, Bosset JF, Milan C, et al. Randomized trial comparing monthly low-dose leucovorin and fluorouracil bolus with bimonthly high-dose leucovorin and fluorouracil bolus plus continuous infusion for advanced colorectal cancer: a French intergroup study. J Clin Oncol 1997;15(2):808–15.

[9] Jager E, Heike M, Bernhard H, et al. Weekly high-dose leucovorin versus low-dose leucovorin combined with fluorouracil in advanced colorectal cancer: results of a randomized multicenter trial. Study Group for Palliative Treatment of Metastatic Colorectal Cancer Study Protocol 1. J Clin Oncol 1996;14(8):2274–9.

[10] Iyer L, Ratain MJ. Clinical pharmacology of camptothecins. Cancer Chemother Pharmacol 1998;42(Suppl):S31–43.

[11] Cunningham D, Pyrhonen S, James RD, et al. Randomised trial of irinotecan plus supportive care versus supportive care alone after fluorouracil failure for patients with metastatic colorectal cancer. Lancet 1998;352(9138):1413–8.

[12] Rougier P, Van Custem E, Bajetta E, et al. Randomised trial of irinotecan versus fluorouracil by continuous infusion after fluorouracil failure in patients with metastatic colorectal cancer. Lancet 1998;352(9138):1407–12.

[13] Saltz LB, Cox JV, Blanke C, et al. Irinotecan plus fluorouracil and leucovorin for metastatic colorectal cancer. Irinotecan Study Group. N Engl J Med 2000;343(13):905–14.

[14] Douillard JY, Cunningham D, Roth AD, et al. Irinotecan combined with fluorouracil compared with fluorouracil alone as first line treatment for metastatic colorectal cancer: a multicentre randomised trial. Lancet 2000;355(9209):1041–7.

[15] Patt YZ, Liebmann J, Diamandidis D, et al. Capecitabine (X) plus irinotecan (XELIRI) as first-line treatment for metastatic colorectal cancer (MCRC): final safety findings from a phase II trial. Presented at the 2004 American Society of Clinical Oncology Annual Meeting. New Orleans, June 5–8, 2004.

[16] Van Custem E, Twelves C, Cassidy J, et al. Oral capecitabine compared with intravenous fluorouracil plus leucovorin in patients with metastatic colorectal cancer: results of a large phase III study. J Clin Oncol 2001;19(21):4097–106.

[17] Hoff PM, Ansari R, Batist G, et al. Comparison of oral capecitabine versus intravenous fluorouracil plus leucovorin as first line treatment in 605 patients with metastatic colorectal cancer: results of a randomized phase III study. J Clin Oncol 2001;19(8):2282–92.

[18] Raymond E, Faivre S, Chaney S, et al. Cellular and molecular pharmacology of oxaliplatin. Mol Cancer Ther 2002;1(3):227–35.

[19] de Gramont A, Figer A, Seymour M, et al. Leucovorin and fluorouracil with or without oxaliplatin as first-line treatment in advanced colorectal cancer. J Clin Oncol 2000;18(16): 2938–47.

[20] Giacchetti S, Perpoint B, Zindani R, et al. Phase III multicenter randomized trial of oxaliplatin added to chronomodulted fluorouracil-leucovorin as first-line treatment of metastatic colorectal cancer. J Clin Oncol 2000;18(1):136–47.

[21] Grothey A, Deschler B, Kroening H, et al. Phase III study of bolus 5-Fluorouracil (5-FU)/ folinic acid (FA) (Mayo) vs weekly high-dose 24h 5-FU infusion/FA + oxaliplatin (OXA) (FUFOX) in advanced colorectal cancer (ACRC). Presented at the 2002 American Society of Clinical Oncology Annual Meeting. Orlando, May 18–21, 2002.

[22] Rothenberg ML, Oza AM, Bigelow RH, et al. Superiority of oxaliplatin and fluorouracil-leucovorin compared with either therapy alone in patients with progressive colorectal cancer after irinotecan and fluorouracil-leucovorin: interim results of a phase III trial. J Clin Oncol 2003;21(11):2059–69.

[23] Goldberg RA, Sargent DJ, Morton RF, et al. A randomized controlled trial of fluorouracil plus leucovorin, irinotecan, and oxaliplatin combinations in patients with previously untreated metastatic colorectal cancer. J Clin Oncol 2004;22(1):23–30.

[24] Kabbinavar F, Hurwitz HI, Fehrenbacher L, et al. Phase II, randomized trial comparing bevacizumab plus fluorouracil (FU)/leucovorin (LV) with FU/LV alone in patients with metastatic colorectal cancer. J Clin Oncol 2003;21(1):60–5.

[25] Hurwitz H, Fehrenbacher L, Novotny W, et al. Bevacizumab plus irinotecan, fluorouracil and leucovorin for metastatic colorectal cancer. N Engl J Med 2004;350(23):2335–42.

[26] Hochster HS, Welles L, Hart L, et al. Safety and efficacy of bevacizumab (Bev) when added to oxaliplatin/fluoropyrimidine (O/F) regimens as first-line treatment of metastatic colorectal cancer (mCRC): TREE 1 and 2 studies. Presented at the 2005 American Society of Clinical Oncology Annual Meeting. Orlando, May 13–17, 2005.

[27] Giantonio BJ, Catalano PJ, Meropol NJ, et al. High dose bevacizumab improves survival when combined with FOLFOX4 in previously treated advanced colorectal cancer: results from the Eastern Cooperative Oncology Group (ECOG) study E 3200. Presented at the 2005 American Society of Clinical Oncology Annual Meeting. Orlando, May 13–17, 2005.

[28] Saltz L, Rubin M, Hochster H, et al. Cetuximab (IMC-C225) plus irinotecan (CPT-11) is active in CPT-11 refractory colorectal cancer (CRC) that expresses epidermal growth factor receptor (EGFR). Presented at the 2001 American Society of Clinical Oncology Annual Meeting. San Francisco, May 12–15, 2001.

[29] Cunningham D, Humblet Y, Siena S, et al. Cetuximab monotherapy and cetuximab plus irinotecan in irinotecan-refractory metastatic colorectal cancer. N Engl J Med 2004;351(4): 337–45.

[30] Diaz Rubio E, Tabernero J, van Cutsem E, et al. Cetuximab in combination with oxaliplatin/ 5-fluorouracil (5-FU)/folinic acid (FA) (FOLFOX-4) in the first-line treatment of patients with epidermal growth factor receptor (EGFR)-expressing metastatic colorectal cancer: an international study Presented at the 2005 American Society of Clinical Oncology Annual Meeting. Orlando, May 13–17, 2005.

[31] Seufferlein T, Dittrich C, Riemann J, et al. A phase I/II study of cetuximab in combination with 5-fluorouracil (5-FU)/folinic acid (FA) plus weekly oxaliplatin (L-OHP) (FUFOX) in the first-line treatment of patients with metastatic colorectal cancer (mCRC) expressing epidermal growth factor receptor (EGFR). Preliminary results. Presented at the 2005 American Society of Clinical Oncology Annual Meeting. Orlando, May 13–17, 2005.

[32] Tournigand C, Andre T, Achille E, et al. FOLFIRI followed by FOLFOX6 or the reverse sequence in advanced colorectal cancer: a randomized GERCOR study. J Clin Oncol 2004;22(2):229–37.

[33] Kabbinavar FF, Hambleton J, Mass RD, et al. Combined analysis of efficacy: the addition of bevacizumab to fluorouracil/leucovorin improves survival for patients with metastatic colorectal cancer. J Clin Oncol 2005;23(16):3706–12.

[34] Greene FL, Balch CM, Fleming ID, et al, editors. AJCC cancer staging handbook. 6th edition. New York: Springer-Verlag; 2002.

[35] Greene FL, Stewart AK, Norton HJ. A new TNM staging strategy for node-positive (stage III) colon cancer: an analysis of 50,042 patients. Ann Surg 2002;236(4):416–21.

[36] NIH Consensus Conference. Adjuvant therapy for patients with colon and rectal cancer. JAMA 1990;264(11):1444–50.

[37] Health tools: adjuvant systemic therapy for resected colon cancer. Available at: http:// www.mayoclinic.com/calcs. Accessed February 1, 2006.

[38] Adjuvant! for colon cancer. Available at: http://www.adjuvantonline.com. Accessed February 1, 2006.

[39] Laurie JA, Moertel CG, Fleming TR, et al. Surgical adjuvant therapy of large-bowel carcinoma: an evaluation of levamisole and the combination of levamisole and fluorouracil. The North Central Cancer Treatment Group and the Mayo Clinic. J Clin Oncol 1989;7(10): 1447–56.

[40] Moertel CG, Fleming TR, Macdonald JS, et al. Levamisole and fluorouracil for adjuvant therapy of resected colon carcinoma. N Engl J Med 1990;322(6):352–8.

[41] Haller DG, Catalano PJ, Macdonald JS, Mayer RJ. Fluorouracil (FU), leucovorin (LV) and levamisole (LEV) adjuvant therapy for colon cancer: four-year results of INT-0089. Presented at the 1997 American Society of Clinical Oncology Annual Meeting. Denver, May 17–20, 1997.

[42] de Gramont A, Banzi M, Navarro M, et al. Oxaliplatin/5-FU/LV in adjuvant colon cancer: results of the international randomized MOSAIC trial. Presented at the 2003 American Society of Clinical Oncology Annual Meeting. Chicago, May 31–June 3, 2003.

[43] Andre T, Boni C, Mounedji-Boudiaf L, et al. Oxaliplatin, fluorouracil, and leucovorin as adjuvant treatment for colon cancer. N Engl J Med 2004;350(23):2343–51.

[44] de Gramont A, Boni C, Navarro M, et al. Oxaliplatin/5FU/LV in the adjuvant treatment of stage II and stage III colon cancer: efficacy results with a median follow-up of 4 years. Presented at the 2005 American Society of Clinical Oncology Annual Meeting. Orlando, May 13–17, 2005.

[45] Sargent DJ, Wieand S, Benedetti J, et al. Disease-free survival (DFS) vs. overall survival as a primary endpoint for adjuvant colon cancer studies: individual patient data from 12,915 patients on 15 randomized trials. Presented at the 2004 American Society of Clinical Oncology Annual Meeting. New Orleans, June 5–8, 2004.

[46] Wolmark N, Wieand HS, Kuebler JP, et al. A phase III trial comparing FULV to FULV + oxaliplatin in stage II or III carcinoma of the colon: results of NSABP protocol C-07. Presented at the 2005 American Society of Clinical Oncology Annual Meeting. Orlando, May 13–17, 2005.

[47] Saltz LB, Niedzwiecki D, Hollis D, et al. Irinotecan plus fluorouracil/leucovorin (IFL) versus fluorouracil/leucovorin alone (FL) in stage III colon cancer (intergroup trail CALGB C89803). Presented at the 2003 American Society of Clinical Oncology Annual Meeting. Chicago, May 31–June 3, 2003.

[48] Van Cutsem E, Labianca R, Hossfeld D, et al. Randomized phase III trial comparing infused irinotecan/5-fluorouracil (5-FU)/folinic acid (IF) versus 5-FU/FA (F) in stage III colon cancer patients (pts). (PETACC 3). Presented at the 2005 American Society of Clinical Oncology Annual Meeting. Orlando, May 13–17, 2005.

[49] Ychou M, Raoul J, Douillard J, et al. A phase III randomized trial of LV5FU2 + CPT-11 vs. LV5FU2 alone in adjuvant high risk colon cancer (FNCLCC Accord02/FFCD9802). Presented at the 2005 American Society of Clinical Oncology Annual Meeting. Orlando, May 13–17, 2005.

[50] Twelves C, Wong A, Nowacki MP, et al. Capecitabine as adjuvant treatment for stage III colon cancer. N Engl J Med 2005;352(26):2696–704.

[51] International Multicentre Pooled Analysis of B2 Colon Cancer Trials (IMPACT B2) Investigators. Efficacy of adjuvant fluorouracil and folinic acid in B2 colon cancer. J Clin Oncol 1999;17(5):1356–63.

[52] Mamounas E, Wieand S, Wolmark N, et al. Comparative efficacy of adjuvant chemotherapy in patients with Dukes' B versus Dukes' C colon cancer: results from four National Surgical Adjuvant Breast and Bowel Project adjuvant studies (C-01, C-02, C-03, and C-04). J Clin Oncol 1999;17(5):1349–55.

[53] Gray RG, Barnwell J, Hills R, et al, for the QUASAR Collaborative Group. QUASAR: a randomized study of adjuvant chemotherapy (CT) vs. observation including 3238 colorectal cancer patients. Presented at the 2004 American Society of Clinical Oncology Annual Meeting. New Orleans, June 5–8, 2004.

[54] Benson AB III, Schrag D, Somerfield MR, et al. American Society of Clinical Oncology recommendations on adjuvant chemotherapy for stage II colon cancer. J Clin Oncol 2004; 22(16):3408–19.

[55] Engstrom P. Update: NCCN colon cancer clinical practice guidelines. J Natl Compr Canc Netw 2005;3(Suppl 1):S25–8.

[56] Gryfe R, Kim H, Hsieh ET, et al. Tumor microsatellite instability and clinical outcome in young patients with colorectal cancer. N Engl J Med 2000;342(2):69–77.

[57] Shibata D, Reale MA, Lavin P, et al. The DCC protein and prognosis in colorectal cancer. N Engl J Med 1996;335(23):1727–32.

[58] Choti MA, Sitzmann JV, Tiburi MF, et al. Trends in long-term survival following liver resection for hepatic colorectal metastases. Ann Surg 2002;235(6):759–66.

[59] Langer B, Bleiberg H, Labianca R, et al. Fluorouracil (FU) plus l–leucovorin (l-LV) versus observation after potentially curative resection of liver or lung metastases from colorectal cancer: results of the ENG (EORTC/NCIC CTG/GIVIO) randomized trial. Presented at the 2002 American Society of Clinical Oncology Annual Meeting. Orlando, May 18–21, 2002.

[60] NCCN practice guidelines on treatment of colon cancer, version 2. 2006. Available at: http://www.nccn.org/professionals/physician_gls/PDF/colon.pdf. Accessed January 15, 2006.

[61] Kemeny N, Huang Y, Cohen AM, et al. Hepatic arterial infusion of chemotherapy after resection of hepatic metastases from colorectal cancer. N Engl J Med 1999;341(27): 2039–48.

[62] Delaunoit T, Alberts SR, Sargent DJ, et al. Chemotherapy permits resection of metastatic colorectal cancer: experience from Intergroup N9741. Ann Oncol 2005;16(3):425–9.

[63] Bilchik AJ, Poston G, Curley SA, et al. Neoadjuvant chemotherapy for metastatic colon cancer: a cautionary note. J Clin Oncol 2005;23(36):9073–8.

[64] Fernandez FG, Ritter J, Goodwin JW, et al. Effect of steatohepatitis associated with irinotecan or oxaliplatin pretreatment on resectability of hepatic colorectal metastases. J Am Coll Surg 2005;200(6):845–53.

[65] Ribic CM, Sargent DJ, Moore MJ, et al. Tumor microsatellite instability status as a predictor of benefit from fluorouracil-based adjuvant chemotherapy for colon cancer. N Engl J Med 2003;349(3):247–57.

[66] Desch CE, Benson AB III, Somerfield MR, et al. Colorectal cancer surveillance: 2005 update of an American Society of Clinical Oncology practice guideline. J Clin Oncol 2005;23(33): 8512–9.

SURGICAL
CLINICS OF
NORTH AMERICA

Surg Clin N Am 86 (2006) 1045–1064

New Therapies for the Treatment of Inflammatory Bowel Disease

Bruce E. Sands, MD, MS[a,b]

[a]MGH Crohn's and Colitis Center, Gastrointestinal Unit, Massachusetts General Hospital,
165 Cambridge Street, 9th Floor, Boston, MA 02114, USA
[b]Harvard Medical School, Boston, MA

Progress in medical therapies for the inflammatory bowel diseases (IBD) has been brisk over the last decade, beyond the 5-aminosalicylates introduced in the 1930s and refined in the 1980s, and corticosteroids in the 1950s. These agents, although beneficial for many patients, were not effective for the majority of patients over the long term. Steroids in particular presented new safety concerns. Further therapeutic leaps were made with the introduction of the thiopurine analogs mercaptopurine and azathioprine, and still later methotrexate. In the mid-1990s, biologic agents came to the fore. Infliximab, a chimeric anti-tumor necrosis factor alpha (TNF) antibody, was the first biologic response modifier indicated for the treatment of Crohn's disease (CD). This was followed over the next decade by the development of a host of other anti-TNF agents, broadening of the indication for infliximab to ulcerative colitis (UC), as well as agents directed at virtually every known pathophysiologic mechanism. The large number of new agents presents a bewildering challenge to practitioners anticipating their use in the clinic, and more than ever requires an understanding of immune mechanisms related to these diseases. This article is intended to introduce the reader to the breadth of new agents that have been studied over the last 10 years as novel therapies for the treatment of CD and UC. Fig. 1 has an overview of pathophysiologic targets discussed in this article.

The author has received research grants, or has received honoraria as a member of speakers' bureaus, scientific advisory boards, or as consultant for the following entities: Abbott Immunology, Centocor, UCB Pharma, Procter & Gamble Pharmaceuticals, Protein Design Labs, Prometheus Laboratories, Otsuka America Pharmaceuticals Inc., Wyeth, Berlex, Amgen, Genentech, Human Genome Sciences, Millenium Pharmaceuticals, Elan, and BiogenIDEC.

E-mail address: bsands@partners.org

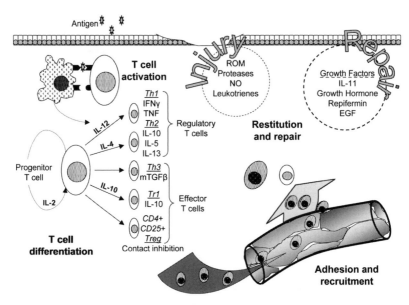

Fig. 1. Therapeutic targets in the pathogenesis of inflammatory bowel disease, counterclockwise from the top left. (*T cell activation*) Luminal antigens, most likely bacterial in origin, are presented by an antigen presenting cell in the context of MHC Class II to a T cell via CD3, T cell receptor. In the presence of a second, costimulatory signal, the T cell is activated. With blockage of the costimulatory signal, anergy or apoptosis occurs. (*T cell differentiation*) Upon activation, progenitor T cells produce IL-2 as an autocrine growth factor. Differentiation occurs as a T effector or T regulatory cell. T effector cells are classically divided into T helper 1 (Th1) or T helper 2 (Th2) cells. Th1 is associated with cell-mediated immunity, and is characteristic of Crohn's disease. Th1 differentiation is facilitated by interleukin-12 (IL-12) and characterized by elaboration of tumor necrosis factor α (TNF) and interferon γ (IFN γ). Th2 is associated with humoral immunity, facilitated by IL-4, and characterized by production of IL-4, IL-5, IL-10 and IL-13. Ulcerative colitis is incompletely characterized as a Th2 response, and natural killer T cells (NK-T cells) appear to predominate. T regulatory cells are more recently recognized, and include Tr1 cells, which elaborate IL-10, Th3 cells that produce the downregulatory cytokine transforming growth factor beta (TGF β), and CD4 + CD25 + Treg cells, which inhibit responses through cell to cell contact. (*Adhesion and recruitment*) The process by which inflammatory and immune cells are attracted to and locate within inflamed tissue in the gut occurs through the coordinated expression of a series of adhesion molecules on leukocytes and vascular endothelium, and the elaboration of various chemokines and chemoattractants in a gradient. Upon diapedesis into the inflamed tissue, cells become activated and further amplify the inflammatory response. (*Restitution and repair*) The final event is injury to the mucosa, with damage inflicted directly by various cell populations, and by soluble mediators of injury, including reactive oxygen metabolites (ROM), nitric oxide (NO), proteases, and leukotrienes. Restitution is the immediate process by which the intestinal epithelium spreads to cover the defect, and repair is the longer-term process by which injury is reversed and tissue remodeled. Various growth factors, including epidermal growth factor (EGF) and interleukin-11 (IL-11) may contribute to this process of recovery.

Infliximab

Before demonstrating the efficacy of anti-TNF antibody in clinical trials, TNF was considered to be but one of numerous cytokines and small molecules shown to be disproportionately expressed in active IBD. Earlier studies had shown that TNF was present at increased levels in the stool of children who had active UC, and to a greater extent in CD than in UC [1]. In addition, tissue expression was known to be elevated, and lamina propria mononuclear cells from patients who had IBD were shown to produce significantly higher levels of TNF when stimulated by lipopolysaccharide [2]. Nevertheless, little was known as to whether TNF was a central cytokine in the inflammatory cascade, or simply one of many proinflammatory molecules elaborated in IBD, and whether inhibiting TNF would produce therapeutic benefit.

Crohn's disease

The logic behind inhibiting TNF was rooted in the knowledge that granulomas are associated with Crohn's disease, and that TNF is essential to the formation of granulomas. By this logic, blocking TNF might provide benefits in treating the granulomatous inflammation of Crohn's disease. An early case series of the chimeric anti-TNF antibody infliximab (then called cA2) [3] showed benefit in 8 of 10 patients treated, with remarkable evidence of mucosal healing even within 4 weeks of treatment. Subsequent studies confirmed both efficacy and rapid onset of effect, with as many as 81% of patients responding to a single intravenous infusion of 5 mg/kg body weight in as little as 2 to 4 weeks, as compared with 17% of patients assigned to placebo [4]. Approximately half of responding patients have a response robust enough to be called remission, essentially a return to a normal state of well-being. Incidentally noted in the course of clinical trials was cessation of drainage and discomfort from perianal fistulas. Studies in both fistulizing and nonfistulizing disease, however, suggested that short-term treatment did not produce durable response, raising the need for long-term treatment strategies [4,5].

The ACCENT I (nonfistulizing CD) [6] and ACCENT II (fistulizing CD) [7] studies were designed to establish whether maintenance dosing could maintain response among those patients who respond to induction treatment. Maintenance dosing was given every 8 weeks, and patients were followed to week 54. In the ACCENT I study [6], among the 59% of patients who responded at week 2 to a single infusion, 28% assigned to 5 mg/kg every 8 weeks and 38% of those given 10 mg/kg every 8 weeks were in clinical remission at week 54, compared with 14% who had received only a single 5 mg/kg infusion at week 0 and placebo every 8 weeks thereafter. The differences between 5 mg/kg and placebo ($P = 0.007$) and 10 mg/kg and placebo ($P < 0.001$) were highly statistically significant. The comparison between the two treatment groups was not significantly different; however, this analysis was not prespecified and the study was of insufficient power to detect a difference of small magnitude. Other observations included significant steroid-sparing effect of infliximab, and benefit to health-related quality of life. Patients who lost their response while on placebo were able to resume dosing at 5 mg/kg no more frequently than every 8 weeks, as needed for recurrent symptoms, whereas patients who had loss of response while on 5 mg/kg maintenance dosing were able to increase to 10 mg/kg [6]. The majority of patients who flared on placebo maintenance were able to be brought into control on resuming episodic dosing on flare; however, the overall efficacy appeared to be somewhat less than with scheduled maintenance dosing. Patients who lost response to 5 mg/kg were also observed usually to respond to dose escalation to 10 mg/kg [6].

ACCENT II studied maintenance dosing in patients who had enterocutaneous fistulas [7]. Approximately 90% of fistulas were perianal fistulas, though some abdominal wall fistulas were also present. Women who had rectovaginal fistulas were included, provided a fistula to skin was also present. Patients were given induction dosing of infliximab 5 mg/kg at weeks 0, 2, and 6. Patients who had achieved a response, defined as a reduction in the number of actively draining fistulas by 50% or more in a given patient, were randomized to maintenance dosing of infliximab 5 mg/kg or placebo every 8 weeks and followed to week 54. Initial response occurred in 69% of patients [7]. Time to loss of response, the primary analysis, was significantly longer in patients randomized to infliximab maintenance compared with placebo. Complete fistula response (closer of all fistulas) at week 54 was achieved by 36% of initial responders assigned to infliximab, as compared with 19% of initial responders assigned to placebo ($P = 0.009$) [7]. Patients who did not respond to induction treatment were unlikely to respond to continued infusions of infliximab: 16% on 5 mg/kg infliximab every 8 weeks compared with 10% on placebo maintenance ($P = $ n.s.) [7]. As with patients who had nonfistulizing disease in the ACCENT I study, patients in ACCENT II who lost their response while on placebo responded well to resuming infliximab 5 mg/kg every 8 weeks (61%) [7]. Similarly, 57% of patients who lost their response to 5 mg/kg and escalated to 10 mg/kg regained their response to infliximab [7]. When categorized by location, 97.2% of perianal fistulas were noted to have closed at any time during follow-up, compared with 79.5% of abdominal wall fistulas and only 64.0% of rectovaginal fistulas [8].

The lessons of ACCENT I and II have had a significant impact upon the treatment of Crohn's disease. These studies demonstrated that complete and durable remission and fistula closure is possible for a subset of patients given maintenance dosing, albeit not a majority of patients. Patients may respond to infliximab even if they have been resistant to other therapies, including immunosuppressant agents. In addition, infliximab was shown to be steroid-sparing. There is a suggestion that responding, as opposed to non-responding, patients may have distinct pathophysiology underlying their symptoms, because those who do not respond to induction treatment are very unlikely to respond to longer term treatment. Finally, it is apparent that patients who lose their response to infliximab may regain response upon dose escalation.

Many physicians have questioned the need for long-term maintenance dosing with infliximab, as opposed to using the drug episodically, or in the case of patients who are flaring but have not yet been tried on immunosuppressive agents, as a short-term bridge to maintenance with azathioprine or mercaptopurine. The desire to limit exposure to infliximab relates to its direct costs (cost of administering the drug and the cost of the drug itself), and concern about long-term, potentially serious side effects. These include acute or delayed infusion reactions; infection, including rare but life-threatening opportunistic infections and tuberculosis; autoimmune phenomena such as positive antinuclear antibody (ANA), and anti-double–stranded DNA antibodies. Rarer side effects include drug-induced lupus, very rare demyelinating disease, worsening of congestive heart failure and increased mortality among those who have congestive heart failure, and lymphoma [9].

Certainly, response over the near long-term of 6 to 12 months suggests that episodic or bridging strategies may be effective for some patients. Data from ACCENT I on patients who de facto underwent episodic treatment indicate that they did not fare as well as patients receiving either 5 or 10 mg/kg infliximab as scheduled maintenance [10]. The overall response rate in the episodic strategy over 54 weeks was approximately 5% to 10% lower than scheduled maintenance dosing strategies [10]. Still, some might view this as a reasonable tradeoff in efficacy, considering the economic and safety concerns raised above.

Although these data might suggest that episodic or bridge strategies with infliximab may be effective in the near long-term, other lines of evidence argue against these strategies. The first concern is that episodic dosing strategies have been clearly associated with development of antibodies to infliximab (ATI), infusion reactions, and loss of response. In one study [11], episodic dosing was associated with ATI in 61% of patients. This compares unfavorably to ATI in 16% to 17% of patients in ACCENT I and II [6,7]. Conversely, ATI are associated with reduced serum infliximab concentrations and shorter duration of response [11]. Factors other than scheduled maintenance dosing that may play a role in reducing ATI include: concomitant steroids, or steroid pretreatment (typically hydrocortisone 200 mg intravenous [IV] immediately preceding infliximab) [12]; concomitant immunosuppressive therapy with AZA, 6-mercaptopurine or methotrexate; and three-dose induction therapy rather single-dose induction. Another line of evidence in favor of scheduled maintenance dosing over episodic dosing is the demonstration that scheduled maintenance dosing is associated with significantly fewer hospitalizations and surgeries [10,13]. This has been shown to be true in both fistulizing and nonfistulizing patients. These results suggest not only improved long-term outcomes of great significance to patients' quality of life, but also potential cost savings that may more than offset the cost of the medication itself. Finally, long-term observational data suggest that steroids, rather than infliximab itself, may be the prime offender in serious infections in Crohn's disease, although infliximab and other anti-TNF agents are clearly implicated in serious infections with intracellular pathogens such as tuberculosis [14], making TB screening mandatory for all patients about to begin treatment and annually thereafter. At present, the preponderance of evidence supports scheduled maintenance treatment with infliximab, primarily because of the concerns of loss of response and inferior disease outcomes with episodic therapy. A reasonable algorithm also takes into account the interpatient variability in duration of response (Fig. 2).

Ulcerative colitis

The preclinical rationale for anti-TNF therapy in UC was not considered to be as strong as in CD. Levels of TNF in blood and stool were thought to be lower in UC than in CD. In addition, CD is thought to be a disease of cell-mediated immunity, associated with T helper 1 (Th1) subsets driven by interleukin (IL)-12 and characterized by production of interferon γ and TNF. By contrast, UC was considered to be characterized by a forme

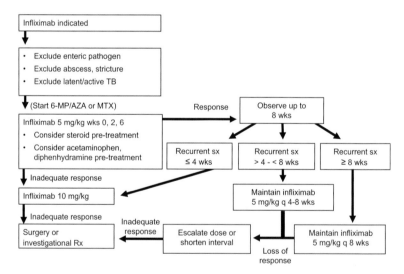

Fig. 2. Infliximab treatment algorithm. Once a decision to treat with infliximab has been made, infectious complications need to be first guarded against by diagnosing and treating enteric pathogens, abscess, tuberculosis, or other infectious issues. Concurrent treatment with an immune modulator is desirable to minimize risk of antibodies to infliximab and subsequent loss of response. Similarly, once a course of treatment has been begun, maintenance dosing at regular intervals of 8 weeks or less should ensue, again to minimize the formation of antibodies to infliximab. Patients who do not respond to 5 mg/kg may respond to dose escalation, whereas patients who require treatment intervals of less than 8 weeks may be maintained at shorter intervals.

fruste of T helper 2 (Th2) responses driven by IL-4 and leading to elaboration of the classic downregulatory cytokine IL-10. According to this evidence, anti-TNF agents were expected to be ineffective in UC.

Indeed, early studies presented conflicting evidence. The earliest reported double-blind, randomized, placebo-controlled trial [15] sought to treat patients who had UC and who were hospitalized and refractory to IV steroids. Five of 8 patients assigned to infliximab (dosed at 5, 10, or 20 mg/kg) had a short-term response, whereas all 3 patients assigned to placebo underwent early colectomy [15]; however, the study was terminated prematurely because of slow enrollment. In a second double-blind study [16], 43 patients who had steroid-resistant UC were randomized to infliximab 5 mg/kg or placebo at weeks 0 and 2. Remission rates were indistinguishable between the two groups at week 6. Open-label infliximab 10 mg/kg at week 6 in nonresponders also did not produce significant benefit [16].

Subsequently, three double-blind, randomized controlled trials [17,18], have clearly demonstrated efficacy of infliximab in UC. ACT 1 and ACT 2 included over 800 patients who had active disease despite a variety of treatments that may have included 5-aminosalicylates, oral corticosteroids, and AZA or mercaptopurine [17]. Nonhospitalized patients were randomized to infliximab 5 or 10 mg/kg or placebo at weeks 0, 2 and 6, and every 8 weeks thereafter to week 30 (ACT2) or week 54 (ACT 1). At week 8, response rates were 65% in the infliximab groups, compared with 35% in the placebo group [17]. Remission was achieved in 35% on infliximab, compared with 15% on placebo [17]. Benefit extended to 30 and 54 weeks as well. As in Crohn's disease, other benefits could be demonstrated, including improved quality of life, steroid-sparing, and reductions in hospitalization and surgery rates. Mucosal healing was also achieved in a significant percentage of patients [17].

Another study was performed in hospitalized patients refractory to intravenous steroids [18]. After randomization to infliximab 5 mg/kg or placebo, colectomy occurred by 90 days in 29% of patients given infliximab, compared with 67% of patients given placebo ($P = 0.017$). These data suggest results comparable to what has been expected with cyclosporine [19], and in clinical practice may be adopted by community practitioners who have never embraced the latter drug because of its potential for immediate and serious toxicities.

Together, these studies clearly show that infliximab is as effective in UC as it is in CD. Attention needs to turn back to basic investigation to elucidate the mechanisms whereby TNF inhibition is effective in UC, and whether those mechanisms are any different from those operative in CD.

Other anti-tumor necrosis factor alpha biologic agents

With the success of infliximab has come a raft of other anti-TNF biologic agents intended to improve upon the original of the class. Two attributes of infliximab—its immunogenicity and its intravenous administration—have been targeted as areas of potential improvement. One approach has been to create antibodies with more human protein sequence. These have included CDP571, a humanized anti-TNF antibody with approximately 95% human sequence [20,21], and adalimumab, reported to be a fully human anti-TNF antibody. A second approach has been to create soluble receptor constructs, which recombine the native p75 or p55 TNF receptor with an immunoglobulin Fc segment (etanercept [22] and onercept [23], respectively) to create a novel TNF binding molecule. A third approach has been to raise Fab′ fragments against TNF and to pegylate this construct to increase its half life (CDP870, or certolizumab pegol) [24]. Fig. 3 reviews structural differences. All the new agents other than CDP571 are delivered by subcutaneous dosing rather than intravenously.

The success of these agents has been variable. Etanercept proved to be ineffective in Crohn's disease at doses known to be effective in rheumatoid arthritis [22], and the p55 soluble receptor, onercept, initially thought to be effective in Crohn's disease [23], also proved to be ineffective. At present

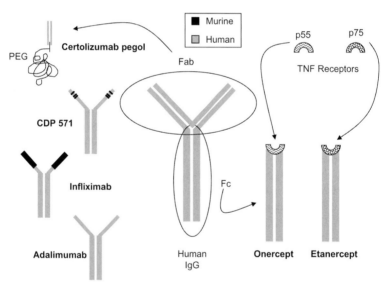

Fig. 3. Anti-tumor necrosis factor biologic agents. Current biologic agents directed against tumor necrosis factor α are based upon the structure of gammaglobulin (IgG). Native human IgG possesses two heavy and two light chains. The molecule is divided into the Fab′ fragment, with its two antigen binding sites, and the Fc portion. Soluble TNF receptor constructs consist of the Fc portion with either the p55 TNF receptor (onercept) or the p75 TNF receptor (etanercept). Neither agent has been shown to be effective in IBD, however. Infliximab is a chimeric monoclonal anti-TNF antibody, with approximately 25% murine sequence in the antigen-binding regions. CDP 571 is a humanized anti-TNF antibody, with 5% murine sequence remaining in the complementarity determining regions. Adalimumab is a human anti-TNF antibody, whereas certolizumab pegol is an Fab′ fragment bound to PEG (polyethylene glycol) to extend its biologic half-life.

it is uncertain if this lack of efficacy relates to mechanistic differences between Crohn's disease and rheumatoid arthritis, or to differences in dosing required for the two diseases.

In contrast to the soluble TNF receptors tried in IBD, some of the newer anti-TNF antibodies have been effective, and others not. CDP571, after initial promising studies, did not demonstrate efficacy in larger trials [21]. Adalimumab has been shown to be effective in induction therapy of Crohn's disease at 4 weeks, with remission rates of 36% at a dose 160 mg to load and 80 mg at week 2 to maintain, compared with a remission rate of 12% for placebo [25]. Subsequent studies have provided preliminary evidence that continued treatment may be effective as a maintenance regimen [26]. Thus far, the demonstrated immunogenicity of this agent has been relatively low, but remains to be fully defined in long-term studies.

Certolizumab pegol has also been shown to be effective as an inductive and maintenance agent. A Phase II study showed treatment to be effective at week 2, but with no significant benefit over placebo at the primary end point measure at week 12 [24]. Three doses (100 mg, 200 mg, and 400 mg given subcutaneously every 4 weeks) were compared with placebo. At week 12, the placebo response rate of 36% was relatively high compared with previous studies, and the 44% response rate at the 400 mg dose was not significant by comparison. A post hoc exploratory analysis of the subgroup of patients who had baseline C-reactive protein 10 mg/L or higher (118 of the original 159 patients studied) provided greater contrast in treatment effect, with response rates at week 12 of 52% for 400 mg, compared with 18% for placebo ($P < 0.01$) [24]. Two subsequent Phase III studies have reportedly demonstrated efficacy regardless of baseline C-reactive protein [27], and it is likely that certolizumab will be approved in the United States sometime in the next year.

Another anti-TNF agent under active investigation is a rationally designed peptide, designated RDP58, consisting of a 9 D-amino acid peptide [28]. This agent has been shown to inhibit synthesis of TNF as well as the expression of interferon γ and IL-12, by disrupting cell signaling at the pre-MAPK MyD88-IRAK-TRAF6 protein complex, critical for downstream activation of the proinflammatory transcription factor nuclear factor kappa B (NFκB). Uniquely, the peptide is delivered to the intestinal mucosa upon oral intake, with no detectable peptide found in circulation, ostensibly providing a purely topical effect. A study in patients who had active UC compared doses of 200 mg and 240 mg orally every day with placebo, and showed a P value of 0.003 for the trend along increasing doses against placebo [28]. Confirmatory studies are ongoing.

Small molecule inhibitors of tumor necrosis factor alpha

Given the repeated demonstration that blocking TNF with biologics can provide effective therapy for IBD, it is not surprising that efforts have also turned to developing small molecules capable of inhibiting TNF. Thalidomide has been studied in open-label series in Crohn's disease [29,30]. It is moderately effective at inhibiting TNF, but perhaps more importantly, it has anti-angiogenic properties that may be quite important for its efficacy. Although open-label studies have reported impressive efficacy, use of this agent is difficult because of the highly restrictive prescribing program in the United States, designed to prevent exposing pregnant woman and the known severe birth defects that can result from exposure. Other dose-limiting toxicities include potentially severe and irreversible peripheral neuropathy, dermatitis, leukopenia, sedation, and obstipation.

Semapimod (CNI-1493) is a mitogen activated protein (MAP) kinase inhibitor capable of preventing downstream activation of NFκB [31]. A pilot study of two different doses in 10 patients who had active Crohn's disease yielded promising results, although phlebitis and abnormal liver function tests were observed in some patients [31]. Another approach has been to inhibit phosphodiesterase 4 (PDE4) [32]. Phosphodiesterases are ubiquitously distributed in various tissues, and nonspecific inhibitors include caffeine, aminophylline, and theophylline. PDE4 is present on immune cells, and inhibition of PDE4 may result in increased levels of cyclic AMP and decreased inflammation. OPC-6535 is a PDE4 inhibitor being studied in active ulcerative colitis [33]. A preliminary study showed 25 mg/d and 50 mg/d doses given orally to reduce disease activity [33]. Large Phase III studies in UC are ongoing.

Other anticytokine therapies

Other cytokines are thought to play a central role in the inflammation of IBD, and have been considered as rational targets for therapy. These include the quintessential Th1 cytokines IL-12, produced mainly by activated macrophages, and interferon γ, elaborated by activated T cells and some populations of NK-T cells. ABT-874 is a humanized anti-IL-12 antibody explored in a Phase IIa study in active Crohn's disease [34]. This small study's primary end point was safety, but efficacy results were also reported. A total of 80 patients were enrolled in two sequential groups. In Group I, 40 patients were randomized to ABT-874 1 mg/kg (n = 16), 3 mg/kg (n = 16), or placebo (n = 8), and given study drug subcutaneously at days 1, 29, 36, 43, 50, 57, and 64. In Group II, the same number of subjects was assigned to the same dose levels, but received the study drug weekly for 7 doses over 6 weeks. No significant efficacy was observed in Group I, but in Group II, 75% of patients assigned to the 3 mg/kg group achieved a clinical response and 38% a clinical remission at week 7, compared with 25% and 0% assigned to placebo, respectively ($P = 0.32$ and $P = 0.066$) [34]. These results are initial confirmation of the hypothesized pivotal role of IL-12 in Crohn's disease, and at least in this small study showed no important safety concerns.

Fontolizumab is a humanized anti-interferon γ antibody. In a relatively large Phase IIb, double-blind study conducted in active Crohn's disease, patients were randomized to fontolizumab 4 or 10 mg/kg or placebo [35,36]. The drug was administered intravenously every 4 weeks. In a post hoc analysis of patients who had C-reactive protein 10 mg/L or higher, response and remission rates in the fontolizumab groups were significantly better than placebo. At 4 and 10 mg/kg, clinical response were 77% and 71%, compared with 14% for placebo, and clinical remission rates were 54% and 57% compared with 0% for placebo [35,36]. Treatment was well-tolerated.

Another cytokine of interest is IL-6, an important inflammatory cytokine that is elaborated at least in part in response to TNF. A pilot study of a humanized anti-IL-6 receptor antibody, tocolizumab, showed response rates at 6 weeks approaching 70%, compared with 30% for placebo [37]. Additional studies are needed to confirm this very small Phase II study.

Agents that disrupt T cell activation

T cells have long been known to be central to the highly activated adaptive immune responses observed in IBD. A critical juncture in T cell activation is when the naïve T cell is presented with antigen in the context of MHC (major histocompatibility complex) Class II on the surface of an antigen-presenting cell. The latter cell type may include macrophages, dendritic cells, B cells, and potentially intestinal epithelial cells. A second, costimulatory signal is required at the T cell surface. Without this second signal, which is not antigen-specific, the T cell presented with antigen will either become inactive (anergic) or may be deleted by apoptosis (programmed cell death). Finally, upon T cell activation, IL-2 is elaborated and is essential as an autocrine growth factor for the activation of other T cells in the local milieu. Thus, therapeutic strategies may interfere with the antigen-specific binding step, the costimulation step, or at the level of IL-2 activation [38].

Cyclosporine has been thought to exert its beneficial effects in ulcerative colitis by inhibiting T cell activation in response to IL-2 binding. Daclizumab is a humanized anti-IL-2 receptor antibody that is effective in the setting of organ transplantation [39]. A small, open-label study in 10 patients who had UC [40] appeared to show excellent efficacy, with response in over 70% of patients; however, a subsequent, larger blinded, randomized controlled trial did not confirm this efficacy. A second agent, basiliximab, a chimeric antibody to the high-affinity IL-2 receptor (CD25) has been explored in a 10-patient, open-label study of patients with steroid-resistant ulcerative colitis [41]. Patients received a 40 mg intravenous bolus of basiliximab. Symptomatic improvement occurred by 1 week, with 9 of 10 patients achieving clinical remission by 8 weeks. Seven patients were in clinical remission at week 24, with 5 of these off steroids [41]. Although promising, these results require confirmation in a larger, blinded, randomized controlled trial.

Visilizumab is a humanized antibody to the CD3, the T cell receptor [42]. This highly potent agent has been explored in a relatively large, early phase, open-label study in severe, steroid-refractory UC. Doses ranging from 5 to 12.5 mcg/kg were administered as two sequential daily intravenous boluses. Remission rates, including endoscopic healing, ranged from 12% to 54% at day 30. A profound but temporary drop in CD8+ T cells is observed almost immediately after treatment, with recovery over a 2- to 4-week period, associated with a rise and return to normal of Epstein-Barr virus counts. In addition, some patients experience a cytokine release syndrome, consisting of chills, headache, fever, arthralgias, back pain, and occasionally hypotension. Both efficacy and safety of this agent need further study in blinded trials.

Adhesion molecule inhibitors

Although small numbers of inflammatory cells reside in the mucosa, ready to respond to infection and insult, IBD is characterized by a massive influx of inflammatory and immune cells from the peripheral circulation. The recruitment of these cells from the periphery to the mucosa is regulated by the coordinate expression of adhesion molecules and their ligands on the endothelial surface. Interrupting these interactions by inhibiting the expression of adhesion molecules or interfering with binding is a key target in both major forms of IBD. The alpha 4 integrins, primarily alpha 4 beta 1, expressed on all inflamed endothelium, and alpha 4 beta 7, found only on intestinal epithelium, are considered prime targets in IBD.

Natalizumab is a humanized anti-alpha 4 integrin antibody that has been investigated as a treatment for Crohn's disease [43]. A Phase II, double-blind, randomized controlled trial in mild to moderately active Crohn's disease [43] demonstrated beneficial effect of natalizumab 3 mg/kg given intravenously 4 weeks apart compared with placebo, although the study was not successful in meeting its primary end point, clinical response (decrease in Crohn's disease activity index of ≥ 70 points from baseline) at week 10. A large pivotal trial of 300 mg given intravenously every 4 weeks [44] also barely missed achieving its primary end point in inducing response at week 10, with a P value of 0.051 and a treatment benefit over placebo of approximately 8% (56.4% for natalizumab and 48.6% for placebo); however, as with other recent studies, the placebo response rate in this study was quite high, and post hoc analysis limited to the population with elevated C-reactive protein (CRP)-demonstrated response rates of 57.6% with natalizumab and 44.8% with placebo ($P = 0.007$) [44]. Results in a study of maintenance of remission were more robust, with remission maintained in 43.8% on natalizumab compared with 25.8% on placebo over 9 months of follow-up in the population that achieved remission in the 12-week induction study mentioned above [44].

Initial safety data on natalizumab were also quite promising; however, shortly after the drug was introduced to the US market as a groundbreaking treatment for multiple sclerosis, three cases among approximately 3000 patients treated for either multiple sclerosis or Crohn's disease were recognized to have developed the extremely rare and most often fatal complication of progressive multifocal leukoencephalopathy (PML) [45,46]. Two of these patients died, and one of the deceased was a patient with Crohn's disease, the nature of whose brain lesion was only recognized post mortem. PML is extremely rare in the general population, and although relatively more common in patients with profound immunosuppression from AIDS, has not been reported with pharmacologic immune suppression for the treatment of IBD. Because patients treated with natalizumab do not appear to have a general state of immune suppression and do not otherwise appear to have greatly increased risk of conventional or opportunistic infection, it is presumed that these cases of PML observed in association with natalizumab may be a consequence of its unique mode of action. One hypothesis is that the agent inhibits immune surveillance of both the gut, which may be a reservoir of JC virus, the causative agent of PML, and the central nervous system. Hypothetically, under certain conditions, JC virus may therefore be released into circulation, and from there into the immune-privileged space of the central nervous system [45]; however, because the complication of PML was still only rarely observed, there are likely to be contributing factors to the occurrence of PML that have yet to be recognized.

According to the line of reasoning just outlined, an agent that more specifically inhibits the interaction of alpha 4 beta 7 with mucosal addressin cellular adhesion molecule 1 (MAdCAM-1), which targets leukocyte adhesion in the gut alone, might avoid the complication of PML. As a proof of principle, a humanized anti-alpha 4 beta 7 antibody (MLN-02) has been demonstrated to be effective in Phase II clinical trials in active Crohn's disease, as well as in UC [47]. Whether PML can be avoided by this more selective adhesion molecule inhibitor needs to be assessed carefully in clinical trials and observational studies should the drug reach the market.

Small molecules inhibitors of adhesion and recruitment have also been studied. Alicaforsen is an antisense oligonucleotide to intercellular adhesion molecule 1 (ICAM-1). Antisense oligonucleotides are a class of agents that abrogate expression of a specific protein by binding in a highly specific way to a species of messenger RNA, and inhibiting its translation, most likely by facilitating its destruction by RNAses. After promising early studies of intravenous infusions of this agent (then called ISIS 2302) in Crohn's disease [48], subsequent blinded, randomized controlled trials failed to demonstrate efficacy [49]. It was not clear if the drug had been delivered at effective doses, and attention turned to alternative means of delivery capable of introducing high concentrations topically to inflamed mucosa [49–51]. Alicaforsen enemas were explored as a means of treating distal UC, and in a small blinded, randomized controlled trial [52], the agent appeared to effect durable response over a 6-month period after 6 weeks of active treatment. Though promising, these results need confirmation in a larger study.

In summary, agents that interfere with the adhesion and recruitment of leukocytes to the inflamed bowel mucosa hold great promise in the treatment of IBD. It is likely that agents with greater specificity for the gut, either through targeted delivery or more focused mode of action, will hold benefits with regard to the safety of this approach, and in particular for risk of infection.

Growth factors

In response to damage inflicted by proteases, reactive oxygen metabolites, and various other destructive species, the intestinal mucosa has mechanisms by which restitution and repair of the epithelium occurs. Various growth factors have been considered as possible agents to promote healing of the mucosa in IBD, and therefore to reduce signs and symptoms of the disease. In addition, promoting mucosal integrity would have theoretical benefits in reducing exposure of the lamina propria to the multitude of antigens present in the lumen that might perpetuate the immune and inflammatory response. Interleukin-11 has cytoprotective effects in various animal models, but exhibited only modest benefit in randomized controlled trials in Crohn's disease [53]. Growth hormone (somatropin) has a host of downstream effects on various tissues, including the gut. A small, blinded, randomized controlled trial of human recombinant growth hormone in combination with a high protein diet showed impressive reduction of disease activity compared with placebo [54]. These results require replication in a larger study before being adopted in clinical practice, because excess growth hormone exposure could have negative health consequences. Epidermal growth factor (EGF) was explored as a topical therapy for distal ulcerative colitis. A small, blinded, randomized controlled trial of EGF enemas showed promising results [55]. A study of repifermin (keratinocyte growth factor 2) administered parenterally in ulcerative colitis did not demonstrate efficacy despite positive effects in various animal models of IBD [56]. Thus, although growth factors remain of interest as potential therapy for IBD, data mostly remain preliminary.

Novel therapies with unique mode of action

The majority of treatments for IBD work by suppressing the adaptive immune responses and inflammation that are known to be activated in these conditions. This is the basis of most accepted therapies, including 5-aminosalicylates, corticosteroids, immune modulators (azathioprine, mercaptopurine, methotrexate), and biologic response modifiers such as infliximab. A number of more unusual therapies have been investigated as alternate ways of modifying the immune response in IBD.

Recently, Korzenik and Dieckgraefe [57] hypothesized that in a subset of patients with Crohn's disease, a defect in neutrophil function may be a key feature of the condition. Data from the 1980s demonstrated possible neutrophil defects in Crohn's disease, but these effects could not be disentangled from the possible confounding effects of concurrent medications. A number of more rare conditions, however, exist in which defects in neutrophil function have been associated with a Crohn's disease-like phenotype. These include chronic granulomatous disease, Chediak-Higashi syndrome, Hermansky-Pudlak syndrome, glycogen storage disease Type Ib [58], and common variable immunodeficiency. Dieckgraefe and Korzenik hypothesized that neutrophil defects might also be the basis of disease in some individuals with Crohn's disease, and reasoned that agents that enhance neutrophil function might be effective.

In an open-label study of G-CSF (filgrastim) in CD [59], 20 patients with a mean Crohn's disease activity index (CDAI) of 307 were treated for 8 weeks. Fifteen patients completed 8 weeks of treatment, at which time a mean CDAI of 196 (range, 36–343) was noted. Thirteen patients completed the study to week 12, with mean CDAI of 162 (range: 20–308). Five patients had a sustained remission, and 55% of patients experienced a drop in CDAI by 70 points or more [59]. Some patients experienced bone pain in the course of treatment.

A second open-label study with GM-CSF (sargramostim) produced similar benefits [60]. Fifteen patients were given GM-CSF 4 to 8 mcg/kg/day subcutaneously for 8 weeks. Adverse events included injection site reactions and bone pain. The mean CDAI decreased by 190 points, with 12 of 15 patients experiencing a decrease in CDAI by 100 points or more, and 8 entering into clinical remission [60].

A double-blind, randomized, placebo-controlled trial of sargramostim in Crohn's disease further explored this treatment in 124 patients [61]. Subjects were randomized 2:1 to sargramostim 6 mcg/kg/d or placebo subcutaneously for 8 weeks. Patients were not permitted to have concomitant treatment with immune suppressants or corticosteroids, in keeping with the hypothesis that sargramostim should work by immune stimulation, which might be inhibited broadly by these agents. The prespecified primary end point of clinical response (drop in CDAI by ≥ 70 points) was not achieved (54% sargramostim versus 44% placebo, $P = 0.28$) [61]; however, secondary end points of clinical response, defined as decreased CDAI by at least 100 points from baseline (48% sargramostim versus 26% placebo, $P = 0.01$), and remission, defined as CDAI 50 or lower (40% sargramostim versus 19% placebo, $P = 0.01$), were reached [61]. Sargramostim was associated with injection site reactions and bone pain, and was treatment-limiting for some patients.

Although G-CSF and GM-CSF hold promise for the treatment of CD, it is not clear whether the mode of action is related to stimulation of neutrophil function as previously hypothesized, or whether other effects of these pleiotropic cytokines are more important. Other questions concern the tolerability of treatment, given the frequent occurrence of bone pain and injection site reactions and the need for daily subcutaneous injection with the current formulation.

Another unusual treatment that has been explored in clinical trials is the therapeutic use of helminthic infestation in IBD [62–64]. The theoretical underpinnings relate to the millennia-old symbiosis between helminths and humans. As part of the hygiene theory of immune mediated diseases, enteric infestation by helminths has historically modified mucosal and systemic immune responses to foster downregulated responses [65]. Over the last century, the prevalence of helminthic infestation has greatly decreased through improved hygiene. Therefore, lack of helminthic infestation during the education of the immune system may play a permissive role in the overly aggressive mucosal immune responses seen in IBD [65].

Extending this line of reasoning, in a single-center investigation of iatrogenic infestation with *Trichiuris suis* (pig whipworm) as treatment for UC and CD was conducted [63]. In the CD study, 29 patients who had active disease (CDAI from 220 to 450) were enrolled in an open-label study in which they took 2500 *T. suis* ova every 3 weeks for 24 weeks. At week 12, 76% of patients experienced a clinical response (decreased in CDAI by ≥ 100 points) and 66% achieved clinical remission (CDAI <150 points). The clinical response rate at week 24 was 79%, and the clinical remission rate was 72%. No adverse effects were noted [63].

A double-blind, placebo-controlled trial of *T. suis* in patients with UC also appeared to demonstrate benefit [62]. Overall, 54 patients who had active UC received placebo or 2500 *T. suis* ova every 2 weeks for 12 weeks. In the active arm, 43% of patients experienced improvement (decrease in the UC disease activity index by ≥ 4 points), compared with 17% for placebo ($P < 0.04$) [62]. Although these results hold promise in both UC and CD, these results need to be replicated in larger, multicenter, blinded, randomized, placebo-controlled trials. The results, if positive, would clearly point investigators toward important interactions in the mucosal immune response that, if elucidated, could further unravel the mystery of IBD.

Medical devices are also making inroads into the treatment of IBD. In particular, leukocytapheresis using various proprietary systems is being investigated as therapies for both CD and UC [66,67]. One such device is a granulocyte-monocyte leukocytapheresis system using a column packed with cellulose acetate beads. Blinded, randomized, sham-controlled trials in CD and UC are under way using this system. A second system accomplishes leukocyte apheresis using a non-woven polyester fiber filter [68]. In theory, such devices might work by selectively adsorbing activated populations of leukocytes that might otherwise be effector cells in the inflamed gut.

Summary

Medical therapy of IBD has made remarkable progress in recent years, driven forward by new knowledge about mechanisms of disease and advances in biotechnology. As we continue to learn about how best to use the agents currently in our hands, the addition of new drugs will further improve outcomes, and will bring new insights into the fundamental causes of these diseases.

References

[1] Braegger CP, Nicholls S, Murch SH, et al. Tumour necrosis factor alpha in stool as a marker of intestinal inflammation [see comment]. Lancet 1992;339(8785):89–91.

[2] Reinecker HC, Steffen M, Witthoeft T, et al. Enhanced secretion of tumour necrosis factor-alpha, IL-6, and IL-1 beta by isolated lamina propria mononuclear cells from patients who have ulcerative colitis and Crohn's disease. Clin Exp Immunol 1993;94(1):174–81.

[3] van Dullemen HM, van Deventer SJ, Hommes DW, et al. Treatment of Crohn's disease with anti-tumor necrosis factor chimeric monoclonal antibody (cA2). Gastroenterology 1995; 109(1):129–35.

[4] Targan SR, Hanauer SB, van Deventer SJ, et al. A short-term study of chimeric monoclonal antibody cA2 to tumor necrosis factor alpha for Crohn's disease. Crohn's Disease cA2 Study Group. N Engl J Med 1997;337(15):1029–35.

[5] Present DH, Rutgeerts P, Targan S, et al. Infliximab for the treatment of fistulas in patients with Crohn's disease. N Engl J Med 1999;340(18):1398–405.

[6] Hanauer SB, Feagan BG, Lichtenstein GR, et al. Maintenance infliximab for Crohn's disease: the ACCENT I randomised trial [see comment]. Lancet 2002;359(9317):1541–9.

[7] Sands BE, Anderson FH, Bernstein CN, et al. Infliximab maintenance therapy for fistulizing Crohn's disease [see comment]. N Engl J Med 2004;350(9):876–85.

[8] Sands BE, Blank MA, Patel K, et al. Long-term treatment of rectovaginal fistulas in Crohn's disease: response to infliximab in the ACCENT II Study. Clin Gastroenterol Hepatol 2004; 2(10):912–20.

[9] Colombel JF, Loftus EV Jr, Tremaine WJ, et al. The safety profile of infliximab in patients with Crohn's disease: the Mayo clinic experience in 500 patients. Gastroenterology 2004; 126(1):19–31.

[10] Rutgeerts P, Feagan BG, Lichtenstein GR, et al. Comparison of scheduled and episodic treatment strategies of infliximab in Crohn's disease [see comment]. Gastroenterology 2004;126(2):402–13.

[11] Baert F, Noman M, Vermeire S, et al. Influence of immunogenicity on the long-term efficacy of infliximab in Crohn's disease [see comment]. N Engl J Med 2003;348(7):601–8.

[12] Farrell RJ, Alsahli M, Jeen YT, et al. Intravenous hydrocortisone premedication reduces antibodies to infliximab in Crohn's disease: a randomized controlled trial [see comment]. Gastroenterology 2003;124(4):917–24.

[13] Lichtenstein GR, Yan S, Bala M, et al. Infliximab maintenance treatment reduces hospitalizations, surgeries, and procedures in fistulizing Crohn's disease. Gastroenterology 2005; 128(4):862–9.

[14] Keane J, Gershon S, Wise RP, et al. Tuberculosis associated with infliximab, a tumor necrosis factor alpha-neutralizing agent [see comment]. N Engl J Med 2001;345(15):1098–104.

[15] Sands BE, Tremaine WJ, Sandborn WJ, et al. Infliximab in the treatment of severe, steroid-refractory ulcerative colitis: a pilot study [see comment]. Inflamm Bowel Dis 2001;7(2):83–8.

[16] Probert CS, Hearing SD, Schreiber S, et al. Infliximab in moderately severe glucocorticoid resistant ulcerative colitis: a randomised controlled trial. Gut 2003;52(7):998–1002.

[17] Rutgeerts P, Sandborn WJ, Feagan BG, et al. Infliximab for induction and maintenance therapy for ulcerative colitis. N Engl J Med 2005;353(23):2462–76.

[18] Jarnerot G, Hertervig E, Friis-Liby I, et al. Infliximab as rescue therapy in severe to moderately severe ulcerative colitis: a randomized, placebo-controlled study [see comment]. Gastroenterology 2005;128(7):1805–11.

[19] Lichtiger S, Present DH, Kornbluth A, et al. Cyclosporine in severe ulcerative colitis refractory to steroid therapy [see comment]. N Engl J Med 1994;330(26):1841–5.

[20] Sandborn WJ, Feagan BG, Hanauer SB, et al. An engineered human antibody to TNF (CDP571) for active Crohn's disease: a randomized double-blind placebo-controlled trial. Gastroenterology 2001;120(6):1330–8.

[21] Sandborn WJ, Feagan BG, Radford-Smith G, et al. CDP571, a humanised monoclonal antibody to tumour necrosis factor alpha, for moderate to severe Crohn's disease: a randomised, double blind, placebo controlled trial. Gut 2004;53(10):1485–93.

[22] Sandborn WJ, Hanauer SB, Katz S, et al. Etanercept for active Crohn's disease: a randomized, double-blind, placebo-controlled trial [see comment]. Gastroenterology 2001;121(5): 1088–94.

[23] Rutgeerts P, Lemmens L, Van Assche G, et al. Treatment of active Crohn's disease with onercept (recombinant human soluble p55 tumour necrosis factor receptor): results of a randomized, open-label, pilot study. Aliment Pharmacol Ther 2003;17(2):185–92.

[24] Schreiber S, Rutgeerts P, Fedorak RN, et al. A randomized, placebo-controlled trial of certolizumab pegol (CDP870) for treatment of Crohn's disease [see comment]. Gastroenterology 2005;129(3):807–18.

[25] Hanauer S, Sandborn WJ, Rutgeerts PJ, et al. Human anti-tumor necrosis factor monoclonal antibody (adalimumab) in Crohn's disease: the CLASSIC-I Trial. Gastroenterology 2006;130(2):323–33.

[26] Sandborn WJ, Hanauer S, Lukas M, et al. Maintenance of remission over 1 year in patients with active Crohn's disease treated with adalimumab: results of CLASSIC II, a blinded, placebo-controlled study. Gut 2005;54(Suppl VII):A81.

[27] Schreiber S, Khaliq-Kareemi M, Lawrance IC, et al. Certolizumab pegol, a humanized anti-TNF pegylated Fab' fragment, is safe and effective in the maintenance of response and remission following induction in active Crohn's disease: a phase III study (PRECISE). Gut 2005;54(Suppl VII):A82.

[28] Travis S, Yap LM, Hawkey C, et al. RDP58 is a novel and potentially effective oral therapy for ulcerative colitis. Inflamm Bowel Dis 2005;11(8):713–9.

[29] Ehrenpreis ED, Kane SV, Cohen LB, et al. Thalidomide therapy for patients with refractory Crohn's disease: an open-label trial [see comment]. Gastroenterology 1999;117(6): 1271–7.

[30] Vasiliauskas EA, Kam LY, Abreu-Martin MT, et al. An open-label pilot study of low-dose thalidomide in chronically active, steroid-dependent Crohn's disease [see comment]. Gastroenterology 1999;117(6):1278–87.

[31] Hommes D, van den Blink B, Plasse T, et al. Inhibition of stress-activated MAP kinases induces clinical improvement in moderate to severe Crohn's disease [see comment]. Gastroenterology 2002;122(1):7–14.

[32] Katz S. Update in medical therapy of ulcerative colitis: newer concepts and therapies. J Clin Gastroenterol 2005;39(7):557–69 [erratum: J Clin Gastroenterol 2005;39(9):843].

[33] Hanauer SB, Miner PB, Keshavarzian A, et al. Randomized, double-blind, placebo-controlled, parallel arm, safety and efficacy trial of once-daily, oral OPC-6535 in the treatment of active ulcerative colitis (UC). Gastroenterology 2004;126(4, Suppl 2):A112–3.

[34] Mannon PJ, Fuss IJ, Mayer L, et al. Anti-interleukin-12 antibody for active Crohn's disease [see comment]. N Engl J Med 2004;351(20):2069–79 [erratum: N Engl J Med 2005;352(12): 1276].

[35] Hommes D, Mikhajlova T, Stoinov S, et al. Fontolizumab (HuZaf), a humanized anti-IFN-gamma antibody, has clinical activity and excellent tolerability in moderate to severe Crohn's disease. Gastroenterology 2004;127(1):332.

[36] Kotsev I, de Villiers WJS, Katz S, et al. Fontolizumab (HuZAF), a humanized anti-IFN-gamma antibody, in patients with moderate to severe Crohn's disease (CD), is active and well tolerated in a multi-dose study. Gut 2005;54(Suppl VII):A19.

[37] Ito H, Takazoe M, Fukuda Y, et al. A pilot randomized trial of a human anti-interleukin-6 receptor monoclonal antibody in active Crohn's disease. Gastroenterology 2004;126(4): 989–96 [discussion: 947].

[38] Sands BE. Therapy of inflammatory bowel disease. Gastroenterology 2000;118(Suppl 1): S68–82.

[39] Jacobsohn DA, Vogelsang GB. Anti-cytokine therapy for the treatment of graft-versus-host disease. Curr Pharm Des 2004;10(11):1195–205.

[40] Van Assche G, Dalle I, Noman M, et al. A pilot study on the use of the humanized anti-interleukin-2 receptor antibody daclizumab in active ulcerative colitis. Am J Gastroenterol 2003;98(2):369–76.

[41] Creed TJ, Norman MR, Probert CS, et al. Basiliximab (anti-CD25) in combination with steroids may be an effective new treatment for steroid-resistant ulcerative colitis. Aliment Pharmacol Ther 2003;18(1):65–75.

[42] Panaccione R, Ferraz JG, Beck P. Advances in medical therapy of inflammatory bowel disease. Curr Opin Pharmacol 2005;5(6):566–72.

[43] Ghosh S, Goldin E, Gordon FH, et al. Natalizumab for active Crohn's disease [see comment]. N Engl J Med 2003;348(1):24–32.

[44] Sandborn WJ, Colombel JF, Enns R, et al. Natalizumab induction and maintenance therapy for Crohn's disease [see comment]. N Engl J Med 2005;353(18):1912–25.

[45] Berger JR, Koralnik IJ. Progressive multifocal leukoencephalopathy and natalizumab—unforeseen consequences [comment]. N Engl J Med 2005;353(4):414–6.

[46] Van Assche G, Van Ranst M, Sciot R, et al. Progressive multifocal leukoencephalopathy after natalizumab therapy for Crohn's disease [see comment]. N Engl J Med 2005;353(4): 362–8.

[47] Feagan BG, Greenberg GR, Wild G, et al. Treatment of ulcerative colitis with a humanized antibody to the alpha4beta7 integrin [see comment]. N Engl J Med 2005;352(24):2499–507.

[48] Yacyshyn BR, Bowen-Yacyshyn MB, Jewell L, et al. A placebo-controlled trial of ICAM-1 antisense oligonucleotide in the treatment of Crohn's disease. Gastroenterology 1998;114(6): 1133–42 [erratum: Gastroenterology 2001;121(3):747].

[49] Yacyshyn BR, Chey WY, Goff J, et al. Double blind, placebo controlled trial of the remission inducing and steroid sparing properties of an ICAM-1 antisense oligodeoxynucleotide, alicaforsen (ISIS 2302), in active steroid dependent Crohn's disease. Gut 2002;51(1):30–6.

[50] Yacyshyn BR, Barish C, Goff J, et al. Dose ranging pharmacokinetic trial of high-dose alicaforsen (intercellular adhesion molecule-1 antisense oligodeoxynucleotide) (ISIS 2302) in active Crohn's disease. Aliment Pharmacol Ther 2002;16(10):1761–70.

[51] Miner P, Wedel M, Bane B, et al. An enema formulation of alicaforsen, an antisense inhibitor of intercellular adhesion molecule-1, in the treatment of chronic, unremitting pouchitis. Aliment Pharmacol Ther 2004;19(3):281–6.

[52] van Deventer SJ, Volfova M, Flisiak R, et al. A phase 2 dose ranging, double-blind, placebo-controlled study of alicaforsen enema in subjects with acute exacerbation of mild to moderate left-sided ulcerative colitis. Gastroenterolgy 2005;128(Suppl 2):A74.

[53] Sands BE, Winston BD, Salzberg B, et al. Randomized, controlled trial of recombinant human interleukin-11 in patients with active Crohn's disease. Aliment Pharmacol Ther 2002; 16(3):399–406.

[54] Slonim AE, Bulone L, Damore MB, et al. A preliminary study of growth hormone therapy for Crohn's disease [see comment]. N Engl J Med 2000;342(22):1633–7.

[55] Sinha A, Nightingale J, West KP, et al. Epidermal growth factor enemas with oral mesalamine for mild-to-moderate left-sided ulcerative colitis or proctitis [see comment]. N Engl J Med 2003;349(4):350–7.

[56] Sandborn WJ, Sands BE, Wolf DC, et al. Repifermin (keratinocyte growth factor-2) for the treatment of active ulcerative colitis: a randomized, double-blind, placebo-controlled, dose-escalation trial. Aliment Pharmacol Ther 2003;17(11):1355–64.

[57] Korzenik JR, Dieckgraefe BK. Is Crohn's disease an immunodeficiency? A hypothesis suggesting possible early events in the pathogenesis of Crohn's disease. Dig Dis Sci 2000;45(6): 1121–9.

[58] Dieckgraefe BK, Korzenik JR, Husain A, et al. Association of glycogen storage disease 1b and Crohn disease: results of a North American survey. Eur J Pediatr 2002;161(Suppl 1): S88–92.

[59] Korzenik JR, Dieckgraefe BK. An open-labelled study of granulocyte colony-stimulating factor in the treatment of active Crohn's disease. Aliment Pharmacol Ther 2005;21(4): 391–400.

[60] Dieckgraefe BK, Korzenik JR. Treatment of active Crohn's disease with recombinant human granulocyte-macrophage colony-stimulating factor [see comment]. Lancet 2002; 360(9344):1478–80.

[61] Korzenik JR, Dieckgraefe BK, Valentine JF, et al. Sargramostim in Crohn's Disease Study G. Sargramostim for active Crohn's disease. N Engl J Med 2005;352(21):2193–201.

[62] Summers RW, Elliott DE, Urban JF Jr, et al. Trichuris suis therapy for active ulcerative colitis: a randomized controlled trial [see comment]. Gastroenterology 2005;128(4):825–32.

[63] Summers RW, Elliott DE, Urban JF Jr, et al. Trichuris suis therapy in Crohn's disease [see comment]. Gut 2005;54(1):87–90.

[64] Summers RW, Elliott DE, Qadir K, et al. Trichuris suis seems to be safe and possibly effective in the treatment of inflammatory bowel disease [see comment]. Am J Gastroenterol 2003; 98(9):2034–41.

[65] Elliott DE, Summers RW, Weinstock JV. Helminths and the modulation of mucosal inflammation. Curr Opin Gastroenterol 2005;21:51–8.

[66] Sawada K, Kusugami K, Suzuki Y, et al. Leukocytapheresis in ulcerative colitis: results of a multicenter double-blind prospective case-control study with sham apheresis as placebo treatment. Am J Gastroenterol 2005;100(6):1362–9.

[67] Hanai H, Watanabe F, Yamada M, et al. Adsorptive granulocyte and monocyte apheresis versus prednisolone in patients with corticosteroid-dependent moderately severe ulcerative colitis. Digestion 2004;70(1):36–44.

[68] Kawamura A, Saitoh M, Yonekawa M, et al. New technique of leukocytapheresis by the use of nonwoven polyester fiber filter for inflammatory bowel disease. Ther Apher 1999;3(4): 334–7.

ELSEVIER
SAUNDERS

SURGICAL
CLINICS OF
NORTH AMERICA

Surg Clin N Am 86 (2006) 1065–1092

Palliating Patients Who Have Unresectable Colorectal Cancer: Creating the Right Framework and Salient Symptom Management

Geoffrey P. Dunn, MD

*Department of Surgery and Palliative Care Consultation Service, Hamot Medical Center,
2050 South shore Drive, Erie, PA 16505, USA*

Over 56,000 individuals succumb to colorectal cancer each year in the United States [1], and many more thousands carry psychological, social, and spiritual burdens associated with all stages of this illness. Despite the availability of effective therapies for cancer pain, recognition of the importance of a patient-centered approach, and increasingly effective therapies for advanced disease, care for individuals who have advanced colorectal cancer has been acknowledged as a difficult problem in several reviews by colorectal surgeons [2,3]. Numerous reports have documented that medical care of those who have serious and advanced illness suffers from poor symptom control, conflicts in decision-making, lack of direction, and erosion of the patient family's physical, mental, and economic health [4–8]. The discrepancy between what is considered ideal care and what is often done suggests a much more profound barrier to successful palliation than simple lack of knowledge, technology, or interest on the part of surgeons. Nevertheless, there has been growing recognition by major surgical organizations of the importance of good palliative care [9–11], not only to patients and their families, but to surgical staff participating in their care. The key elements of palliative care—effective communication, diligent symptom control, and continuity of care—are well within the reach of practitioners and medical institutions, given a clear vision of the framework and context of palliative care. This article discusses the framework of palliative care for patients who have advanced colorectal malignancy, as well as specific interventions for selected symptoms and problems associated with it.

E-mail address: gpdunn1@earthlink.net

0039-6109/06/$ - see front matter © 2006 Elsevier Inc. All rights reserved.
doi:10.1016/j.suc.2006.05.008
surgical.theclinics.com

Palliation has been defined as making less serious, to make less severe without curing, to reduce the pain or intensity of, to mitigate, and alleviate. It comes from the Latin palliare, "to cloak or cover." Unfortunately, the adjective form, palliative, has been used in contrasting ways in surgical literature, reinforcing the deep-seated ambivalence many surgeons have towards palliative situations [12]. It has been used to describe: (1) surgery to relieve symptoms, knowing beforehand that all of the tumor could not be removed; (2) surgery in which microscopic or gross disease was knowingly or unknowingly left behind; and (3) surgery for recurrent or persistent disease after primary treatment failure (ie, "salvage surgery"). In addition to these discrepancies, the term is usually used as a description of the surgeon's intent, not a measurable result from the patient's perspective. The surgical literature, similar to the literature on palliative chemotherapy [13], offers scant guidance about the effectiveness of palliative interventions because of the lack of prospective, randomized controlled studies and the tendency to measure only survival and morbidity outcomes. Unlike survival, the only one who can truly answer if palliation has been achieved is the patient.

In a symposium on surgical palliative care [14], surgical oncologist Blake Cady succinctly outlined the rules of engagement for major palliative resections. The principles and considerations he discussed can be just as usefully applied to all palliative interventions, including nonsurgical therapies. He prefaced these by noting that one of the major reasons for continued follow-up in clinic and office after a initial curative treatment is for the continuation of emotional and psychological support of the patients. He discouraged "technical" follow-up—the routine post-treatment procession of tumor markers, blood studies, radiographs, and scans that contribute nothing to the long-term success of patients after initial curative multidisciplinary measures. While cautioning against overlooking opportunities for cure (ie, resection of a solitary liver metastasis from a colorectal cancer with favorable biological characteristics), he noted that the decision to intervene for cure recognizes that recurrent disease is a pattern- and not a time-dependent phenomenon. Recognizing this, ongoing searches for asymptomatic metastases are not useful. If the patient is asymptomatic, palliation is not needed. Pre-emptive palliation assumes suffering is as predictably preventable as disease. This may be true in some cases, but it will require a methodology of proof that has not yet been developed.

For surgeons seeking perspective when making management decisions for palliative care, Cady commented, "It is easier to make day-to-day surgical decisions in the framework of some overall surgical philosophy. Certainly if you have a mature surgical philosophy that understands the vicissitudes of life, you're better equipped to deal with some of these situations than a surgeon who thinks that 'I can cure all problems'" [14]. To proceed with palliative interventions, the surgeon must understand three key elements: (1) the psychology of the particular patient, (2) the biology of the disease, and (3) the effectiveness of the particular operation. Each of these elements is considered through weighing alternative examples. A summary of his approach to decision making with some expansion is tabulated in Table 1.

Cady completed his advice on cautioning not to allow the patient to think we [surgeons] are magicians. Good guidance for palliation will always include some type of nonsurgical therapy. The goals of palliation must be clearly and honestly explained to your patient, your team, and especially your residents and referring physicians.

Palliative care needs assessment

The immediate goal of patient assessment in end-of-life care is to permit the relief of suffering, though an additional goal is the identification of sources of strength that may be helpful for the patient and family. Trauma care has shown how well surgeons can make assessments of complicated situations in an emotionally charged atmosphere. Making a palliative assessment can foster enough trust that the surgeon may be asked by the previously hesitant patient for information about prognosis and what symptoms to expect as a result of progressing disease. A useful palliative assessment must reflect more than the physical problems, even if they dominate the immediate picture. Each surgeon has his own comfort level for the degree to which he explores the nonphysical concerns, but with experience and reinforcement, the

Table 1
Decision making for palliative interventions

Element of decision making	Considerations
Psyche of the patient	Active versus passive
	Mature versus panicked
	Realistic versus magical thinking
Physiology of the patient	Functional versus debilitated
	Actual age versus chronologic age
	Preserved nutrition versus hypoalbuminemic
Biology of the disease	Single disease versus multiple comorbidities
	Slow-growing versus aggressive
Nature of the intervention	Evidence-based versus "N of one" (personal anecdotal experience)
	Routine versus uncommon
	Low versus high morbidity risk (physical, financial, social)
	Straight-forward versus difficult procedure
	One of many options versus no other option
Profile of the surgeon	Empathic healer versus technician
	Experienced versus inexperienced
	Cautious versus "cowboy"
	Realistic versus magical thinking or projecting
	Collegial versus isolated and dominating

Modified from Cady B, Easson A, Aboulafia A, et al. Part 1: Surgical palliation of advanced illness—what's new, what's helpful. J Am Coll Surg 2005;200(1):115–27.

surgeon will experience an increased sense of satisfaction with his increasing depth of participation in discussion about the other dimensions.

Assessment for palliative care can be seen as a staging procedure for the dimensions of distress, analogous to the approach used to stage the extent of disease. Along with the stepwise procedure for giving bad news, it should be considered part of the surgeon's cognitive operative repertoire. Following the general guidelines for communication outlined by Buckman in his land-mark book, *How to Break Bad News* [15], a thorough assessment for palli-ative care can be done in the amount of time it takes to do a secondary survey using advanced trauma life support (ATLS) protocol.

Staging for palliative care not only provides a reliable patient-centered platform for further interventions, but also creates a unique bond between the practitioner making the assessment and the individual assessed, not un-like that which forms between a surgeon and an individual she has operated on. Because of the inherent vulnerability of a patient revealing his innermost fears and yearnings while in a physically precarious condition, this interven-tion is as invasive as any physical operation, and deserves the same attention and skill. The procedure of exploring and staging an individual's perception of life is based on many small, careful steps and a few big steps, any one of which could be irreversible.

Delivery models of palliative care

There are two formal delivery models of palliative care in the US medical system that surgeons should be aware of in their capacities of consultant and primary physician. The first of these is hospice, which has been recognized and compensated through Medicare legislation since 1983; the other model is palliative care support (eg, consult services, clinics, and designated in-hos-pital units), which can be seen as an application of the hospice model to a wider spectrum of illness without the restraint of prognostic consider-ations. Both delivery models share the following features: (1) patient/family is the unit of care, (2) relief of distress and promotion of quality of life is the clinical goal, and (3) care is provided using an interdisciplinary approach. A hospice program provides palliative care for terminally ill patients and their families. All hospice programs are palliative care programs, but palliative care is not limited to terminally ill patients. Palliative care consultation in hospitals and in outpatient settings has became increasingly available since the later 1990s because of increasing public interest in improved end-of-life care and the favorable impact on patient care made by hospice programs in this country since its introduction to this country in the later 1970s. Pallia-tive care can be given concurrently with all other appropriate medical care.

Palliative care programs have proliferated rapidly in the United States since 2000 [16], numbering about 1,027 (in 25% of hospitals) in 2003. Some of these programs are directed by and actively supported by surgeons. Palliative care programs were more likely to be offered in larger hospitals, teaching hospitals, veterans' hospitals, and hospitals designated as American College of Surgeons' Commission on Cancer approved cancer hospitals.

Multiple reviews [17–21] have documented improved pain and non-pain symptom management, improved patient and family satisfaction, reduced critical care unit and hospital stay, decreased in-hospital deaths, and significant cost reductions. A high rate of implementation of recommendations from palliative care teams has been noted [22]. Currently, fewer than 2000 physicians are certified in palliative care in the United States—far fewer than necessary to staff existing and future palliative care and hospice programs. Participation by surgeons as medical consultants, volunteers, and referral sources would greatly help in bridging this gap.

Criteria for palliative care referral include: (1) patient/family request, (2) "triggered" referrals (ie, protocols that initiate a referral of any patient in an intensive care setting over a defined period of time, or any patient who has a Karnofsky status of less than 50), or (3) by clinician judgment for a given patient. Palliative care consultation referral criteria are listed in Box 1. Some hospitals have designated units for palliative care; others use a consultative model, often in conjunction with pain management services, with or without a designated unit.

For any individual whose treatment is palliative and no longer life-prolonging, hospice referral from the hospital or outpatient setting should be considered if there is a physician-certified prognosis of less than 6 months

---

Box 1. Indications for palliative care consultation

- Patient has an illness typified by progressive deterioration and worsening symptoms, often ending fatally.
- Patient has limiting/threatening conditions with declining functional status, mental or cognitive function.
- Suboptimal control of pain or other distressing symptoms
- Patient/family would benefit from clarification of goals and plan of care, or resolution of ethical dilemmas.
- Patient/surrogate declines further invasive or curative procedures, preferring comfort-oriented symptom management only.
- Patients on medical/surgical or critical care units who are expected to die imminently or shortly following hospital discharge
- Bereavement support of hospital workers, particularly after the death of a colleague

Courtesy of Robert A. Milch, MD, Buffalo, NY

if the disease pursues its usual course. Eligibility requirements for Medicare hospice benefit are listed in Box 2. Any terminal diagnosis is appropriate as long as its prognosis of 6 months or less is confirmed by two physicians. A do not (attempt to) resuscitate order (DNR or DNAR) is not required for enrollment into a hospice program, nor is it allowed to be under Medicare regulations. The presence of a DNR order has been mistakenly used as a marker for preferences about end-of-life care [23]. As a practical matter, most patients or surrogates who have had appropriate counseling prior to election of hospice care are prepared to discuss and authorize a DNR order.

Another inaccurate belief about hospice and palliative care is that it emphasizes withdrawal of burdensome care and usage of sedatives and opioids. Theoretically, no treatments are automatically excluded from consideration by hospices as long as the criterion for a treatment rests on its proven ability to achieve symptom control, regardless of its impact on the underlying disease process. Depending on the resources and size of the hospice program (Medicare reimbursement is only $125 per day per patient under its capitated system [24]), services vary. Hospice benefit team members and services are listed in Box 3. Benefits may include the options of intravenous (IV) and total parenteral nutrition (TPN) therapy, chemotherapeutic agents, and transfusion. Despite the effectiveness of some surgical procedures such as gastrointestinal (GI) tract stenting, video-assisted thoracoscopy (VATS), and open fixation of pathologic fractures, they are not usually considered for patients enrolled in hospice. Possible reasons for this include: (1) lateness of hospice referrals, with survival of only a few weeks to days, despite the hospice admission criterion that allows patients who have up to 6 months life expectancy; (2) cost of the interventions that is prohibitive given the limited resources of many hospice programs; and (3) hospice professionals' lack of familiarity with palliative surgical techniques.

Although a consulting surgeon may not be in a position to make a direct referral to palliative care or hospice services, the surgeon's interest and support for these interventions on behalf of a patient, when indicated, will be deeply appreciated by the patient and his family. Recommendations made

---

Box 2. Eligibility for Medicare hospice benefit

- Patient is eligible for Medicare Part A.
- Two physicians must certify that patient has a condition whose prognosis is associated with a survival of 6 months or less if the illness pursues its natural course.
- Patient (surrogate if patient not competent) must sign form electing hospice benefit.
- Hospice care must be provided by a Medicare-certified hospice program.

Box 3. Medicare hospice benefit team and services

Core team members
- Physician
- Registered nurse
- Social worker
- Pastoral (spiritual) or other counselor
- Minimum percentage of volunteer hours required

Services
- Pain and non-pain symptom management
- Assistance of patient and family with the emotional, social, and spiritual aspects of dying
- Provides medications for control of symptoms, medical supplies, and durable medical equipment.
- Education of family on care of the patient
- Specialized therapy services (speech, massage, and physical therapy)
- Short-term inpatient care (respite care) when pain or symptoms are unmanageable at home, or when caregiver needs respite
- Bereavement care for surviving family and friends for 1 year from the date of the death

---

for these interventions are quite likely to be heeded if the surgeon's relationship with them has been positive.

Symptoms management of advanced colorectal cancer

Symptom burden is high with advanced cancer, and an increasing number of symptoms correlates with higher degrees of psychologic distress and poorer quality of life [25]. Symptoms are classified as cancer-related, cancer treatment-related, and non-cancer–related. As a general rule, physical symptoms that are immediately distracting are addressed before nonphysical symptoms, which may ultimately be more significant for the individual if not mitigated. Intervention is not deferred until definitive diagnosis and treatment plan is made, but should begin promptly while the evaluation is initiated, especially when symptoms are severe. Symptoms from comorbid illness can trump cancer-related symptoms and should be triaged accordingly (ie, severe dyspnea from advanced chronic obstructive pulmonary disease [COPD] triages to a higher priority of treatment than mild cancer-related pain).

Most of the symptoms of advanced colorectal cancer are encountered in non-GI cancers, with the important exceptions of GI tract obstruction and fistula. Symptom management is the work of palliative care, but not its goal.

Although new assessment scales for specific symptoms and quality of life are continuously being introduced and revised, validated and culturally specific instruments should be used whenever possible, especially in the setting of clinical research. Well-known and validated assessment scales include the Functional Assessment of Cancer—General Version (FACT G) [26] and the Edmonton Symptom Assessment System (ESAS) [27].

The Karnofsky scale, well known to oncologists, assesses physical function, not degree of distress or success of palliation. Numerous studies have correlated low Karnofsky scores with shortened survival in advanced cancer. It has been used, sometimes naïvely, as an index of quality of life because of this association; however, loss of physical function does not necessarily preclude quality of life, and preservation of physical function does not guarantee it.

Pain

The incidence of pain in advanced colorectal cancer is not known, though up to 90% of individuals in some categories of advanced cancer report pain [28], often severe [29], and often undertreated [30,31]. Barriers to effective pain management have been extensively discussed. Fears shared by all participants in the patient encounter have created many of these. Some of these fears are based on lack of information or exaggeration of known risks, whereas others are based on the psychology of life-limiting disease. Fear of addiction, fear of respiratory suppression, and fear of scrutiny by regulatory agencies have been consistently identified as barriers. More subtle barriers are rooted in the association of opioids with imminent demise, because of medical practice in the past ("They got the morphine out when he only had a few days left.") and the reluctance of a patient (or caregiver) to acknowledge progressing disease as the reason for escalation of dose. The differential diagnosis for "refractory" cancer pain includes denial or avoidance of the recognition of progressing disease by either patient or care giver.

Pain is classified into acute or chronic, nociceptive (somatic and visceral) or neuropathic. Some pain syndromes are a mix of each of these groupings. The classification has therapeutic implications because of the differing underlying physiologic mechanisms of each class. The potential causes of pain in patients who have advanced colorectal cancer include pain from cancer, pain from cancer-related treatments, and pain unrelated to cancer. Mechanisms of pain include tumor infiltration, including direct infiltration of nerves; malignant bowel obstruction (MBO); inflammatory changes; chemotherapy or surgically induced neuropathy; hepatic capsular distention; and nonmalignant causes.

The clinical expression and the psychology of chronic pain differs from acute pain. The visible signs of increased sympathetic discharge—grimacing, pallor, tachycardia, and high blood pressure—observable and measurable in acute pain, are muted or absent in chronic pain, giving the misleading impression that "He does not look like he is in pain." The psychological and existential impact of acute pain that has evolved to chronic pain can be summarized as the distress of having an unpleasant sensory-emotional experience that has outlived its purposefulness. For some unfortunate individuals, chronic pain becomes a metaphor for life itself, which may in some way be linked to their increased risk of depression and suicide.

Improved cancer pain management is an institutional responsibility as well as the surgeon's individual moral and professional responsibility. In the summary of the American Pain Society Recommendations for Improving the Quality of Acute and Cancer Pain Management [32], the authors, based on a systematic review of quality improvement in pain management from 1994 to 1994, recommend that "all care settings should formulate a structured, multilevel systems approach (sensitive to the type of pain and setting of care) that focuses on five primary areas: (1) prompt recognition and treatment of pain, (2) involvement of patients in the pain management plan, (3) improved treatment patterns, (4) regular reassessment and adjustment of the pain management plan as needed, and (5) measurement of processes and outcomes of pain management."

Physicians believe that their failure to manage pain effectively is related to their inability to assess it properly [29]. Twycross [33] proposed a mnemonic, modified by Ray [34]: PQRSTU (think of an EKG of a hypokalemic patient!). Table 2 outlines this mnemonic for initial and subsequent pain assessment. Pain assessment should include some acknowledgement of the three nonphysical types of pain: (1) psychological, (2) social (economic), and (3) spiritual. The sum of physical and nonphysical pain has been frequently referred to in the palliative care literature as "total pain" [35].

The numerous mechanisms of cancer-related pain provide numerous targets for pharmacotherapy and other types of intervention for the relief of pain. Depending on the nature of the symptoms and the tolerances and wishes of the patient, any single agent or combination of agents can be used for the management of pain, in addition to achieving other goals of therapy such as prolonged survival (chemotherapy), improved appetite (steroids), or control of fever (nonsteroidals). Cytotoxic chemotherapy, nonsteroidal anti-inflammatory agents (NSAIDs), steroidal agents, antidepressants, and opioid analgesics, have been used singly or in combination for the relief of cancer pain or cancer treatment-related pain.

All of these modalities have the potential for major side effects, including death, which have to be anticipated in this vulnerable patient population that frequently has major comorbidities. Therapeutic nihilism, often directed towards the "terminal" patient in the hospital, nursing home, and hospice setting, should not discourage the surgeon from pursuing uncommonly used pain management strategies known to be highly effective for certain pain syndromes when simpler approaches are inadequate (eg, using axial analgesia via an epidural catheter instead of high-dose systemic opioids with debilitating side-effects). By contrast, caution must be exercised when

Table 2
PQRSTU mnemonic for assessment of pain

Provoked or palliated by	What makes pain better? Worse? Effect of position, climate, company, prayer, meditation, procedures

Quality of pain	Have patient describe quality of pain in own words:
	• Nocioceptive
	  Somatic (skin, muscle, bone): described as achy, stabbing, throbbing.
	  Visceral (bowel, bladder): described as crampy, gnawing, achy, sharp
	• Neuropathic (nerve damage)
	  Burning, tingling, sharp, shooting, electric shock-like
	  Quality of pain can give clue to etiology and guide selection of analgesic:
	• Nociceptive pain generally responds to opioids and anti-inflammatory agents.
	• Neuropathic pain is less responsive to opioids and may require addition of an adjuvant agent (tricyclic antidepressant or anticonvulsant).

Region and referral	Guides imaging and regional therapies
Severity	Visual analogue scale (VAS): 0–10. Patient is asked to rank pain: 0=no pain, 10=worst pain imaginable • Mild pain=1–3 • Moderate pain=4–6 • Severe pain=7–10, pain emergency Severity ranking can be used to guide pace of titration; eg, if pain is "severe," opioid dose can be increased up to 50%–100% over a 24-hour period.
Temporal	Need to know for identifying end-of-dose failure of analgesic
Utilized medications	What has worked or not worked and why. Opportunity to clarify confusion of "allergy" with drug side-effects

Adapted from Ray JB. Pharmacologic management of pain. Surg Onc Clin N Am 2001;10(1):73–4.

prescribing the familiar: NSAIDs such as ibuprofen, available over the counter, can lead to renal compromise, GI hemorrhage, and platelet dysfunction.

NSAIDS are effective in the management of cancer pain [36]. They are included in the first step of the World Health Organization (WHO) step-ladder for cancer pain control [37], outlined in Box 4. They can be given concurrently with opioids, but should not be given to patients receiving corticosteroids or anticoagulants, or to thrombocytopenic patients. NSAIDs should be avoided in patients who have renal impairment, congestive heart failure, and liver disease. Extreme caution is also advised in the treatment of the elderly. The risk of renal impairment from NSAIDs is increased in patients of advanced age, those with pre-existing renal impairment, heart failure, hepatic dysfunction, or hypovolemia; those with concomitant therapy with other nephrotoxic agents (including diuretics); and those with elevated angiotensin II or catecholamine levels [38]. Toxicity is the most significant factor limiting long-term use [39]. Major complications are not necessarily preceded by minor ones.

Box 4. World Health Organization's analgesic ladder: "By mouth, by the clock, by the ladder, with attention to detail"

Step 1: mild pain, visual analogue scale (VAS) 1–3
- Acetaminophen, aspirin, NSAIDs
- May add a nonopioid analgesic or an adjuvant agent. Adjuvant or coanalgesic agents are drugs that enhance analgesic efficacy of opioids, treat concurrent symptoms that exacerbate pain, or provide independent analgesia for specific types of pain [36] (eg, a tricyclic antidepressant for treatment of neuropathic pain).

Step 2: moderate pain, VAS 4–6
- Acetaminophen or aspirin compounded with hydrocodone, codeine, oxycodone, dihydrocodeine
- NSAIDs as used in Step 1
- May add a nonopioid analgesic or an adjuvant agent

Step 3: Severe pain, VAS 7–10, pain emergency
- Morphine: "gold standard"; most flexibility in dosing forms
- Hydromorphone: useful in renal failure patients and for subcutaneous infusions
- Oxycodone: no IV form; growing stigma due to illicit use
- Fentanyl: extremely fast-acting, transcutaneous dosing available
- Methadone: cheap and effective; not a first-line agent
- Levorphanol (rarely used)
- NSAIDs as used in Step 1
- May add a nonopioid analgesic or an adjuvant agent

Opioids are the mainstay of steps two and three of the WHO ladder (Table 3). Initiating them does not preclude ongoing use of nonopioid agents. Reassurance that use of opioids for the management of pain will not cause addiction is frequently necessary to encourage compliance. It is helpful to distinguish physical dependence from addiction to reinforce this. This also educates patients about the dangers of voluntary or unintended sudden withdrawal of opioids. Physical dependence is neuroadaptation to exogenous opioids, usually occurring after continuous dosing over 7 to 10 days. Sudden termination of exogenous opioids or administration of opioid-reversing agents (naloxone) precipitates an abstinence syndrome that is, somewhat misleadingly, the very picture of the popular stereotype of the heroin addict: bodily aches, abdominal pain, cutis anserina (goose flesh), sweating, nausea, vomiting, diarrhea, psychosis, hallucinations, diarrhea, tachycardia, and hypertension. Precipitation of the abstinence

Table 3
Approximate opioid equivalences for management of moderate to severe pain. This conversion chart is a guideline only. Inter- and intra-individual variability of response to opioids requires the dose to be individualized and titrated to effect.

Analgesic	IM, SC, IV route (mg)	PO route (mg)	Comments
Morphine	10	30	Immediate and controlled-release formulation available. Analgesic metabolite, M6G, can accumulate with renal impairment, producing prolonged analgesia. Accumulation of analgesically inactive metabolite M3G may cause neurotoxicity (myoclonus, hyperalgesia, cognitive dysfunction).
Fentanyl	10 mcg IV ≈ 1 mg IV morphine 25 mcg/hr patch q72h ≈ 50 mg oral morphine/24h		Short half-life, but at steady state, slow elimination from tissues can lead to prolonged half-life (up to 12 hours). Opioid-naïve patients should not be started with more than 12 mcg/hr transdermally.
Hydromorphone	1.5	7.5	Useful alternative to morphine, but oral dosing impractical for very high doses because of tablet burden/dose. Tolerated by patients with renal impairment.
Methadone [87]	Ratios relative to methadone depend on the dose of the previous opioid		If daily morphine dose before switch is 30–90 mg, estimated dose ratio (EDR) = 4:1 (ie, 4 mg morphine = 1mg methadone); 90–300 mg morphine, EDR = 8:1; above 300 mg morphine, EDR = 12:1. Methadone has a variable and long half-life. Dosing interval every 8–12 hours.
Oxycodone	–	20	Immediate and controlled-release formulation available. Used for moderate pain when combined with nonopioid (Step 2, WHO Analgesic Ladder). Can be used like oral morphine for severe pain when used as a single entity. (Step 3, WHO Analgesic Ladder)

Dosing information adapted from Principles of analgesic use in acute pain and cancer pain, 5th edition. American Pain Society; Glenview, Illinois. 2003. p. 1–74.

syndrome should be anticipated when rapidly withdrawing opioids following procedures that significantly reduce pain (anesthetic blockade).

The converse of this situation is the syndrome of opioid overdosage that can emerge as the result of marked opioid sparing following a pain-reducing procedure without a reduction of the previous opioid dose.

Both of these scenarios can occur in a patient who has a painful sacral recurrence of rectal cancer and who has been treated with high doses of systemic opioids, and then undergoes a successful anesthetic block. Close monitoring with frequent and careful evaluation is necessary for a period of 12 to 24 hours following pain-ablating procedures done to patients receiving chronic opioid therapy.

True addiction has been defined as "a primary, chronic, neurobiological disease, with genetic, psychological, and environmental factors influencing its development and manifestations. It is characterized by behaviors that include one or more of the following: impaired control over drug use, compulsive use, continued use despite harm, and craving" [40]. Drug dependence is physiologic and adaptive; drug addiction is pathologic.

Whenever opioid doses are adjusted, it is important to explain the reason to patients, especially when death appears imminent. Patients often erroneously assume that the reason for dose escalation is tolerance to the drug instead of progressing disease, almost always the real reason. It is critical that patients near death and their caregivers understand that the purpose of the opioids is the relief of pain (or dyspnea), not deliberate hastening of death; however, according to the US Supreme Court's 1997 opinion in Vaco v Quill [41], the hastening of death resulting from the use of opioids for palliation of pain should not be a deterrent to their use.

When initiating opioid therapy, common side effects should be anticipated and discussed. Counseling about and prophylaxis for possible opioid side effects increases compliance. Constipation is a universal opioid side effect to which tolerance does not develop (the "other" neurologic crisis besides unrelieved pain!). Prophylaxis for constipation should be started at the commencement of opioid therapy using a stool softener and a stimulant laxative such as senna. Bulk-forming agents such as psyllium or methylcellulose should be avoided, because of their propensity to form impactions with decreased fluid intake. Nausea is a frequent side effect of opioids; tolerance usually develops within a few days. Opioid-induced nausea can be pre-empted by use of an antiemetic, a useful maneuver in patients who have a history of opioid-induced nausea. Stimulants (methylphenidate) can be used for persistent opioid-induced sedation, another opioid side-effect to which tolerance normally develops fairly quickly.

The most feared opioid side effect is respiratory depression. Tolerance to this, fortunately, develops quickly, making it an uncommon problem with chronic usage. The risk of respiratory depression is greatest in the opioid-naïve, the elderly, patients who have impaired renal function, and those receiving sedating medications. Because respiratory depression is always preceded by increasing sedation with opioid overdosage, careful monitoring provides the opportunity to stop the agent until it is metabolized, and then resume it at a lower dose. This is much less traumatic then full opioid reversal, which can precipitate opioid withdrawal syndrome and abrupt return of severe pain. When opioid reversal is necessary, dilute a 0.4 mg ampoule of naloxone with 10 ml saline and give 1 ml of this solution every 5 minutes until partial reversal has occurred [42]. This may need to be repeated.

Because of the potential for dose-limiting side effects and reluctance of many patients to escalate opioid doses, a strategy using the least amount of opioid necessary for relief of pain is employed. Nonopioids and other treatment modalities can be used with opioids for "opioid sparing" to accomplish this. An example of this is the concurrent use of systemic opioids in conjunction with regional therapies such as external beam radiation or epidural anesthesia.

Although many patients and surgeons are familiar with oxycodone as a component of frequently prescribed compound medications for postoperative pain, they may not be aware that the acetaminophen content of compound drugs (usually 325 mg) limits their use for cancer pain management. The maximum 24-hour allowance for acetaminophen in an adult who had no liver disease or heavy alcohol consumption is 3000 mg. The amount would be even less in the elderly. In a compound containing 325 mg of acetaminophen and 5 mg of oxycodone, the maximum daily amount of oxycodone that could be given as an agent compounded with acetaminophen without incurring acetaminophen toxicity would be less than 50 mg—far short of what is often required for the effective relief of cancer pain. In instances where oxycodone is prescribed, using the uncompounded form is recommended to avoid potential acetaminophen toxicity and to provide greater flexibility in dosing for breakthrough pain and conversion to long-acting forms.

Two other medications encountered commonly in surgical practice, dolophine and meperidine, have no role in cancer pain management because of potential side-effects of their metabolites that can occur in the presence of renal compromise, particularly in the elderly.

Codeine is of limited usefulness in cancer pain management for several reasons. Codeine is metabolized to morphine, accounting, in part, for its analgesic property, though 7% of Caucasians genetically lack this capacity [43]. It has unpredictable intramuscular absorption and cannot be given intravenously. It is sold compounded, limiting its use to the ceiling dose of acetaminophen in the compound. Some studies have shown increasing untoward side-effects for doses above that, yet diminishing returns for analgesic effect [44].

Use of codeine for cancer patients should be restricted to perioperative pain control for procedure-related pain that will resolve (eg, laparoscopy, hernia repair; as an induction analgesic agent for mild to moderate cancer pain; and control of cough and diarrhea).

The pronounced anti-inflammatory properties of steroids (hydrocortisone, dexamethasone) have made them useful as adjuvants to management of cancer pain complicated by neural compromise, especially if there are other symptoms such as anorexia, nausea, and generalized malaise that may also respond to them. Future palliative care research should look more closely at the relationship between tumor necrosis factor (TNF) levels and palliation outcomes, based on the suppressive property steroids are known to have upon TNF production and the presence of TNF in many of the cytokine mediated metabolic pathways generating systemic symptoms of advanced cancer. Activation of some of the same pathways can also result from systemic cancer treatments.

The use of steroids must be considered in light of several possible significant side-effects that include immunosuppression, peptic ulceration, hypergylcemia, psychological disturbances, and myopathy. Prophylaxis against peptic ulceration is provided by concurrent use of a proton pump inhibitor.

Although the large majority (>80%) of patients who have cancer pain will have their pain well-controlled using the WHO stepladder approach [45], some patients will require procedural interventions for control of pain because of failure to respond or presence of unacceptable side-effects with pharmacotherapy. These interventions run the spectrum from direct approaches correcting, reducing, or bypassing pathology to approaches directed towards the neural basis of pain. Interventions can be operative or minimally invasive operative procedures, percutaneous interventions, and radiation therapy.

The description of specific interventions is beyond the scope of this article.

Amersi and colleagues have recently written an excellent review [46] of operative and "minimally invasive" interventions for the palliation of symptoms from advanced colorectal malignancy. They point out that studies have previously been nonrandomized, case-control descriptions or case series that may have an inherent selection bias. Despite the diverse menu of operative interventions reviewed, they conclude that the best approach to palliation is one that is individualized, interdisciplinary, and incorporates surgical and nonsurgical modalities. Recent evidence has shown that formal education in palliative care significantly influences surgical judgment [47].

Radiation therapy has been used to mitigate symptoms of pain, bleeding, obstruction, and fistula in advanced colorectal malignancy. The morbidity of treatment is related to the anatomic position of the region treated, the radiation field, and dose. A standard treatment regimen for symptomatic recurrent rectal disease, a particularly anguishing problem, consists of 40 Gy in 20 fractions to 54 Gy in 30 fractions, often with systemic cytotoxic chemotherapy to enhance radiation response [48]. Morbidity from radiation, immediate and delayed, include strictures, fistula, bleeding, and ulcers. Pharmacologic palliation of side effects from palliative radiation therapy is usually possible. Endoscopic and surgical interventions are reserved for more extreme complications in patients who have better prognosis.

Bonica and Benedetti [49] have proposed two additional steps to the WHO analgesic stepladder for "very severe" and "excruciating" categories of pain, which, if present at presentation, allow for immediate bypassing of steps for control of pain. These additional steps, in addition to potent opioid analgesics and coanalgesics, include neurolytic blocks, central nervous system (CNS) stimulation procedures, and neurosurgery.

Nausea and vomiting

Nausea and vomiting is a common symptom complex in advanced cancer [50], with a prevalence reported at 40% during the last 6 weeks of life [51]. It can occur as a symptom with an identifiable etiology (opioids, bowel obstruction) or as a chronic syndrome characterized by some authors as a manifestation of autonomic failure [52]. Similar to pain management, knowledge of the physiology of nausea and vomiting allowing targeting of specific receptors is helpful in the selection of therapy. Though closely related, nausea should be seen as a separate entity from vomiting, because each is a distinct subjective experience and has an anatomically distinct locus in the CNS associated with it. The central mediation of nausea and vomiting is located in two centers—the chemoreceptor trigger zone (CTZ), which senses distress; and the vomiting center (VC), which responds to the distress. Both of these areas are extensively integrated with the rest of the central nervous system, with far-ranging sympathetic and parasympathetic input. In addition, the metabolic milieu of the body is continuously presented to the exquisitely sensitive chemosensors of the CTZ through their direct contact with cerebrospinal fluid. The psychological and practical implications of the two centers differing roles (nausea center = distress, vomiting center = "fighting back") are helpful in counseling patients about the management of nausea and vomiting, particularly in the nonoperative management of MBO [53].

The VOMIT acronym (Vestibular, Obstruction, Motility, Inflammatory, Toxins) [54] is a somewhat graphic way of classifying the etiologies of nausea and vomiting. For each etiologic class, specific receptors for nausea are implicated providing the rationale for the use of the blockers specific for the receptors (Table 4). The identification of activity in the inferior frontal gyrus of the cortex (association cortex) during the sensation of nausea [55] demonstrates the importance of cortical input for this perception, and suggests a rationale for therapies directed towards this region of the central nervous system (eg, anxiolytics for anticipatory nausea).

Although the management of nausea and vomiting in the setting of advanced colorectal cancer is heavily weighted towards pharmacotherapy, nonpharmacologic approaches, pending formal evidence-based confirmation of their efficacy, should be encouraged if the therapy is not known to induce harm. Chronic nausea is a psychologically debilitating symptom. Anything that fosters a sense of hope, even openness to trials of complementary therapies, is welcomed by patients. Openness develops the basis of trust

Table 4
VOMIT acronym. Nausea and vomiting: etiologies, receptors, drugs

Etiology	Receptors	Blockers/stimulants
Vestibular autonomic failure, hypovolemia	Cholinergic, histaminic	Scopolamine patch, promethazine
Obstruction constipation, but not mechanical obstruction	Cholinergic, histaminic, 5HT3	Senna products (stimulate myenteric plexus)
Motility Upper intestinal tract dysmotility	Cholinergic, Histaminic, 5HT3	Metoclopropamide (contraindicated in mechanical bowel obstruction)
Inflammatory Infection, inflammation (radiation therapy)	Cholinergic, Histaminic, 5HT3. Neurokinin 1	Promethazine
Toxins Opioids, chemotherapy, uremia, digitalis	Dopamine 2, 5HT3	Prochlorperazine, haloperidol, odansetron (no established superiority as first-line agent, expensive)

Adapted from Hallenbeck J. Fast fact and concept #5: Causes of nausea and vomiting (V.O.M.I.T.). August 2005, 2nd edition. End-of-Life Physician Education Resource Center. Available at: www.eperc.mcw.edu.

necessary to encourage consideration of more aggressive approaches, including operative and chemotherapy interventions.

Bowel obstruction

The management of MBO from advanced cancer is the paradigmatic challenge of surgical palliative care (Table 5). Surgeons who have opened the abdominal cavity and have been greeted by straw-colored ascites and the tactile sensation of diffuse tumor studding of the peritoneum know the sinking feeling: "What am I doing here? I wish I could have avoided this. Now what am I going to do?"

Colorectal cancer accounts for approximately 10% to 28% of instances of MBO [56]. MBO is a heterogeneous clinical syndrome whose management is influenced by the levels of obstruction, the pattern of disease, clinical features of the disease related to prognosis, prior treatment, and patient preferences. Management decisions must also account for the possibility of a benign etiology for bowel obstruction in the patient who have previously diagnosed malignancy; the incidence of benign causes of obstruction in these patients approaches 50% in some series [57].

Plain film radiography remains the initial evaluation of patients who have suspected bowel obstruction. It can accurately diagnose small bowel obstruction up to 60% of the time [58]. The diagnostic findings of bowel obstruction, dilated loops of small bowel, multiple air fluid levels on upright

Table 5
Pharmacotherapy of malignant bowel obstruction (MBO)

Drug	Action	Dose
Opioids (morphine, hydromorphone)	Antiperistaltic effect reduces cramping, targets pain from bowel distention or tumor invasion.	Titrate to relief of pain. Both can be given PO, SC, IV, or SL (see Table 4 for PO to IV or SC conversion ratios).
Antisecretory agents (octreotide, scopolamine, glycopyrrolate)	(1) Octreotide minimizes volume of emeses (2) Minimize gut distention by reducing gastrointestinal secretions. (3) Anticholinergic antisecretory agents slow gut peristalsis, making them effective for abdominal cramping.	Octreotide: 0.3 mg/day SC. Can betitrated up to 0.6 mg/day. Can be given as infusion or scheduled BID dosing. Favored for rapid reduction of GI secretions. Expensive. Scopolamine: 1–2 patches every 3 days. Anticholinergic side effects include dry mouth, urinary retention, confusion. Convenient. Glycopyrrolate: start at 0.1 to 0.2 mg Q6hr SC PRN adjusted to renal and hepatic function [86]. Some anticholiergic side-effects, though no CNS effects, unlike scopolamine
Central-acting antiemetics (haloperidol chlorpromazine, hydroxyzine)	Relief of nausea	Haloperidol: 5 to 15 mg/day SC, IV, or PO. Chlorpromazine: 25 to 100 mg TID PO, PR, or IV. Use if sedation desired. Avoid above in patients with Parkinsonism or patients taking other drugs with potential Parkinsonian side-effects (ie, metoclopropamide). Dystonia can be reversed with diphenhydramine 1 mg/kg or benztropine 0.02–0.05 mg/kg/ dose, (maximum = 4 mg IV) Hydroxyzine: 100–200 mg/day PO, SC, or IV.
Steroids (dexamethasone)	(1) Central antiemetic effect (2) Reduces inflammatory component of tumor causing mechanical bowel obstruction (3) Appetite stimulant	Dexamethasone: 12–16 mg/day. Discontinue if no relief after 5 days. Helpful for concommitant pain from hepatic distention from metastases or symptomatic CNS metastases.
Propulsive agents (metoclopropamide, amidorizoate)	Increase peristaltic activity. Contraindicated in complete obstruction, but may have use in partial MBO.	Metoclopramide: 60 mg/day PO, SC, IV. Also can act as a centrally active antiemetic in higher doses. Can worsen colic and may not be used with anticholinergics.

views, and absent or minimal intraluminal gas distal to the point of obstruction, may be muted or misinterpreted in patients who have malignant obstruction. Tumor can encase the bowel, preventing distention, can cause bowel dilatation from paresis due to infiltration of the mesentery and autonomic nerves, and can obstruct at more than one point.

Because of the limitations of plain film radiography, CT imaging has increasingly become the gold standard for diagnosis, especially for suspected malignant obstruction. It is sensitive, particularly for high-grade obstruction, and can identify the cause of obstruction in over 95% of cases [59]. Because of its specificity, it is the preferred initial screening modality for patients presenting with suspected bowel obstruction who have abdominal tenderness, leukocytosis, or fever [60].

Adjuncts to the primary imaging modalities include oral small bowel follow-through with barium or water-soluble contrast agent, enteroclysis, and contrast enema. These can be helpful in identifying low-grade obstructions and in establishing the diagnosis of carcinomatosis [61]—generally a sign of nonoperability.

Based on accumulating data, Krouse and colleagues [62] recommend the use of CT in the evaluation of suspected MBO, especially if invasive treatment approaches are being considered, because there are no comparative studies comparing cost, patient comfort, and accuracy of current radiographic diagnostic modalities.

At presentation of MBO, nasogastric drainage is routinely initiated before plain radiographs are obtained. This controls nausea and vomiting promptly, but at the cost of having a nasogastric tube inserted and left in place. Nasogastric drainage should be used only as a temporizing measure for the relief of obstructive symptoms in patients who have advanced or terminal colorectal cancer. No one needs to "have a tube in until they die" anymore when satisfactory control of symptoms is almost always possible with operative intervention, minimally invasive procedures, or pharmacotherapy. Although bowel obstruction in the setting of advanced malignancy will spontaneously resolve during a trial of nasogastric suction in some cases, a course of either operative or nonoperative management should be planned for durable relief of symptoms. Consultation with palliative care services, when available, is helpful to assist in framing the context of future care through skilled communication, pharmacologic management of obstructive symptoms, and attention to social, psychologic, and spiritual aspects of progressing life-limiting illness.

Surgeons are familiar with operative approaches for the relief of MBO, as well as some of the other technically difficult problems encountered in the setting of intra-abdominal malignancy (ie, radiation enteritis and bowel fistulas); however, because of the unique nature of an individual's suffering and the reasons for it, prospective randomized trials of palliative surgical interventions have not been performed in the past, and will only be conceivable when research methodologies used in the social sciences are employed in addition to those used in the natural sciences.

Mortality and morbidity are sobering when considering operation for MBO: operative mortality has been reported to be as high as 32% [63] and morbidity as high as 42% [64], with reobstruction rates up to 50% [65]. In a review of 823 palliative surgical procedures by Cady and colleagues [66], a major postoperative complication reduced the probability of symptom relief to 17%, and the combination of a complication-free palliative procedure and symptom resolution until death (their ideal outcome) occurred in only 16% of patients.

Relative contraindications to surgery for malignant obstruction are many and include: diffuse intraperitoneal carcinomatosis, palpable multiple intra-abdominal masses, liver metastases, extra-abdominal metastases, pleural effusions, multiple sites of partial obstruction or prolonged transit time of contrast on intestinal radiographs, ascites, cachexia or hypoalbuminemia, advanced age, poor performance status, recurrence following recent laparotomy for malignant obstruction, previous abdominal radiation therapy, and disease refractory to chemotherapy. Reports of success and patterns of failure are inconsistent: one study demonstrated that multiple sites of obstruction by colorectal cancer did not correlate with failure to resume bowel function or postoperative death [67]. In weighing options for surgery in the obstructed patient who has known malignancy, it must be remembered that a certain percentage of these (up to 48%) are due to benign causes [68].

Operation is preceded by the process of informed consent, in which it is clearly understood by patient, surrogates, and family that the primary goal of treatment is improvement or preservation of quality of life, without necessarily having any impact on the disease process itself. Nonabandonment by the surgeon and other members of the care team should be assured; if opportunity allows, the subject of advance directives should be broached. Arrangements for possible postoperative axial analgesia (ie, epidural catheter placement) should be discussed with anesthesiologist consultants.

Spiritual concerns and needs should be assessed for appropriate ministrations.

The principles of operative management outlined by Krouse [69] include liberal use of bypass and stomas (preoperative enterostomal therapist consultation advised) in avoiding extensive dissection and performance of gastrostomy in cases where no resection or bypass for relief of obstruction can be performed. Laparoscopic procedures will inevitably become more commonly performed, though no large series for this indication have been reported.

Intestinal stenting is an attractive alternative to surgery that, in addition to relief of obstruction, can permit bowel preparation for a resection and primary closure. Covered stents have been used for the control of intestinal fistulas. Complications are most likely during or immediately after insertion. These include perforation, bleeding, malpositioning, or migration. Tumor ingrowth with reobstruction can occur from days to months after insertion. Laser therapy, usually with Nd:Yag lasers, can be used for recanalization through intraluminal malignancy, but not for extrinsically compressing or completely obstructing lesions. Usually several treatments are required. Relief has been reported in 75% to 80% of patients [70].

Although 20 years have elapsed since Baines and colleagues reported successful management of symptoms of inoperable MBO using pharmacotherapy alone [71], nonoperative approaches other than nasogastric tube drainage have been slow to find their way into surgical practice. Lack of this information and knowledge of its satisfactory outcomes have probably led to many unnecessary laparotomies. Several studies documenting a very low incidence of strangulation secondary to malignant obstruction [72,73] can reassure the surgeon that a nonoperative approach to its management will not hazard intrabdominal septic catastrophe.

The goal of pharmacotherapy for MBO is relief of symptoms (pain, nausea, and fewer than two emeses/day), not resolution of obstruction. In some cases, however, relief of obstruction may occur if obstruction is partial. Successful symptom control for MBO can be anticipated using combination therapy with an opioid, an anticholinergic (or antisecretory agent such as octreotide), and an antiemetic without intestinal drainage tubes, surgery, or intravenous fluids [74]. A prospective randomized study of patients receiving antisecretory therapy for inoperable MBO [75] demonstrated that patients receiving octreotide had a more rapid reduction in GI secretions (allowing for earlier removal of a nasogastric tube) than patients receiving an anticholinergic antisecretory drug (scopolamine butylbromide). All patients studied were assessed for pain, nausea, dry mouth thirst, abdominal distention, dyspnea, and drowsiness. A significant observation, given the emotional issue of hydration at end of life, was the lack of difference in the daily thirst and dry mouth intensity in relation to the amount of parenteral hydration or the treatment provided. Also observed was that patients receiving less parenteral hydration presented with significantly more nausea and drowsiness. Pain control was good in all patients studied and most were cared for at home [75].

During pharmacotherapy for MBO, patients will tolerate an occasional emesis as long as nausea is well-controlled. This discrepancy can be used to advantage if the patient desires to eat or drink—as long as nausea is absent many patients are willing to risk or even accept an occasional emesis in order to try a small amount of food or liquid. As a general rule, the more distal the obstruction, the more likely it can be managed successfully with pharmacotherapy alone. For resistant symptoms, high intestinal obstruction, or burdensome MBO-related medication side effects, placement of a percutaneous endoscopic gastrostomy (PEG) tube for drainage should be considered.

Mercadante [76] has reported success in reversing MBO using an aggressive and early multiple agent therapy (dexamethasone, octreotide, metoclopropamide, and gastrografin) that combines propulsive and antisecretory agents. In addition to symptom relief, bowel function probably resumed because treatment was initiated before permanently obstructing impaction and edema developed.

Ascites

Malignant ascites is a harbinger of very limited prognosis, associated with a median survival of roughly 2 months. If no further disease-directed therapy is anticipated, the finding of malignant ascites would satisfy admission criteria for hospice care, following the appropriate course of disclosure and consent of the patient. Malignant ascites is usually caused by diffuse peritoneal and mesenteric tumor infiltration, accounting for its poor prognosis. Knowledge of this pathogensesis is important in understanding the rationale and limitations of therapy. Unless liver involvement with tumor has led to portal hemodynamic changes, diuretics useful in nonmalignant ascites are of limited or no use for the malignant variety, and they may even complicate management of other terminal symptoms by inducing prerenal azotemia, leading to lethargy and confusion from accumulating drug metabolites. Symptoms caused by ascites are fullness, bloating, pain, dyspnea, nausea, and body image-related distress.

Drainage is the definitive symptom management approach, except in patients actively dying, in which case relief of symptoms (pain and dyspnea) is best managed by opioids. Even if chemotherapy is expected to resolve intra-abdominal disease, drainage is still necessary for temporary symptom relief. No particular drainage procedure has emerged as evidence-based best. The simplest approach is paracentesis, which has the advantages of speed, simplicity, flexibility of treatment setting (it can be done in the home or office), and low complication rate. Ultrasound has been increasingly used, especially when loculated ascites is suspected. Drainage of malignant ascites is less likely to be followed by hemodynamic instability than nonmalignant varieties. Volumes of 5 liters drained at a sitting have been reported as safe [77], though larger volumes can be justified to relieve severe distress, especially dyspnea.

More durable drainage approaches include placement of a pigtail catheter, Tenkhoff catheter [78], pleurex catheter [79], or peritoneal port [80]. Peritoneal venous shunting has been used for malignant ascites, though morbidity related to infection, congestive heart failure, coagulopathy, venous thrombosis, and shunt occlusion from protein-rich ascites, as well as the need for hospitalization, are sobering downsides to palliative benefit. Nondrainage approaches for ascites management include systemic or intraperitoneal instillation of chemotherapeutic agents, or intracavitary injection of sclerosing agents, though these approaches may take weeks to realize symptomatic benefit.

Cachexia-anorexia

The incidence of cachexia-anorexia syndrome (or cancer cachexia syndrome) in patients who have advanced colorectal malignancy is not known, though it is most common in solid tumors (pancreas, stomach, lung) except breast [81]. Both anorexia and cachexia are quite common in patients presenting to palliative care or hospice programs.

Cancer cachexia has been defined as "a wasting syndrome involving loss of muscle and fat directly caused by tumor factors, or indirectly caused by an aberrant host response to tumor presence" [82]. Cancer cachexia is characterized by breakdown of skeletal muscle and deranged fat and carbohydrate metabolism, despite adequate or forced nutritional intake. Although the appearance of this syndrome outwardly mimics simple starvation, its metabolic basis is profoundly different. To suggest to patients "you need to eat more" in the face of advanced cancer cachexia overlooks this difference and creates confusion and doubt about medical guidance. Many etiologies for cachexia and anorexia in cancer patients are reversible, however, and a diligent search for these should not be prevented by a sense of resignation about advanced illness. Megesterol acetate, dexamethasone, cannabinoids, and other agents have been used successfully to enhance appetite and sense of well-being, but have not been shown to reverse cachexia-anorexia syndrome. Omega-3 fatty acids found in some fish oil supplements show some promise in the treatment of this syndrome [83,84]. See Box 5 for general recommendations for the management of cancer cahexia syndrome.

The inevitability of appetite and weight loss in patients who have progressing and incurable colorectal cancer requires surgeons to be familiar with this syndrome in order to respond helpfully to the equally inevitable questions from patients and families about what can be done and not done about it. Because the association between feeding and caring is so central to most cultures, the surgeon must walk the delicate line between truthfulness about the limitations of feeding or medication for this condition, and not taking away hope or impugning caregivers' good intentions. The word "starvation" should be used carefully in discussions about weight loss in advanced cancer when one considers the different physiologic and moral connotations of weight loss in starvation, forced starvation, and cancer-induced cachexia. To imply or allow it to be implied that neglect or lack of aggressiveness is the reason for weight loss when it is the result of an irreversible physiologic process risks future bereavement complications. Even in the most far advanced cases of cachexia, surgeons can use their well-earned credibility on matters of nutrition and gastrointestinal function to comfort a family, by clarifying the reasons for weight loss and its implications for care giving. Gently redirecting a family's attention from feeding to other expressions of concern is almost always deeply appreciated by a patient no longer possessing the appetite or strength to consume food. Weight loss in this context does not mean hunger. McCann and colleagues [85] demonstrated that hunger and thirst are uncommon complaints in terminally ill cancer patients. When these symptoms occurred, small amounts of food or water were needed for symptom relief.

Box 5. Recommendations for management of cancer cachexia syndrome

1. Regularly assess weight, change in appetite, food intake.
2. Obtain sHb, sAlbumin, and C-reactive protein as a baseline study.
3. Systematically rule out treatable secondary causes of wasting.
4. Refer for nutritional counseling from a team with special interest in wasting disorders.
5. Encourage patient participation in a rehabilitation program for consideration of the use of specific nutritional and pharmacologic interventions.
6. Follow-up visits should review antitumor therapy, tumor volume, symptom control, weight, appetite, and function.
7. Regular review of the full medication profile of patients who are wasting. These might include drugs that could have a favorable effect on anorexia-cachexia (cardiac agents such as the statins, angiotensin-converting enzyme [ACE] inhibitors) and other agents that may be deleterious (eg, herbal medications laced with corticosteroids).
8. It is reasonable for patients to increase the amount of eicosapentaenoic acid (EPA)-rich omega-3 fatty acids in their diet.
9. Testosterone status should be established in cancer patients who have the anorexia-cachexia syndrome. If clearly reduced, physiologic testosterone supplementation should be considered after discussion with the patient.
10. Patients must be assured of a reasonable intake of amino acids. Protein-containing foods are indicated, and rich sources of both essential and nonessential amino acids will support any anabolic potential.
11. Clinical researchers are encouraged to familiarize themselves with the work of colleagues in sports medicine, AIDS, and geriatrics.
12. Patients should be encouraged to keep active or take part in tailored exercise programs.
13. Surgeon researchers have led the way in studies on acute stress reactions related to surgery and trauma, and the role of nutrients in combating these events. These can guide further anorexia-cachexia trials, and should be expanded to encompass studies on wasting associated with chronic disease.

Adapted from MacDonald N, Easson A, Mazurak V, et al. Understanding and managing cancer cachexia. J Am Coll Surg 2003;197:143–61. 82; with permission.

The surgeon can mitigate his sense of frustration or failure in this and other scenarios of terminal illness by willingness to participate in the process of reframing the problem in a larger and redefined context of meaning. This is the ultimate test of the primary principles of all surgical palliative care: nonabandonment and preservation of hope.

Summary

The last phases of colorectal malignant illness may be the most challenging and saddening for all involved, but they offer opportunities to become the most rewarding. This transformation of hopelessness to fulfillment requires a willingness by surgeon, patient, and patient's family to trust one another to realistically set goals of care, stick together, and not let the treatment of the disease become a surrogate for treating the suffering that characterizes grave illness.

References

[1] American Cancer Society. Cancer facts and figures 2005. Atlanta (GA): American Cancer Society; 2005. Available at: www.cancer.org/docroot/CRI/content/CRI_2_4_1x_what_are_the_key_statistics_for_colon_and_rectum_cancer.asp?rnav-cri. Accessed June 30, 2006.

[2] DeCosse JJ, Cennerazzo WJ. Quality-of-life management of patients with colorectal cancer. CA Cancer J Clin 1997;47:198–206.

[3] Amersi F, Stamos MJ, Ko CY. Palliative care for colorectal cancer. Surg Oncol Clin N Am 2004;13(3):467–77.

[4] The SUPPORT principal Investigators. A controlled trial to improve care for seriously ill hospitalized patients: The study to understand prognoses and preferences for outcomes and risks of treatments (SUPPORT). JAMA 1995;274:1591–8.

[5] Billings JA. Module 1: Gaps in the end-of-life care of cancer patients. Disseminating end-of-life education to cancer cCenters. The National Cancer Institute, 2001.

[6] Emanuel EJ, Fairlough DL, Slutsman J, et al. Understanding economic and other burdens of terminal illness: the experience of patients and their caregivers. Ann Intern Med 2000;132:451–9.

[7] Covinsky KE, Goldman L, Cook EF, et al. The impact of serious illness on patients' families. JAMA 1994;272:1839–44.

[8] Morrison RS, Meier D. Palliative care. N Engl J Med 2004;350:2582–90.

[9] American College of Surgeons. Principles of care at end of life. Bull Am Coll Surg 1998;83:46.

[10] American College of Surgeons. Principles of palliative care. Bull Am Coll Surg 2005;90(8):34–5.

[11] American Board of Surgery, Inc. American Board of Surgery Qualifying Examination. Booklet of information. July 2005–June 2006. Available at: www.absurgery.org/xfer/ABS_BookletOfInfo05.pdf. Accessed January 23, 2006.

[12] Finlayson CA, Eisenberg BL. Palliative pelvic exenteration: patient selection and results. Oncology 1996;10(4):479–84 [Huntingt].

[13] Colorectal Meta-analysis Collaboration. Palliative chemotherapy for advanced or metastatic colorectal cancer. Cochrane Database Syst Rev 2000;2:CD001545.

[14] Cady B, Easson A, Aboulafia A, et al. Part 1: Surgical palliation of advanced illness—what's new, what's helpful. J Am Coll Surg 2005;200(1):115–27.

[15] Buckman R. How to break bad news. Baltimore (MD): Johns Hopkins Press; 1992. p. 65–97.

[16] Morrison SR, Maroney-Galin C, Kralovec PD, et al. The growth of palliative care programs in United States hospitals. J Palliat Med 2005;8(6):1127–34.

[17] Morrison S, Meier DE. Palliative care. N Engl J Med 2004;350:2582–90.

[18] Elsayem A, Swint K, Fisch M, et al. Palliative care inpatient service in a comprehensive cancer center: clinical and financial outcomes. Clin Oncol 2004;22:2008–14.

[19] Meier DE. Palliative care in hospitals: making the case. New York: Center to Advance Palliative Care; 2002.

[20] Higginson IJ, Finlay IG, Goodwin DM, et al. Do hospital-based palliative teams improve care for patients or families at the end of life? J Pain Symptom Manage 2002;23:96–106.

[21] Campbell ML, Guzman JA. Impact of a proactive approach to improve end-of-life care in a medical ICU. Chest 2003;123:266–71.

[22] Manfredi PL, Morrison RS, Morris J, et al. Palliative care consultations: how do they impact the care of hospitalized patients? J Pain Symtom Manage 2000;20(3):166–73.

[23] Beach MC, Morrison RS. The effect of do-not-resuscitate orders on physician decision-making. J Am Geriatr Soc 2002;50:2057–61.

[24] National Hospice and Palliative Care organization. Available at: www.nhpco.org/Files/members/TheCostsofHospiceCare-Millman.pdf. Accessed February 23, 2006.

[25] Portenoy RK, Thaler HT, Kornblith AB, et al. The Memorial Symptom Assessment Scale: an instrument for the evaluation of symptom prevalence, characteristics, and distress. Eur J Cancer 1994;30A(9):1326–36.

[26] Cella DF, Tulsky DS, Gray G, et al. The Functional Assessment of Cancer Therapy Scale; development of and validation of the general measure. J Clin Oncol 1993;11:570–9.

[27] Bruera E, Kuehn N, Miller MJ, et al. The Edmonton Symptom Assessment System. (ESAS): a simple method for the assessment of palliative care patients. J Palliat Care 1991;7(2):6–9.

[28] Larue F, Colleau SM, Brasseur L, et al. Multicentre study of cancer pain and its treatment in France. BMJ 1995;310:1034–7.

[29] Von Roenn JH, Cleeland CS, Gonin R, et al. Physicians' attitudes and practice in cancer pain management: a survey from the Eastern Cooperative Oncology Group. Ann Intern Med 1993;119:121–6.

[30] Cleeland CS, Gonin R, Hatfield AK, et al. Pain and its treatment in outpatients with metastatic cancer. N Eng J Med 1994;330:592–6.

[31] Wolfe J, Grier HE, Klar N, et al. Symptoms and suffering at the end of life in children with cancer. N Eng J Med 2000;342:326–33.

[32] American Pain Society Quality of Care Task Force. American Pain Society recommendations for improving the quality of acute and cancer pain management. Arch Intern Med 2005;165(14):1574–80.

[33] Twycross RG. Pain and analgesics. Curr Med Res Opin 1978;5:497–505.

[34] Ray JB. Pharmacologic management of pain. Surg Oncol Clin N Am 2001;10(1):71–87.

[35] Saunders S, Sykes N. The management of terminal malignant disease. 3rd edition. London: Edward Arnold; 1993.

[36] Levy M. Pharmacological treatment of cancer pain. N Engl J Med 1996;335:1124–32.

[37] World Health Organiztion. Cancer pain relief and palliative care. Report of a WHO expert committee. World health Organization Technical Report Series, 804. Geneva (Switzerland): World Health Organization; 1990. p. 1–75.

[38] Jacox A, Carr DB, Payne R, et al. Mangement of cancer pain. AHCPR publication No. 94-0592: Clinical practice guideline No. 9. Rockville (MD): U.S. Department of Health and Human Services, Public Health Service; March 1994. p. 1–257.

[39] Pace V. Use of non-steroidal anti-inflammatory drugs in cancer. Palliat Med 1995;9:273–86.

[40] Definitions related to the use of opioids for the treatment of pain: a consensus document from the American Academy of Pain Medicine, the American Pain Society, and the American Society of Addiction medicine. 2002. available at: www.painmed.org/productpub/statements/pdfs/definition.pdf. Accessed April 5, 2006.

[41] Vaco v Quill, 521 US 793 (1997).
[42] Storey P, Knight C. UNIPAC three: assessment and treatment of pain in the terminally ill. 2nd edition. Larchmont (NY): Mary Ann Liebert Publishers; 2003. p. 1–91.
[43] Sindrup SH, Brosen K. The pharmacogenetics of codeine hypoalgesia. Pharmacogenetics 1995;5(6):335–46.
[44] Lipman AG, Gauthier ME. Pharmacology of opioid drugs: basic principles. In: Portnoy R, Bruera E, editors. Topics in palliative care, vol. 1. New York: Oxford University Press; 1997. p. 1–316.
[45] Stjernsward J, Colleau SM, Ventafridda V. The World health Organization Cancer Pain and Palliative Care Program: past, present, and future. J Pain Symptom Manage 1996; 12:65–72.
[46] Amersi F, Stamos MJ, Ko CY. Palliative care of colorectal cancer. Surg Oncol Clin N Am 2004;13:467–77.
[47] Galante JM, Bowles TL, Khatri VJ, et al. Experience and attitudes of surgeons toward palliation in cancer. Arch Surg 2005;140:873–80.
[48] Howell D. Radiation therapy in the palliation of gastrointestinal malignancies. Gastroenterol Clin North Am 2006;35:125–30.
[49] Bonica JJ, Benedetti C. Management of cancer pain. In: Moosa AR, Robson MC, Schimpff SC, editors. Comprehensive textbook of oncology. Baltimore (MD): Williams &Wilkins; 1986. p. 462.
[50] Coyle N, Adelhardt J, Foley KM, et al. Character of terminal illness in the advanced cancer patient: pain and other symptoms during the last four weeks of life. J Pain Symptom Manage 1990;5(2):83–93.
[51] Reuben DB, Mor V. Nausea and vomiting in terminal cancer patients. Arch Intern Med 1986;146(10):2021–3.
[52] Ventafridda V, Sbanotto A, Burnhill R. Palliative care. In: Garden OJ, Geraaghty JG, Nagorney DM, editors. Liver metastases. biology, diagnosis, and treatment. London: Springer-Verlag Limited; 1998. p. 1–207.
[53] Mount BM. Bowel obstruction. In: MacDonald N, editor. Palliative medicine. A case based manual. Toronto: Oxford Medical Publications; 1998. p. 1–318.
[54] Hallenbeck J. Fast fact and concept #005; treatment of nausea and vomiting. Available at: www.eperc.mcw.edu/FastFact/ff_005.htm. Accessed February 24, 2006.
[55] Miller AD, Rowley HA, Roberts TPL, et al. Human cortical activity during vestibular and drug-induced detected using M.S.I. In: Highstein SM, Cohen B, Buettner-Ennever JA, editors. New directions in vestibular research. 1996; Ann NY Acad Ser 781. p. 670–2.
[56] Davis MP, Nouneh D. Modern management of cancer-related intestinal obstruction. Curr Pain Headache Rep 2001;5:257–64.
[57] Legendre H, Vahhuyse F, Caroli-Bosc FX, et al. Survival and quality of life after palliative surgery for neoplastic gastrointestinal obstruction. Eur J Surg Oncol 2001;27:364–7.
[58] Maglinte DD, Kelvin FM, O'Connor K, et al. Current status of small bowel radiography. Abdom Imaging 1996;21:247–57.
[59] Maglinte DD, Reyes BL, Harmon BH, et al. Reliability and role of plain film radiography and CT in the diagnosis of small-bowel obstruction. Am J Roentgenol 1996;167(6):1451–5.
[60] American College of Surgeons, Division of Education. Surgical Education and Self-Assessment Program (SESAP) No. 12. Vol. 1. 2004. p. 1–626.
[61] Bundrick T, Cho SR, Ammann A, et al. Intraperitoneal carcinomatosis: incidence of its radiographic findings and description of a new sign. Br J Radiol 1983;56:13–6.
[62] Krouse RS, McCahill LE, Easson AM, et al. When the sun can set on an unoperated bowel obstruction: management of malignant bowel obstruction. J Am Coll Surg 2002;195:117–28.
[63] Averbach AM, Sugarbaker PH. Recurrent intra-abdominal cancer with intestinal obstruction. Int Surg 1995;80(2):141–6.
[64] Makela J, Kiviniemi H, Laitinen S, et al. Surgical management of intestinal obstruction after treatment for cancer. Eur J Surg 1991;157:73–7.

[65] Miner T, Jaques DP, Paty PB, et al. Symptom control in patients with locally recurrent rectal cancer. Ann Surg Oncol 2003;10(1):72–9.

[66] Cady B, Miner T, Morgenthaler A. Part 2: Surgical palliation of advanced illness—what's new, what's helpful. J Am Coll Surg 2005;2005(2):281–90.

[67] Lau PWK, Lorentz TG. Results of surgery for malignant bowel obstruction in advanced, unresectable, recurrent colorectal cancer. Dis Colon Rectum 1993;36:61–4.

[68] Legendre H, Vah Huyse F, Caroli-Bosc FX, et al. Survival and quality of life after palliative surgery for neoplastic gastrointestinal obstruction. Eur J Surg Oncol 2001;27:364–7.

[69] Krouse RS. Surgical management of malignant bowel obstruction. Surg Oncol Clin N Am;13:479–90.

[70] Adler DG, Merwat SN. Endoscopic approaches for palliation of luminal gastrointestinal obstruction. Gastroenterol Clin North Am 2006;35:65–82.

[71] Baines M, Oliver DJ, Carter RL. Medical management of intestinal obstruction with advanced malignant disease: a clinical and pathological study. Lancet 1985;II:990–3.

[72] Butler JA, Cameron BL, Morrow M, et al. Small bowel obstruction in patients with a prior history of cancer. Am J Surg 1991;162:244–9.

[73] Rubin SC. Intestinal obstruction in advanced ovarian cancer: what does the patient want? Gynecol Oncol 1999;75:311–2.

[74] Ripamonti C, Conno FD, Ventafridda V, et al. Management of bowel obstruction in advanced and terminal cancer patients. Ann Oncol 1993;4:15–21.

[75] Ripamonti C, Mercadante S, Groff L, et al. Role of octreotide, scopolamine butylbromide, and hydration in symptom control of patients with inoperable bowel obstruction and nasogastric tubes: a prospective randomized trial. J Pain Symptom Manage 2000;19(1):23–34.

[76] Mercadante S, Ferrera P, Villari P, et al. Aggressive pharmacological treatment for reversing malignant bowel obstruction. J Pain Symptom Manage 2004;28(4):412–6.

[77] Muir JC. Ascites. In: Von Roenn J, Smith TJ, Loprinzi CL, et al, editors. ASCO curriculum: optimizing cancer care. The importance of symptom management, vol. 1. Dubuque (IA): Kendall/Hunt; 2001. p. 1–31.

[78] Lomas DA, Wallis PJ, Stockley RA. Palliation of malignant ascites with a Tenkhoff catheter. Thorax 1989;44:928.

[79] Richard HM, Coldwell DM, Boyd-Kranis RI, et al. Pleurex tunneled catheter in the management of malignant ascites. J Vasc Interv Radiol 2001;2:373–5.

[80] Savin MA, Kirsch MJ, Romano WJ, et al. Peritoneal ports for treatment of intractable ascites. J Vasc Interv Radiol 2005;16:363–8.

[81] Kern KA, Norton JA. Cancer cachexia. J Parenter Enteral Nutr 1988;12(3):286–98.

[82] MacDonald N, Easson A, Mazurak V, et al. Understanding and managing cancer cachexia. J Am Coll Surg 2003;197(1):143–61.

[83] Wigmore SJ, Barber MD, Ross JA, et al. Effect of oral eicosapentaenoic acid on weight loss in patients with pancreatic cancer. Nutr Cancer 2000;36:177–84.

[84] Gogos CA, Ginopoulos P, Salsa B, et al. Dietary omega-3 polyunsaturated fatty acids plus vitamin E restore immunodeficiency and prolong survival for severely ill patients with generalized malignancy: a randomized control trial. Cancer 1998;82:395–402.

[85] McCann RM, Hall WJ, Groth-Juncker A. Comfort care for terminally ill patients. The appropriate use of nutrition and hydration. JAMA 1994;272:1263–6.

[86] Davis MP, Furste A. Glycopyrrolate: a useful drug in the palliation of mechanical bowel obstruction. J Pain Symptom Manage 1999;18(3):153–4.

[87] Ripamonti C, Bianchi M. The use of methadone for cancer pain. Hematol Oncol Clin N Am 2002;16:543–55.

ELSEVIER
SAUNDERS

SURGICAL
CLINICS OF
NORTH AMERICA

Surg Clin N Am 86 (2006) 1093–1101

Index

Note: Page numbers of article titles are in **boldface** type.

0039-6109/06/$ - see front matter © 2006 Elsevier Inc. All rights reserved.
doi:10.1016/S0039-6109(06)00104-6
surgical.theclinics.com